Surgical Roots and Branches

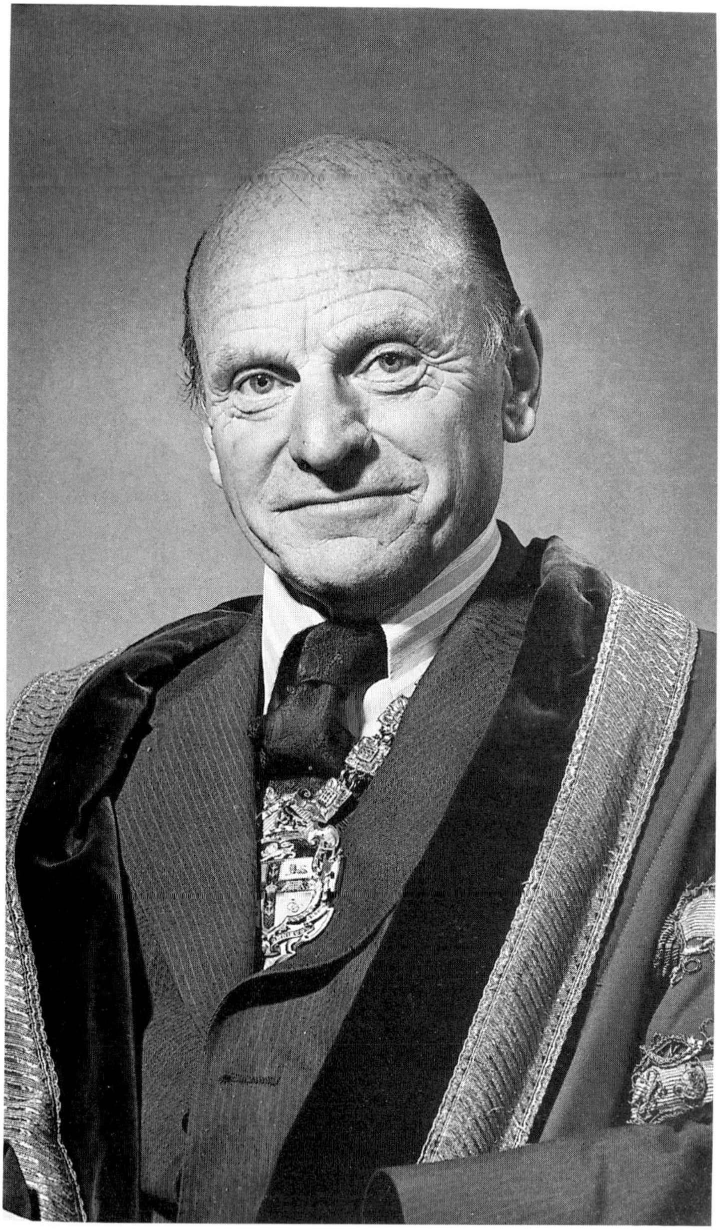

Reginald Murley on Bastille Day, 14 July 1977

REGINALD MURLEY

Surgical Roots and Branches

The
MEMOIR
Club

The British Medical Journal
Tavistock Square, London WC1H 9JR

First published 1990

ISBN 0 7279 0284 9

Typeset in Great Britain by Latimer Trend & Company Ltd, Plymouth
Printed in Great Britain by The University Press, Cambridge

To Daphne

Contents

Preface

When, shortly after I had sent him an entertaining note about how a deceased surgeon's name had come to be double barrelled, Dr Stephen Lock, the editor of the *British Medical Journal*, suggested that I might write a few "*lighthearted* comments for our Memoir Club series" he explained that "the style should be essentially conversational (just as in your note) rather than anything more formal." I thereupon responded by sending him several reminiscences which I had recently written and then recorded on tape for the entertainment of an old medical friend who had become blind. Stephen read those short pieces over Christmas 1987 and surprised me by writing that, although they were not quite in the style he wanted, they "read like very good after dinner speeches" – a use to which I had never thought of putting them. But to give an idea of the genre he had in mind he went on to say, "What we would be after, of course, [is] an account of your career and the people you met, with some homespun philosophy emerging." With this encouragement and guidance I felt prepared to accept the challenge, and so *Surgical Roots and Branches* was begun during 1988 and completed last year.

Having been conceived and born during what came to be known as the Great War, I never in my childhood suspected that I would spend nearly six and a half years of my early adult life in the army. In the event, this period in what might aptly be described as the "univeristy of life" was to prove invaluable for those of us whose education, constrained by strictly professional goals, had been intense and occasionally narrow. Wartime service, despite its sometimes extreme frustrations, gave many of us unrivalled opportunity for overseas travel, as well as the chance to meet unusual people and to cope with situations which we would not have faced in normal conditions. For these reasons, as well as some strictly medical ones, I thought it appropriate to devote a number of the earlier chapters to my army life.

My colleagues have often complimented me on the accuracy of my memory, but I certainly do not flatter myself that it is as reliable as some would seem to think. As the years pass it is common for memories to become less clear; even more important, many people assume that they have the facts at their finger tips when they do not. Fortunately I still possess some of my wartime operation books and unit records; and my study is lined with files of documents and letters covering the postwar period up to the present time. Thus wherever necessary I have been able to check my records carefully to ensure that facts, dates, and the order of events are accurately recounted. And, in accordance with Stephen Lock's early injunctions, I have tried to ensure that what follows is as entertaining and informative as possible – not forgetting a little homespun philosophy. I thank him warmly for his interest and indulgence and trust that this book will meet with his approval.

Finally, I must cordially thank Dorothy Sharp, who has been such an indefatigable, enthusiastic, and good humoured editor, for her careful revision of my own *Amstrad* printout and for helping to select the appropriate illustrations.

REGINALD MURLEY
January 1990

1 Genesis and school days

The Times of 2 August 1916 reported that temperatures had reached 83°F on the previous day and that seven German zeppelins had been seen over England during the night. There is no evidence that either of these factors was in any way responsible for my delivery that day, in a small suburban terraced house at Wandsworth, during the battle of the Somme. My birth was not announced in *The Times* for my parents were neither so well off nor so pretentious as to do that. I was, I am told, delivered by a Dr Lang, the Aberdonian partner of our own Dr Melville Young, another Aberdonian graduate then in the Royal Army Medical Corps, to whom I shall have cause to refer again.

My birth certificate records my father's occupation as "Warehouse superintendent." He was then 30 years of age and my mother was 34. My parents had only one other child, my sister, who was born in 1912. That small family home at 56 Badminton Road was bought by my parents for £400 shortly after their marriage in 1910, and we were there for the first few years of my life. My only clear memories of that period are of Armistice Day, when the flags were hung out, and of having my tonsils removed on the kitchen table by Dr Young, the anaesthetic being administered by Dr Lang. I have a vivid memory of the greenish mask over my face and especially the pungent smell of the anaesthetic agent, presumably chloroform, as I was asphyxiated into temporary oblivion. I know that early recollections can be misleading but I am confident about Armistice Day as my earliest memory, when I was 2 years and 3 months old.

In about 1920 we moved to a larger house, 10 Hillbury Road. It was in a pleasant situation overlooking Tooting Bec

Common and with lawn tennis courts opposite. The house was officially located in Balham – later to be made famous by Peter Sellers as "the gateway to the south." I recall that rather than admit to a domicile in either Tooting or Balham I was snobbish enough in my boyhood usually to claim that we lived on the edge of the then more fashionable Streatham. But that, of course, was before Streatham finally lost its superior cachet with the recent press revelations about "Madam Sin" and her brothel.

There was only a small garden at the back of our house, but we were lucky enough to have the large common, which was well maintained by smartly uniformed keepers of the London County Council. Despite that relatively green ambience I could then recognise only a handful of birds and even fewer trees. Our neighbours, with whom we enjoyed good relations but had no close contact, were all middle class business or professional people on the Heaver estate, with Mr Heaver, the builder, living at no 1. He was a member of the Surrey County cricket club and later, when I was at preparatory school, he was occasionally kind enough to take me to Kennington Oval in his chauffeur driven car. Those were the days of P G H Fender's captaincy, with Strudwick as wicketkeeper and Hobbs and Sandham as opening batsmen.

When I was 5 I excitedly enrolled at Wickhambreaux kindergarten, only five minutes' walk from my home; it was run by two elderly ladies, Miss Law and Miss Pearson – at least they looked elderly to me in those far off days. I much enjoyed writing neat numbers and letters with my coloured crayons; rapidly progressed with my reading and spelling; and stayed there until the age of 7. I left a little before the end of what would have been my last term through being expelled – as one of my colleagues later so succintly described the event – for having "displayed an offensive weapon." I well remember that a boy called Maurice Patrick had dared me to stick out my penis under the class room table. This I did and, as far as I am aware, he, peeping under the other end of the table, was the only child to confirm this rude display. However, I soon learnt that the little blighter had sneaked on me to Miss Law. Without bothering to apprehend me in any way, the same evening she called on my mother and presumably demanded my removal lest I should expose myself to any of the small girls in my class.

Although I felt slightly guilt ridden, my parents made no mention of the matter. The next term they moved me to the Mayfair preparatory school (locally known as "the black and white school" because of the distinctive caps worn by the pupils – peak and crown alternately and distinctively halved), which operated in the downstairs rooms of a suburban house only two streets away from my first school. The headmaster, Mr F H Dickson, was a Cambridge graduate and an excellent all round teacher. He ran the school virtually single handed with some part time help from his two sons. The front and back classrooms were separated by a sliding division, which was opened for morning assembly and then closed for the subsequent classes. Dickson taught us English, Latin, Greek, mathematics, geography, general knowledge, and French. He was especially strong on the basics of learning and always inspired the respect and enthusiasm of his pupils. Looking back on it all now, I realise I was fortunate to be in the hands of such a pleasant and gentlemanly teacher.

That preparatory school in a suburban road had only a small garden, but every week Dickson would hire a charabanc (a single decker soft top bus) to take the whole school – about 30 boys – to a sports ground at Mitcham. There we learnt the elements of cricket and soccer, and of good sportsmanship. I was not meant to play football for during one of my childhood illnesses Dr Young had detected a heart murmur and told my mother that I should avoid strenuous games. But no one had told the school and so, quite unknown to my dear mother, I took part in all sports. Incidentally, I still have the same harmless heart murmur, which is of no material significance.

Quite early in my life I began to suffer from intermittent severe headaches, which later occurred mostly at the weekends. This was a fairly classical migraine, characterised by a preliminary well marked fortification spectrum in one half of the visual field succeeded by intense headache on the opposite side. On such occasions the doctor recommended my confinement to a darkened room with a cooling vinegar cloth across my aching forehead. These attacks could last for several hours, or even a whole day, and were eventually relieved by vomiting. How I hated vomiting. So I have always tried to suppress it by repeated swallowing, but usually without success. I have fond memories of the kindness of Dr Young when he visited me during those migraine attacks. In his pleasant Scottish voice he would say, "It's just a wee liver attack, Mrs Murley." I also remember the occasion of another visit, not for migraine, when he thrashed me for being rude to my mother. Although I cannot recall what I had said to her, I thought I deserved that punishment and I always had the greatest respect and affection for Melville Young.

By contrast my contact with dentists was none too happy. I had poor teeth because I ate too many sweets and neglected my dental hygiene. But my mother fondly attributed my dental caries to the fact that I was "a war baby." Around the age of 7 I was taken to Mr Cox, in Balham, with a fairly recently erupted and acheing lower right molar. This had to be removed but, with my vivid memory of tonsillectomy on the kitchen table, I refused to have gas. Inferior dental blocks were rarely used in those days and I suspect that Mr Cox may have been unfamiliar with the technique, or reluctant to use it in the presence of a dental abscess. Faced with my adamant rejection of nitrous oxide he said, "Very well then, I shall remove it without gas." He told me to open my mouth and promptly proceeded to yank out the tooth. The pain was frightful and my screams must have been heard in the high street. But at least I know how bad it was in the days before anaesthesia.

My parents decided that when I was 11 they would send me to Dulwich College. It was predominantly a day school of more than 800 boys (there are nearly 1400 now) with just 120 boarders. Although the college was only four miles from my home, as my sister had already boarded at Northwood for several years it was decided that I should do likewise at Dulwich. The annual fee was then £150, and I do not think that it changed during the six years I was there. Once the decision was made I sat for the entrance examination at the age of 11 and was accepted. The housemaster of my boarding house, Elm Lawn, was Alfred Taylor, the head of the engineering side, always affectionately known as "Lanky." He always called me "George." He was a large, handsome man and a superb precision engineer. He had a splendid workshop and specialised in making fine clocks. He also made a large reflecting telescope through which we were occasionally invited to study the moon and the stars. His wife was very good looking and they had three attractive daughters, but we had no "Young Woodley" in the house and I am not aware of any serious problems arising in regard to these four ladies.

I moved into Elm Lawn in September 1928 and settled down happily. About a dozen of us in the junior common room would fag for the house prefects, but the atmosphere was in no way oppressive. A number of the boys were domiciled overseas and a few had parents in the services. There were none that I strongly disliked. A few formed close friendships but I never encountered a trace of overt homosexuality during my six years at the school. The junior and senior common rooms included wall lockers for each boy but were bare in all other respects. We always had a blazing fire there in the winter at which we toasted bread and chestnuts or converted tins of condensed milk into rich caramel. The three house prefects shared a study which was immediately adjacent to the door leading into Lanky's own comfortable study. About half a dozen boys in my house were killed in the second world war, and two of the survivors – one in Zimbabwe, the other in England – still keep in touch with me.

Boarding house food was neither better nor worse than might be expected. The Taylors always had breakfast with us in the boys' dining room; on Sundays they would join us for lunch, often with one or other of their daughters. Like many a schoolboy I often suffered from what I thought to be constipation and trotted off to the house matron for a "dose." Having a bowel which now works with clockwork-like precision each day, I can only presume that my school problems were largely due to lack of dietary roughage. The only time I was ill enough to require admission to hospital, rather than the school sanatorium, was in my first summer term of 1929. After cricket nets one hot evening I was astonished and frightened to pass dark reddish-black urine. I told nobody, but I awoke in the night with acute pain in the back. My bed was moved into matron's surgery, where I was seen by Dr Stewart, the school practitioner, and given a shot of morphine. The following morning they took me into Victoria and Albert ward at King's College Hospital, under the care of John Everidge. Once free from pain I loved every minute of my hospital stay. I was intrigued when a man in the next bed disappeared in the night. Sister was reluctant to answer my over eager inquiry as to whether he had died, which indeed he had, though she tried to bluff me into believing that he had been moved to another ward.

That spell in King's was towards the end of my first year in the upper II form. My form master, who always wore a dark suit and butterfly collar, was the exceptionally kindly Mr Taylor-Jones, and I was most touched when he came to visit and read me a book. "T-J," as we called him, was a good teacher but not a strong disciplinarian and I am afraid that some of us behaved badly in class. When he came to see me I felt guilty about some of my recent behaviour. His son was then house surgeon with one of the other consultants, and he regularly attended in my ward; his daughter went into medical practice in Highbury where many years later, at the Royal Northern Hospital, I had cause to exchange letters with her about a number of patients. The ward sister was a pleasant woman. One of the staff nurses later married Dr Cove-Smith, the distinguished England rugby captain. In later life I came to know both of them well. One feature of hospital procedure at that time, which persisted until quite recently, was the regular nightly inquiry as to whether each patient had "one for the book." A negative answer invariably led to a dose of a foul black mixture. In this connection I made two mistakes: firstly, I gave too many truthful answers; and secondly I was imprudent enough to dispose of these purges by opening my bedside locker and tipping them on to the woodwork. A few telltale leaks I deftly wiped away, but I had not reckoned with the periodic check on the lockers. Sister opened mine a few days later and, seeing the dark stain on the wood, said, "Oh, you naughty boy, you haven't been taking your mixture."

I have another vivid memory of the spell in King's. That was when I had an intravenous urogram. This method of investigation had been introduced in 1926, just three years before. Uroselectan was used to give an *x* ray outline of the collecting parts of the kidneys and ureters, and this iodine containing compound was injected intravenously by my house surgeon, Dr Sheldon, who came of a large medical family. Within a few minutes I developed violent headache and repeated vomiting. Having suffered severe migraine from an early age, I was not too disturbed, but Sheldon and the *x* ray staff were alarmed by this severe reaction to the Uroselectan.

I know nothing of what those *x* rays revealed. But shortly afterwards I was cystoscoped under general anaesthetic by John Everidge. I waited on a trolley in the anaesthetic room for a long time, amusing myself by talking to a nurse and watching the heads of the operating team through the small round window in the anaesthetic room door. When all was ready I was put to sleep by inhalation anaesthesia, of which I have much happier memories than the tonsillar session on the kitchen table in Wandsworth. In the succeeding 60 years I have had about four severe attacks of ureteric colic, usually without any bleeding. A month after my last and most severe attack, in January 1974, I had the satisfaction of painlessly passing a stone just before starting an operation list.

When I returned to school for the rest of the summer term after that first attack I had no thought of becoming a doctor. Yet I have little doubt that it was during that short spell in King's that the seeds of interest in medicine, which matured a few years later, were first sown. In the autumn of 1929 I left the kindly T-J's form and entered the upper second under the dreaded Treadgold junior. His father was then the senior master and in marked contrast to his son was a benign man. But "Tready junior" was a sadist and a year with him was the most miserable of many a young life. Those who excelled at translating his long Latin sentences, which stretched across several wall blackboards, were his favourites. Those who did badly were regularly kept in for an hour or so after class. Maurice Kinmonth, who later became a plastic surgeon at Leicester, shared a similar fate to mine and I think that we were the most punished boys in our year. We took our revenge by wrecking Tready's class room desk on Founder's Day 1930, and I have photographs of the desk in my old school album. Luckily we were not found out.

My next two years were spent successively with form masters Hamilton and Bovill. I had one enjoyable 10 day school trip to Rouen, Paris, Chartres, and Fontainebleau. A party of more than a dozen boys was accompanied by two masters, Jack Rubie and J A (later Sir Jack) Westrup. The latter, an excellent musician and teacher of classics, became musical correspondent for the *Daily Telegraph* shortly before the war and then professor of music at Birmingham before taking the chair at Oxford. Though I had coped moderately well with foreign languages, in advanced mathematics I was largely defeated by differential calculus, despite the excellent teaching of Mr Jackson. Before I was 15 I had begun to lose interest in the modern side and had firmly made up my mind to do medicine. I regret the relative idleness and indecision of those earlier years; and I also regret that I gave up violin lessons when I went to Dulwich. Later, however, I did teach myself to play the piano, rather badly. When auditioned for the choir I had deliberately sung out of tune, but I always enjoyed singing in chapel at morning and evening service each Sunday.

On switching to the science upper fifth in 1932 I promptly moved to the top of the form in most of the fortnightly and end of term "lists," much to the astonishment of my parents as I had generally been among the lowest half dozen on the modern side. Only then did I dare tell my father that I wanted to study medicine. He expressed concern, as this was during the depression. He sadly explained that he did not think he could support me all the way through as he was threatened with bankruptcy. I should explain that he had been apprenticed at the age of 15 to the London fur trade firm of Blatspiel, Stamp & Heacock and worked there until 1909; he then joined the fur auction house of A & W Nesbitt and, as already mentioned, was their warehouse superintendent when I was born. In 1920, just before we moved to our larger house, he left Nesbitt's to start up as a fur broker in Garlick Hill, first in partnership and then on his own. He was a hardworking and conscientious man and although he had left school so early had managed to learn enough French and German, as well as a little Russian, for business use.

Meanwhile I completed the Oxford and Cambridge school certificate – though I only scraped through in physics. When I went home for the summer vacation my mother told me that Dr Young would like me to visit him, preferably at the end of an evening surgery. I duly arranged this and attended his surgery in Nightingale Lane, Wandsworth, just a short way from my birthplace. When his last patient had gone my general practitioner for the last 16 years welcomed me into his consulting room. He told me how pleased he was that I had decided to be a doctor; that I was entering a great profession; and that I must remember that all the great discoveries were made by relatively young men. He thereupon gave me a copy of Paul de Krief's *Men Against Death*, perhaps one of the early popular works concerning the great discoveries of some of the most oustanding medical scientists up to the 1930s. I left his surgery under the distinctly false impression that I too might join those ranks one day. Only years later, when reading Sir James Howie's presidential address to the British Medical Association, did I learn that it had been traditional in Aberdeen for the family doctor there to meet any aspiring medical student in his practice, to welcome him into the profession, and speed him on his way. What a delightful tradition.

The next term I went into the science remove to spend my last year preparing for the London University first MB examination. Among my classmates were Noel Glover, later a surgeon at Guy's, and Maurice Kinmonth, who became a plastic surgeon at Leicester. The teaching of biology by W C Crowther and chemistry by A J Oldham was excellent, but physics was less well taught by Walter Booth, the headmaster – at Dulwich always known as "The Master." "Wallie" was a cheerful man who had thrice caned me during my days in

Treadgold's form. Though I certainly held nothing against him for those beatings, and he was clearly convinced of the good he had done me, he was a little too fond of whisky, the distinctive odour of which was sometimes discernible in class. I worked hard during those last two years at Dulwich and was encouraged by my unexpected success. This also greatly improved my performance and sense of responsibility in other ways. Ever since then I have realised that, apart from the relatively few natural scholars, it is essential for most of us to have real motivation towards a clear cut goal.

I was in the Officers' Training Corps for six years, serving in the bugle band as a side drummer, but I never rose above the rank of corporal. The only award I ever won, but failed to collect, was the Kittermaster prize (named after a master who was killed in the first world war). By some miracle I was top in the training corps certificate A examination. My sports record was patchy. I shot in the school VIII without ever winning my colours, but I once had a "possible" on the 500 yards at Bisley. I also played intermittently in the school squash rackets team as well as the second rugby fives IV. I played in my athletic house as well as my boarding house cricket and rugby teams; but I had no success in the school teams apart from the odd appearance as a wing forward in the third XV. I think I had a slightly cavalier attitude to team games because I felt so overshadowed by near contemporaries like Denis Wilcox, Billy Griffith, and Hugh Bartlett, all of whom became county cricketers. Billy Griffith, like Hugh Bartlett, was a day boy who lived only a couple of hundred yards from my home. Whereas Hugh was a cricket blue in each of his three years at Cambridge, Billy won his blue as wicketkeeper only in his last season – but he went on to keep wicket for England, and made a century in his first test match.

In May 1934, during my last term, I sat the first MB examination as an external student at the Central School of Art in Southampton Row. The psychological pressure during the three days of papers was more intense than I realised. Every morning I was smitten by migraine and had difficulty in seeing my writing because of the intense visual fortification figures. The headache was not too severe, and mercifully I was not sick. Each lunch hour I went to a nearby chemist's shop (still identifiable by its prominent displays of Durex and related products) where I purchased a daily dose of APC (aspirin, phenacetin, and caffeine) for one shilling, or was it sixpence? I had been tempted to write on each of my papers, "I have frightful migraine," but I wisely desisted. A few weeks afterwards I travelled to Bloomsbury to read the pass list. How relieved I was to be safely through. I arrived at West Dulwich station, and while walking back to Elm Lawn I met Mrs Taylor and her youngest daughter, Agatha, on their way to the station. I excitedly told them of my success and they seemed astonished, as was "Lanky" when I gave him the glad news a few minutes later.

Although my school days were not the happiest of my life, my six years at Dulwich were certainly never unhappy. Considering my rather wasted earlier years, and my slowness in recognising the joys of scholarship and hard work, I feel that I owe much to some of my teachers. Although by no means among the worst in the school, I was often rash and naughty. Was it in that last summer term, or the year before, that some of us broke into the masters' common room, collected a number of their mortarboards, and then decorated the statues in the library and around the roof of James Barry's rather baroque Italianate buildings? I cannot remember. But I do know that it was during my last term that we hoisted a china chamberpot up the flagmast of a local girls school – fitting preparation for my early days as a prewar medical student at Barts.

This chapter would be incomplete if I did not confess that St Thomas's Hospital Medical School turned me down. Maurice Kinmonth was later accepted even though he failed his first MB at school and then passed in the following year after attending Borland's, the crammers, where William Joyce (the notorious wartime "Lord Haw-Haw") was one of his tutors. But Maurice's older brother, John (who many years afterwards became a close friend of mine), had passed first MB the year before me and then gone to St Thomas's, where he later became professor of surgery. John served on the council of the Royal College of Surgeons when I was president; and he eventually faced up to a punishing terminal illness with patience and fortitude.

It was after studying the student handbooks of Barts, Guy's, the London, Middlesex, and St Thomas's, that I had hopefully presented myself to Dr Thompson, the St Thomas's Medical School dean. Stupidly, I was a little narked when he asked me first about my sporting accomplishments. Being unfamiliar with interviewing techniques I failed to establish rapport and, on the basis of that interview, he was probably right to reject me. Shortly afterwards my father and I called on the rotund and extrovert surgical dean of Barts, Mr William Girling Ball. After a few minutes he seemed to like the look of me and offered me a place. My father and I were then sent on a tour of the hospital and medical school in the safe hands of Andrews, the medical college head porter. The then comprehensive fee for my five years was £250, which I believe my father paid as a lump sum. Even at prewar prices that was a bargain.

2 Busy times at Barts

I cannot remember where my summer holiday was spent in 1934, but I entered Barts medical college that year in the October term. I had forgotten my father's earlier reference to his financial difficulties; but on 1 January 1935 his firm went into voluntary liquidation. He afterwards became general manager of the old established C M Lampson & Co, a subsidiary of the Hudson's Bay Company since 1928. Too preoccupied with my own life, I had not bothered to inquire about my father's situation, but it is plain that he had gone through a great deal before achieving this appointment, after which he never looked back. I could hardly forget, however, the period a few years earlier, while I was still at school, when he was off work for a week or two with intense headaches. He later confessed that the illness had been due to extreme psychological stress; so we were all lucky that he managed to weather that particular storm. I continued to live at home during my student days, travelling to Barts by underground from Balham or by Southern Electric from Streatham. I believe that my allowance was £5 per month until I qualified.

The medical college was situated both on the hospital site and adjacent to it. One or two of my fellow students had, like me, taken the first MB examination at school, but the rest had started at Barts. About a dozen of my contemporaries were mature students. Of the three South Africans, two had been pharmacists in Durban and the third had been a gold miner in Johannesburg. We had a former dentist, a chartered accountant, an ex-army officer, several who had been in business, and one or two arts and science graduates. Since most of us were only in our late teens it was good to have this leavening of older and more experienced men – in those days there were no women students at Barts. There were also two German Jewish refugees. One of them, Fred Gunz, had only been in the country for two years but had passed the London matriculation after a year at Borland's (like Maurice Kinmonth he too was coached by William Joyce) and had then taken his first MB at Barts. He later became a distinguished haematologist in the United States, New Zealand, and Australia. He is a splendid man and remains a good friend. Frankel, the other German, I later lost trace of.

The next two years were spent in studying anatomy, physiology, organic chemistry, and biochemistry. The anatomy we were taught then was much more detailed than in the modern curriculum, and the department retained a close relationship with some of the hospital staff. It was not unknown for one or two of the consultant surgeons to visit the dissecting rooms if they wanted to refresh their memories before an unfamiliar operation. The demonstrators of anatomy, who supervised our dissections and regularly gave us viva voce examinations on the parts we had dissected, were embryo surgeons who had usually passed, or were due to take, the final FRCS examination. This always gave a distinctly clinical flavour to the subject and most of our demonstrators were good teachers who then moved on to further surgical training. Of those in my time, Harold Rodgers was appointed to the Barts staff but later became professor of surgery in Belfast; John O'Connell, after spending time as a general surgical chief assistant and one year with neurosurgeons in North America, was the first specialist neurosurgeon at Barts; and Oswald Tubbs was later cardiothoracic surgeon to Barts and the Brompton Hospital. My own group demonstrator, Philip Scott, became an ear, nose, and throat surgeon in the west country; Sam Birdsall did ear, nose, and throat work in London, and Vincent Snell went into orthopaedics.

Our anatomy professor, Herbert Henry Woollard, was an Australian graduate of Melbourne University who had served with distinction in an Anzac division at Gallipoli during the first world war. He was small in stature and nearly bald, with grey hair at the sides. Rather surprisingly, he spoke with an Oxford accent. He was a strict disciplinarian, but an excellent lecturer who demanded total silence in the lecture theatre. By his apt choice of word and gesture, his dry humour, and his occasional philosophical digressions, he had no difficulty in holding the rapt attention of his audience. On one occasion, the day after our rugby XV had been defeated by St Mary's in the hospital cup final, as he entered the old Abernethian theatre there was the usual prompt cessation of all conversation on the benches. In that great hush Woollard firmly intoned, "Gentlemen, we have been defeated by the hire purchase system." Everyone collapsed in helpless mirth. His comment was directed at Dr Charles Wilson (later Lord Moran), the dean of St Mary's, who had recently been offering athletic scholarships to promising sportsmen from Oxbridge, thus greatly strengthening the St Mary's teams.

Woollard deserves special mention for a number of reasons. Many of us, and particularly Fred Gunz and I, regard him as the most outstanding character and teacher of our student days. Though he appeared to be an old man he was, in fact, only in his mid-forties when we first met him. He suffered from angina pectoris, due to coronary artery disease, and his pain could easily be provoked by anger and frustration. This largely explained his firm control of his classes and his occasional irascibility. But he was a fine man who had a keen understanding of his students, warts and all. I can remember more than one occasion when his angina occurred during a lecture. He would put a hand on his chest, sometimes slipping a trinitrini tablet under his tongue, and then say, "Angina pectoris, gentlemen, the enemy of mankind: it killed John Hunter and will as surely kill me." Indeed it did. For he shortly succeeded Grafton Elliot Smith at University College and died there of a myocardial infarct in 1939, aged only 49. One other vivid memory of Woollard is of a neat bandage which he had on his left wrist for about a year. Unknown to us he was studying the sensory end organs in the skin and had set out to discover whether regeneration could occur after skin loss. Having mapped out the sites of his pain and temperature end organs on the volar aspect of his wrist, he persuaded Archie (later Sir Archibald) McIndoe to take Thiersch grafts of increasing thickness under local anaesthetic. My recollection of the study is that he then remapped the skin sensation when healing had occurred, and I believe that this study was published in *Brain*.

Organic chemistry, studied for only two terms, was followed by part I of the second MB examination. We were most methodically taught by the kindly Dr Hurtley, and careful attention to his lectures, with use of his notes, was all that one needed for success. I found this an unexpectedly interesting subject. Hurtley was supported by one demonstrator, George Discombe, who was working his passage into medicine and qualified a year or two after us. He became a first class clinical pathologist at Central Middlesex Hospital. One of the laboratory attendants, Francis, later graduated in science and became reader in biochemistry at Barts. The second lab boy, Geoffrey Bond, became a medical student and was an excellent houseman and later general practitioner at Rickmansworth. The relatively cossetted present day students sometimes need reminding how much was achieved by energy and sheer guts in days gone by.

The physiology department was situated on the opposite side of Little Britain, above the White Hart. The proximity of that hostelry offered refreshment to many a thirsty student after a morning session in the adjacent laboratories and lecture rooms. Our professor was Hamilton Hartridge, who in recognition of his important work on colour vision had been elected to fellowship of the Royal Society at an early age. He always wore a rather shiny blue suit and an Old Harrovian tie; never once did we see him without that old school tie. He was a pleasant man but an uninspiring lecturer. One of his senior demonstrators, Mr Haynes, was a friendly man who regularly drank with us in the pub on the corner of Giltspur Street and regaled us with anecdotes and dirty jokes from "The Pink 'un" (the *Sporting Times*). Indeed, there was a plethora of pubs in those parts and I have little doubt that some of us tended to consume a little more than was good for us.

At the end of my first year I sat for the junior scholarship examination, which I was astonished to win. I have a more or less photographic memory and never had any difficulty in mastering anatomy. However, my physiology was not so strong. It so happened that one of the questions in the physiology paper was concerned with the functions of the suprarenal gland. About two years before, while in my last year at school, I had attended a conversazione at Charing Cross Hospital Medical School. One of the pathologists there, Professor Vines, had given us a lucid talk on the role of the suprarenal in relation to the so called sterile freemartin cow. At the time this knowledge was a little in advance of what appeared in our student textbooks and my memory of the lecture was so clear that my examiners were impressed by my wholly serendipitous distinction. Without this physiological snippet I doubt whether the scholarship would have been mine.

Success in that first year inspired me to do my best in the following year. I may have swotted unnecessarily hard but I greatly enjoyed every challenge in the syllabus. Regrettably, I did little general reading and chiefly relaxed by taking violent physical exercise, usually squash and fives during the week and rugby football in our sociable B and extra B teams during the winter weekends. That exercise engendered considerable thirst, which encouraged the consumption of so much beer that, especially during the weekends, I was often too sleepy to work by the time I arrived home. Some of my mature colleagues – notably Dick Grindlay, the ex-chartered accountant; Gerry Schofield, the dentist; and "Pip" Palmer, mature student and father of four children – had enrolled me in a club at Charterhouse Square where we commonly repaired for refreshment. It would be fair to say that I occasionally drank more beer than was good for me, but I did not gain weight and that ale may have been a valuable source of calories. After a year or two I often played squash for the hospital and eventually captained the fives club.

I am compelled to recall an incident concerning the unfortunate "Pip" Palmer. He was one of my group of five students who dissected together. For our first term we had to dissect the abdomen of an exceedingly thin female corpse. Working usually in pairs, it was customary for one to read the dissecting manual while the other wielded the knife. Cunningham's practical manual for the abdomen ordained: "Make a bold incision in the right iliac fossa and expose the shining aponeurosis of the external oblique muscle." I had done just that, but I neither knew my own strength nor the sharpness of my new Bard–Parker blade. To my dismay the abdominal muscles were completely divided as well as a few underlying loops of small gut. A short time later Palmer and I had changed places; I with the book and he with the knife. At that moment Bertie Woollard arrived. After surveying my bold incision with horror he said to Palmer: "Good God, man, have the rats been at it?" I was too dumbstruck to confess and Palmer remained silent, but Woollard continued, "What is your name?" Pip replied, "Palmer, sir, . . ." Woollard responded, "Ah, Palmer, the man who was thrown out of King's; it won't be long before you're thrown out of Barts." Then, as he was about to move off, he added, "Palmer, but yes, *Palmer*, that was the name of the only Barts student to be hanged for murder!" This was indeed true and is mentioned in a celebrated paper by the late Sir James Paget. Perhaps I should add that Barts is the only hospital to have the distinction of having one of its physicians, the Elizabethan Dr Lopez, hanged, drawn, and quartered for alleged high treason. Palmer was gallant to have taken the blame. When I apologised to him for funking the issue he cheerfully responded, "Don't worry chum, I can take it."

Bertie Woollard's intolerance of needless movement, and noise, is well shown by two further incidents. In the first, one of our younger students, Alan Walker, was fidgeting in the back row of the lecture theatre. Woollard was disturbed by the light rhythmical tapping of a foot on the floor, and he observed the movement of the offending leg. Standing still, with pale and tightening countenance, he pointed a finger at the hapless Walker and exploded, "Get out, boy. What are you doing, *masturbating*?" A week or two later a Persian student named Pezesghi, diligently taking notes, dropped his large pencil box on the floor with a loud clatter. Woollard looked up, pale and visibly shaking with anger. Pezesghi grabbed his notebook and beat it up the steep stairs of the ancient lecture theatre and out of the top door without a backward look. The silence was deathly; but as the miscreant disappeared from sight Woollard broke down in helpless laughter, to be joined in relief by the whole class. At his next lecture the projector attendant was missing. Woollard, after starting to talk, picked up a large handful of old glass slides. Looking around the theatre, his resonant voice gently intoned, "Now, which of you gentlemen will have the kindness to work the projector for me?" Keen to make amends, student Pezesghi promptly volunteered for the task. As he handed over the slides Woollard said, "Ah, thank you, Mr Pezesghi." A moment's pause and then he continued to muse aloud, "Mr Pezesghi, my *dear* Mr Pezesghi, the student to whom a beneficent Persian government sent £10 with which to buy a half skeleton – but, alas, who then blued it all on a bird or a tart!" There were peals of good natured laughter all round, and even Pezesghi himself grinned broadly. The story was largely true: the Persian Embassy had sent a cheque to the student and then asked his professor for confirmation that the half skeleton had been bought. Woollard had been much amused when he heard that Pezesghi had spent the money on one of his girlfriends. But he ensured that justice was done by insisting that a half skeleton was purchased and brought to him for confirmation. Despite his periodic irascible outbursts, Herbert Henry Woollard was a fair, friendly, and just man. Those who did not come to love him could assuredly admire him, and I was one of those whom he inspired.

Well, rotten little swot that I was, at the end of the next academic year I won the senior scholarship examination in anatomy and physiology; passed my second MB examination in which I came top in anatomy; and was awarded the Sir William Dunn exhibition of London University. Two of us, Jonathan Gould (who became a psychiatrist) and I, were advised to take the BSc honours course during the next year, as we had both managed to pass the primary FRCS six weeks after the MB examination. The BSc honours degree for medical students had only just been introduced and Gould was keen to take the physiology course. Woollard wanted me to do research on the lymphatics as part of an anatomy BSc. But our contemporaries had already moved on to clinical work and I was anxious to join them; so, perhaps unwisely, I rejected this offer.

Notwithstanding my academic success I am sure that I was mentally exhausted at that time. I had, moreover, narrowly missed another distinction. In those days the primary FRCS examination was confined to anatomy and physiology and could be taken by both undergraduates and postgraduates. But the latter, having been out of touch with these basic subjects for some years, were always given a single extra mark in each part of the examination. Nowadays we let the candidates have their results on the day of their oral examination, but then one's success or failure was not published for two or three weeks. The longer I waited for those results the more convinced I became that I had failed. My state of anxiety compelled me to report miserably to Woollard and confess that I felt sure I had let him down by failing. He looked at me incredulously and said, "Of course you're through, but you have missed the Hallett prize by one mark, you bloody young fool!" He added that the prize had been secured by a much more senior graduate and that graduates always had bonus marks. My relief at having passed was so great that I did not ask who the prizewinner was. Not until 41 years later, when I was president of the Royal College of Surgeons, did I have the records examined. It was exactly as Woollard had told me. The Hallett prizeman was Kenneth Starr, who, in 1963, became president of the Royal Australasian College of Surgeons. I wonder whether our examiners ever anticipated our later success.

Looking back on that period now I think that I may have worked too hard in those first two years at Barts. I certainly neglected my general reading; physical exercise and conversation in the pubs became my main methods of relaxation. Despite a natural disposition to argument I never took an active part in the debates of the Abernethian Society; but in later life I was frequently invited to debate. I often, however, attended meetings of a literary society which had been started by Lionel Grunbaum, one of my Jewish contemporaries. Politically he was distinctly to the left. He had taken an Arts degree at Cambridge before deciding to enter Barts as a medical student. It was because of his known political stance that the dean had refused to authorise Grunbaum's literary society within the medical school, and so most of our meetings took place at the houses of the hospital staff, or of fellow members.

Three of those meetings of the literary society I remember clearly. At the first, held in the house of Dr Geoffrey Evans (a Barts physician who teamed with Lord Horder), Alistair Cooke gave an entertaining talk on contemporary politics. On the second occasion Captain Basil Liddell Hart, the notable military historian, talked on "the next war." He spoke, I believe, of the vulnerability of the Maginot line, but I cannot recall whether he was supportive or dismissive of the concept of *Blitzkrieg*. That meeting in 1935 was at the house of Tim Nelson, a former surgical chief assistant at Barts who had recently been appointed thoracic surgeon to the London and Brompton hospitals. A year later he contracted staphylococcal pyaemia after pricking a finger in the course of an empyema operation. He was admitted to Barts under James Paterson Ross, then our professor of surgery, and treated ineffectually with the newly developed Prontosil rubrum, which was only effective against streptococci. Indeed, Ross tried the new drug out on himself before giving it to Nelson. The following morning Ross's urine was bright red and he told his wife that he had haematuria before recognising that the red colour was due to the drug. There were no antibiotics in those days and antibacterial chemotherapy was only just beginning. Poor Tim had the affected arm amputated at the shoulder joint and died (perhaps fortunately for so gifted a surgeon) a few days later – one of many such fatalities among doctors in the preantibiotic era. Some years later his widow married Liddell Hart.

I have especial cause to remember the third, rather later, meeting of Grunbaum's society. It was addressed by Sinclair Loutit, a Barts student some two years older than me. He had strong communist sympathies and had spent a year in Spain, in opposition to Franco, during the Spanish civil war. He gave a fascinating talk about his war experience, and I remember that the room was decorated with several propaganda posters.

One of these concerned the prevention of venereal disease; but Loutit explained that the high degree of illiteracy made it impossible for the simpler folk to understand the message. He told us that the "early treatment" packages had been made up in paper bags which contained condom, lubricant, cotton wool, and a small tube of mercury ointment. Failure to understand the instructions led to one unfortunate girl being admitted to hospital in extreme discomfort. Examination revealed that the condom, the wool, the discharged tube of ointment, its contents, and, finally, the screwed up paper bag had been stuffed into her vagina by her amorous companion.

I had two happy and successful, if somewhat fatiguing, preclinical years at Barts. Only later did I realise the lack of breadth and depth of my earlier education. But my rather slender intellectual foundations were by no means unusual among young students who single mindedly pursued their cherished goals. That is where some of our mature contemporaries scored over us. But, unknown to me then, I was shortly to remedy many of those earlier deficiencies in the great university of life during a second world war.

3 Walking the wards

Our clinical appointments conformed to a quarterly programme so that, having proceeded to the primary FRCS after the second MB examination and then waited a fortnight for the results, my entry to hospital work was delayed until July 1936. My former London contemporaries were now three months ahead of me, though this did not ultimately prejudice my planned date of graduation in May 1939. A welcome feature of the clinical period then, rather more than nowadays, was the arrival of undergraduates from Oxford and Cambridge. I emphasise this point since neither of these ancient universities then had a clinical school of its own. Indeed it was only after the second world war that the dons in both places, rather reluctantly it seemed, came to accept the respectability of clinical medicine. Before the war both Addenbrooke's at Cambridge and the Radcliffe Infirmary at Oxford had some general practitioner physicians and surgeons on their staffs. There were appreciably more medical students from Cambridge than from Oxford and it was good for all of us to be mixed together at the London teaching hospitals. Among some of my closer Cambridge acquaintances then were Charles Fletcher, Bryan Brooke, Tom Rowntree, Maxwell Bull, and Arthur Levin. Fletcher, a rowing blue and double first, was older than the rest and had spent some six years in physiological research. In later years, when working in the Postgraduate Medical School at Hammersmith, he became well known for his BBC television appearances in *Your Life in Their Hands*. Bryan Brooke and Tom Rowntree were, like me, both intent on surgery. Brooke worked for some years in Birmingham before his appointment to an inaugural full time chair of surgery at St George's Hospital, and Rowntree had a distinguished career at Southampton. Bull became a full time anatomical don at Cambridge and Levin made his mark by persuading the Kayser shipping firm to build the avowedly up market Wellington Hospital at St John's Wood.

My first appointment as a junior surgical dresser involved attendance on casual outpatients – mainly those with infected fingers, boils, carbuncles, and minor injuries – as opposed to those who had been specifically referred to consultant clinics by their general practitioners. We also attended patients in the "septic" wards (Radcliffe for women and Colston for men), most of whom were suffering from severe abscesses, carbuncles, osteomyelitis, tubercular joints, or related problems – conditions that are rarely seen by the students of today.

In the outpatient department we worked from so called casualty boxes – that is, examination and treatment rooms which had the colour of each of the five surgical firms' record cards displayed above their doors. I was attached to the surgical professorial unit, whose patients' cards were dark blue. Each of us had to buy a simple instrument case which contained scissors, dissecting forceps, surgical probe, and sinus forceps. For every dressing we boiled up our instruments in a gas fired water container with any necessary gallipots and kidney dishes and then laid these out on a trolley. Each group of dressers was under the supervision of his firm's casualty house surgeon. The service was primitive, but most of our patients were grateful for what we did for them. We were on friendly terms with cockneys from Dalston, bumarees (meat porters) from Smithfield, and the occasional city clerk – an essentially Anglo-Saxon clientele which would be unusual in most London hospitals today. Under supervision we also attended to sprains and lesser fractures and did minor surgery, generally with nitrous oxide or local anaesthetic.

In the two septic wards we were strictly supervised by the sisters in charge. Sister Colston, on the male ward, was firm and aloof until she had summed each of us up, but was then a good friend to any conscientious dresser. In the female ward Sister Radcliffe, a red faced, rotund, and fierce woman, scared the wits out of most of her probationer nurses and was rarely well disposed to the dressers. But sepsis was commoner in males, so we generally had much more to do in Colston ward. My first three male patients were suffering from chronic osteomyelitis (a persistent relapsing infection of bone), which was a dispiriting condition. It is usually caused by staphylococcal infection; unfortunately there was then no drug to kill or control that organism. An appropriate sulphonamide was to appear two years later, followed by penicillin during the war. The infected bone, often the femur or tibia, had to be drained by a primitive "guttering" process to remove sequestra (dead fragments of bone). There followed a long period of healing as an inpatient. Many of the patients with osteomyelitis were youngsters, who required repeated admission to hospital in their school and early working years. One of our older patients, Detective Serjeant Spink of the City of London police vice squad, was an entertaining raconteur who astonished the more innocent of us with tales of curious homosexual and heterosexual activities within the famous square mile.

In the old septic wards we worked in almost mediaeval conditions which, unknown to us, were shortly to be transformed by the emergence of effective antibacterial chemotherapy and antibiotics. It must seem surprising that fresh from the anatomy rooms, and with no previous introduction to management of the sick, we were then thrown in the deep end: a rude awakening in the realms of blatant pathology. More than one of our teachers urged us to read pathology; indeed, our own casualty surgeon instructor, Bill Underwood (who was appointed to the surgical staff after the war and then moved to a professorial chair in Johannesburg), said, "Study your patients; read about the pathology of their diseases and don't read the surgical textbooks at this stage." That was all very well, but compared with our Cambridge contemporaries we were ill prepared for the clinical transformation. The Cambridge preclinical course included a sound grounding in basic pathology and bacteriology, so that, having completed the natural science tripos, the students were better equipped for the change to clinical medicine. It was only many years later, when I was training young surgeons from different backgrounds and examining in pathology for the much improved English primary FRCS, that I recognised how much better prepared those Cambridge students were. I suspect that much of this was due to "Daddy" Dean's long influence in the Cambridge pathology chair, where he remained until he was in his 90s, having been appointed when there was no statutory retiring age. I cannot speak with any authority about the relative merits of the Oxford tripos in my time as I had only two Oxford contemporaries.

After three months as junior dressers we moved on to senior dresserships in the surgical firms of our choice, provided they were not overbooked. I chose the surgical professorial unit, then under the directorship of James Paterson Ross, with Clifford Naunton Morgan as assistant director. The chief assistants, who would now be called senior registrars or registrars, were Bill Underwood, Michael Boyd, and Alan Hunt. After the war Boyd became professor of surgery at Manchester and Hunt was appointed to the Barts staff, eventually to die of leukaemia in his 50s. The two house surgeons were Gordon Bohn, later surgeon to the Royal Berkshire Hospital at Reading, and Trevor Baynes (a prefect at Dulwich when I was a new boy), who went into obstetrics and gynaecology. Of my eight or so fellow dressers some were contemporaries and others were more senior students who were doing their second spell as senior dressers. The mixture of more advanced and less advanced students meant that it was often possible to pick up useful tips from those who had greater experience.

One of my first patients in Percivall Pott ward was Eustace Bacon, a 55 year old government statistician with pyloric obstruction due to a longstanding duodenal ulcer. Gordon Bohn, having taken me to the bedside and introduced me as Mr Bacon's new dresser, showed me how I was to wash out the patient's stomach on alternate days, using a large bore stomach tube. The tube was about as thick as my forefinger, but my task was simple since Eustace Bacon was able to pop the tube down with the easy accomplishment of a sword swallower. I still have copies of all my record cards of those days and I find that I washed that stomach out with normal saline no less than nine times in the ensuing 18 days. Paterson Ross then did a posterior gastrojejunostomy under a local infiltration anaesthetic and splanchnic block, assisted by the house surgeon and me. The procedure went off smoothly and recovery was uneventful.

In those days a middle class patient, such as Eustace Bacon, would have made a contribution towards his hospital care; the amount would have been determined by one of the lady almoners. Poorer patients were either treated free or paid according to a sliding scale of charges, frequently with support from the Hospital Savings Association, to which many contributed. It is surprising how today many people assume that the sick poor were untreated before the National Health Service. In fact, we had a remarkably efficient voluntary and municipal hospital system; waiting lists for surgery were rarely excessive, and extra beds were often willingly put up to accommodate an unexpected influx of patients. Of course, the pressure of work was of an entirely different pattern to that of today. Nevertheless, judged in the context of those days, the service was both sensitive and responsive to the needs of the times.

One of my other interesting patients in Percivall Pott was Henry Keats, a 26 year old meat porter from Holloway who had a meningioma (a generally benign tumour arising from the covering membrane of the brain) on the right side. For a little over two years he had suffered increasingly troublesome headaches, occasional vomiting, irritability, and lapses of memory, and for six months he had noticed weakness in his left leg and arm with "catching of the toe" on walking. The diagnosis was established on the basis of the history, physical signs, and a plain *x* ray of the skull. Four days after transfer from a medical ward, where he had been admitted under the neurologist, Dr Hinds-Howell, he was operated upon by Professor Ross. A bone flap was turned down on the right side of the skull and as second assistant for some four hours it was my job to drop cooling saline on the steel burr and the Gigli saw which were used to open the skull, and generally to make myself useful for the rest of the operation. Dr John West, the senior resident anaesthetist (who was later consultant in Cardiff), put the patient to sleep with nitrous oxide and oxygen and maintained anaesthesia by adding a trace of chloroform, according to my note. The operation was done on 6 October 1936, and the patient was discharged on 2 November. Although it had been thought prudent to leave a small and less accessible part of the tumour in situ, I see that this man was re-explored in May of the following year when the hospital records show that the residual tumour had entirely disappeared.

I have described the above two cases in some detail for several reasons. Longstanding pyloric obstruction such as Eustace Bacon suffered could cause serious disturbance of the blood chemistry. In those days the laboratory was able to measure the blood electrolyte levels by much more tedious methods than are used today. But the basic principles of the chemical changes in these cases were beginning to be better understood, so that operating on such patients became far safer. The use of the traditional alkaline stomach washout of sodium bicarbonate could do much harm; that is why I had to use normal saline for this purpose. Moreover, since regular checking of the blood electrolytes was not then considered feasible or necessary we dressers were taught to do a daily check on the chloride output in the urine as a rough guide to the patient's chemical state. In the course of the next few years there was to be a notable revolution in our understanding of the blood chemistry in more difficult surgical cases; but considering the state of the art in the 1930s I believe that Mr Bacon was managed in exemplary style.

Turning now to the case of the meat porter with the meningioma, it is worth recalling how simple and cheap were the preoperative tests which established the correct diagnosis. Paterson Ross, as a young chief assistant, had been sent to Harvey Cushing in Boston for one year's neurosurgical training. On returning to Barts, well before the days of specialised neurosurgical departments, he undertook the cranial surgery in his general unit and also had an appointment at the West End Hospital for Nervous Diseases. At that time there was not one "pure" neurosurgeon in the country, but Hugh Cairns, at the London Hospital, was shortly to confine himself solely to that specialty. We prided ourselves on the high standard of anaesthesia at Barts in those days; but, by comparison with the state of the art less than a decade later, Henry Keats, although skilfully put to sleep and well maintained, was really given a quite simple anaesthetic. To his credit, Paterson Ross recognised that he would not be able to provide the required specialist service of the future. Therefore John O'-Connell, then surgical chief assistant to another firm, and formerly senior demonstrator of anatomy in my dissecting days, was sent to work for a year with Dandy and others in North America, returning to Barts only shortly before the outbreak of war. But had it not been for the outbreak of war in 1939 and the need to establish a wide range of specialist surgical services in the main sector hospital at Hill End, St Albans, it is doubtful whether O'Connell would have been able to develop his highly efficient neurosurgical unit so soon.

I much enjoyed that three month dressership on the surgical unit in the last quarter of 1936. On Christmas and Boxing days it was customary for dressers on the surgical and certain other firms to mount ward shows for the entertainment of the patients. Appropriate costumes were designed and assembled by willing female hands and the props for each show were moved around from ward to ward on a trolley. Patients considered too unwell to withstand the more boisterous shows were strategically moved by the ward sister and staff to the side rooms or the back of the ward. The shows were advertised by posters, most of which were extremely well designed and executed. These were displayed at strategic points in the hospital and medical college. Our own show that year had the somewhat ambiguous title of "The Dark Blue Seamen," and we were dressed in sailor suits. Our brilliant pianist, John Beeston, had been at school with me and was later to win the George Medal during the London blitz. Another of my former school friends in the show, who later became a fine and kindly family doctor in Suffolk but who had better remain unnamed, became so drunk on Christmas Day that he had to be resuscitated by the ever resourceful Sister Lawrence (Miss Gimson), who washed out his stomach in the side room of her female ward and restored him to a good enough state to put on a passable performance in the very next ward.

New Year 1937 saw me as a medical clerk on the firm of George Graham. George was a solemn old bachelor who had reputedly ordered a round of cocoa at his golf club after shooting a hole in one. He certainly liked to imbibe a cup of cocoa with the sister of Sol Memorial or Luke wards at the time of his rounds. The assistant consultant, Edward Cullinan, was married to Lord Horder's daughter, Joy, who had recently delivered their third child. Indeed, I can remember Miss Gimson's telling me of the the babe's arrival, adding, with a significant nod, "Of course, he's a Roman Catholic!" Heaven knows what she would have thought had she later learnt that, as non-Catholics, my wife and I had twice that number: doubtless she might have murmured, "Careless protestants!"

John Hunt, chief assistant on the Graham–Cullinan firm, was a superb teacher and an outstanding physician. He was the elder brother of Alan, junior assistant on the surgical professorial unit. John enthused us all mightily with the challenge and excitement of clinical medicine and even though I had been inclined from the start to see my future in surgery I derived tremendous satisfaction from each of my medical appointments. I shall never forget how, having introduced himself to us and stressed the importance of a careful and meticulous medical history, Hunt took us into his wards and said, "Let me show you one or two significant physical signs in a few of our patients before you each attend to your own patients." Thereupon he demonstrated one man with an upper motor neurone lesion; another with Hodgkin's disease; a young boy with renal rickets; and a woman who had been labelled for some time as having disseminated sclerosis but who he believed to have an acoustic nerve tumour. This lady, Mrs Lillian Gaffney, became one of my patients and subsequently had her tumour successfully removed by John O'Connell. Indeed she survived long afterwards, and many years later John O'Connell told me that he had operated on her for two recurrences. As for John Hunt, he was later to marry Elizabeth, the beautiful sister of Kit Evill, one of my fellow students. All three have been good friends of ours for many years; but sadly John died in 1987.

We had assumed that John Hunt would be appointed to the staff of Barts and possibly to the Hospital for Nervous Diseases. After serving in the RAF medical service during the war as medical and neurological specialist, however, he chose to establish a high quality general practice in London. He was chiefly responsible for the founding, and much of the early and vital secretarial support, of the Royal College of General Practitioners, later becoming its president before the ultimate award of a well deserved peerage. He was blind for the last six years of his life, while bravely and patiently suffering from a number of other serious problems. I know that his great enthusiasm for medicine inspired many students of my generation and that we owe much to his example.

After nine months of dressing and clerking in the wards we became involved in medical and surgical outpatient sessions, and in such specialties as ear, nose, and throat work, ophthalmology, dermatology, and venereology. Into the programme were fitted regular lectures and practical classes in pathology and bacteriology. It was also possible to take on voluntary appointments and, in July 1937, I became a solitary dresser to the orthopaedic surgeons, working mainly with Jackson Burrows in the wards and operating theatre and with Derek Coltart and Harold Lee in the outpatient clinics. I helped Coltart and Lee with the manipulations under anaesthesia. I sometimes shudder when I think of the vigour with which spines and joints were manipulated. I was also allowed to do a number of minor operations on the foot. This voluntary orthopaedic appointment gave me a good deal of experience in the management of bone and joint disorders, and there was a fair amount of assisting at operations too. The orthopaedic house surgeon also looked after Sir Harold Gillies, the consultant plastic surgeon. Gillies operated every Wednesday afternoon, generally arriving anything up to an hour or two late but then putting in a long spell of work well into the evening. At that time he had a fellow New Zealander and distant cousin, Archibald McIndoe, as his chief assistant. Using two tables in our largest operating theatre, Gillies would work at the main table assisted by the house surgeon (Percy Jayes, who was later to succeed Gillies at Barts and McIndoe at East Grinstead), while I much enjoyed assisting McIndoe at the second table, where he often gave me some suturing to do.

I remember one notable occasion when Gillies was constructing a penis for an unfortunate man who had lost his in an accident. Using the skin and fat of the abdomen below the umbilicus, he had raised a long tube pedicle which he had then "tubed" again to make the future urethra. While all this was in progress an eager and bespectacled student with bats' wing ears, named Dwyer, had leant forward and inquired, "Excuse me, sir, do you do many of these operations?" Gillies promptly replied, "This is the 360th case in my series." Dwyer made appropriate murmurs of approval to signify his appreciation of the work of the "great man." There was a long pause as Gillies continued stitching; then he added with a snort, "Don't be so damned silly, boy. This is the first I have ever done, but I shall have lots more when the Abyssinian war is over!" Mussolini's fascist forces had invaded Abyssinia a few months earlier and there were rumours about certain revengeful mutilations which some of the Italians were suffering.

I had become especially interested in orthopaedic surgery after reading Frederick Watson's *Life of Sir Robert Jones*, the famous Liverpool surgeon. I planned to visit the accident hospital in Vienna in the coming September and chanced to mention this one morning when I was scrubbing up with Jackson Burrows (J B) to assist him in the theatre. J B said, "Oh, I've always wanted to visit Böhler's accident hospital." I responded, more lightheartedly than seriously, "Why don't you come with me, sir?" To my surprise J B said that he would love to do so. During one of his clinics that afternoon I told an older student contemporary of mine, Christopher Jackson, and he too decided to join us. And so it was that a week or two later we three met on a platform at Victoria station and took the boat train to France, thence to Vienna where we stayed in a comfortable little pension quite near the *Allgemeineskrankenhaus* (general hospital) and the *Unfallkrankenhaus* (Böhler's accident hospital). Even for students like Christopher and me this was a wonderful experience.

Lorenz Böhler had earned a worldwide reputation for his system of fracture management, and his book had been translated into English by Professor Hey Groves of Bristol. His hospital, financed and run by an insurance company, occupied the top two floors of the company's main building. The hospital had been set up to reduce substantially the long period of invalidity suffered by many manual workers after injury. Böhler ruled that institution with Germanic ruthlessness, but there was no denying the excellent results which he achieved and I learnt much from that visit – not least the importance of medical economics.

We had one or two amusing experiences at Böhler's hospital. During our one week visit Dr Roger Anderson, of Seattle, arrived. He had introduced the Roger Anderson pin with which he transfixed the broken parts of a fractured long bone before effecting their reduction with a machine which manipulated the fragments. That philosophy of fracture treatment was about as far removed from Böhler's as possible; so we saw tension developing between the two men. One of Böhler's assistants, who spoke excellent English, whispered to us one day, "Did you know that in Seattle they call him 'get-yer-right-quick Anderson'?" At the accident hospital the reduction of most fractures was done under local anaesthetic. One morning we watched the nailing of a fractured neck of femur in a young woman. Now the Smith–Pedersen nail had only been introduced quite recently and even JB had little experience in its use. Fixed to the central post of the orthopaedic table Lorenz Böhler had a cunning device, which, after reduction of the displacement, enabled him to position the guide wire accurately within the femoral neck. All went well under the local anaesthetic until the nail was driven into the upper fragment. At that point the woman screamed with pain. Böhler promptly shouted, "Haben Sie keine Stolz?" ("Have you no pride?"). The woman was silent for a short time but then cried out again, so one of the assistants was asked to administer inhalation anaesthesia.

The stoicism of many of these Austrian patients was seen also in the general hospital clinics. We did not watch Professor Finsterer operating; but apparently he used local anaesthetic for most of his gastric surgery and his patients usually walked to, and from, the theatre as well as hopping on to, and off, the table. Christopher and I watched Professor Ranzi and his *Dozent* (university lecturer) at work; we were impressed by what we saw, and even more impressed by Ranzi's beautiful embroidered waistcoat, which had been solemnly removed by an attendant nurse before he scrubbed up. In the 1930s Vienna was still a great centre for medical postgraduates, especially those from the United States, and many were to be seen in the town or visiting notables such as Finsterer. The general hospital was a huge place with some 4000 patients. The wards were in pleasant old buildings. One of the wards we visited seemed greatly overcrowded, and I am still haunted by the jaundiced and emaciated faces we saw there. One pavilion which J B visited on his own accommodated the electrical institute of Professor Jellinek, who had made an important study of fractures and burns caused by electric shocks sustained on the Vienna tramways. Until then I had not heard of the interesting fractures caused by the violent muscle action that can result from the passage of a high voltage current through the body. Many years later I met Jellinek's son in London, when he was working at the Hospital for Nervous Diseases. I believe that his father left Vienna before the war. Ranzi, who was bitterly opposed to the Nazis, did not survive, but Lorenz Böhler was reputedly better disposed to the Anschluss with Nazi Germany.

Our Austrian visit in 1936 was just a year before that Anschluss. The only hint of what might be in the air was an occasional man in the street with a red armband which bore a black swastika on a white circle. I have a picture of one such fellow in my photograph album. We were certainly made more aware of the situation through an introduction to Dr Nagel Grunbaum, a cousin of my contemporary who had organised the controversial literary society at Barts. With fellow students like Gunz and Frankel in our year we should have known more about the situation, but they told us very little and we were not well disposed to accepting Lionel Grunbaum's warnings. His cousin Nagel met us one afternoon and we took a tram out of Vienna to one of the Grinzing vineyards, where we sampled the new wines. It was an exceptionally hot day and shortly after boarding the tram I was smitten by the marked fortification figures of one of my periodic migraines. On reaching our destination, just as I was dismounting Nagel remarked, "You have the migraine." I replied, "Yes, I have, but it only started a few minutes ago. How did you know?" Nagel said, "One side of your face is paler than the other." I had never before heard of this particular sign of migraine, even though I had read a great deal of the literature. My attack quickly eased off, despite my sampling of the pale green young wine in the garden of that vineyard.

Nagel Grunbaum like many of his Jewish compatriots was clearly worried about the future and his sombre mood is well shown in a picture which I took that afternoon. It was clear to us that he shared the anxieties of his cousin Lionel in England. However, another of our contemporaries, Peter Gimson, who had spent a year at the University of Heidelberg before entering Barts, always strongly disputed Lionel's warnings since the menace of Hitler had not been so apparent in Heidelberg. Peter eventually became a general practitioner in Aylesbury. Only two months before my visit to Vienna Peter and I had spent a fortnight together walking briskly in the Swiss Alps near Interlaken. But during that summer even the most insensitive and busy of students could sense the gathering shadows.

4 Rumours of war

In October 1937, just after our return from Vienna, I began to realise that I still had a lot of reading to do in preparation for my qualifying examinations. The final MB, BS was to take place early in 1939, but many of us were planning to take the conjoint final (MRCS Eng, LRCP Lond) in December 1938. This not only gave a practice run for the degree examinations but also offered the possibility of taking the MRCP or final FRCS at an earlier date. Having acted on Bill Underwood's advice to "study the patients," I began to realise that I had spent so much time in the wards, the clinics, and the operation theatres that my systematic reading had suffered. I had also learnt that clinical art and science was far more difficult to master than the basic sciences. No longer could one's study be confined to a few standard texts, and no longer could one rely on a photographic memory for immediate recall of anatomical details.

During that autumn and winter I did some serious swotting, often taking the odd Dexedrine tablet to promote cerebral activity by day and by night. The amphetamine drugs had only recently been introduced and I do not think that we knew much of their ill effects. Fortunately, without coming to any serious harm, I quickly discovered these for myself. I certainly stayed wide awake throughout my swotting and my brain *appeared* to be functioning with exceptional clarity as I raced through my books. I was careful to take one tablet in the morning and another in the early afternoon for I had soon learnt that Dexedrine in the evening could make sleep almost impossible. After a month or so on this high pressure regime, however, I realised that what I had been reading was not properly registered in my brain. Although I had no knowledge of drug addiction, and do not recall having been taught anything at all about the subject, I had enough insight to realise that the tablets were doing me no good. I thereupon stopped taking the drug and am glad to report that I have had a healthy repugnance for all tranquillising and stimulating drugs ever since.

In the course of that last year or so I sat for a number of the scholarship examinations. Although I achieved the final shortlist in them all, I did not manage to win one, nor do I feel that I deserved to do so. I continued, however, to enjoy an interesting series of clinical appointments. Great changes were beginning in medicine of which we were only vaguely aware. At the time of my junior medical clerkship the death rate for patients with lobar pneumonia was 20%. I remember seeing one medical sister, in dressing gown and hair curlers, emerge from her bedroom at the end of the ward (where our ward sisters dwelt in those days) to help an anxious junior nurse who was struggling with a patient undergoing a pneumonic "crisis." But soon after the Tim Nelson septicaemia tragedy chemotherapy began steadily to advance. Following Bayer's early manufacture of the sulphonamide Prontosil the British firm of May & Baker had produced sulphapyridine (M&B 693), which was lethal to the pneumococcus. The same firm then produced sulphathiazole, which was effective against the staphylococcus and would almost certainly have been life saving for poor Nelson had it been available in 1936. Those of us who started clinical medicine when virtually the only specific therapeutic agents were Ehrlich's organic arsenical 606 for syphilis, quinine for malaria, insulin for diabetes, and digitalis for the heart were suddenly confronted with truly explosive developments.

We were also suddenly confronted with other explosive developments of which we now knew far more. The war in Abyssinia had seemed a long way away and Benito Mussolini something of a sick joke – like Sir Harold Gillies's reference to his impending penile reconstruction programme. But the Austrian Anschluss a year after our Viennese visit and then the German rape of the Sudetenland of Czechoslovakia, followed by the Munich agreement of September 1938, left us in no doubt about what the future held for us. Indeed at that time the students had been busily occupied with the hasty filling of sandbags in preparation for air raids which never came.

It was beneath those gathering shadows that in the last quarter of 1938 I started my senior clerkship on the medical professorial unit with the young Professor Leslie J Witts. He had come to us from Guy's only two years before, having built a solid reputation for his work on the anaemias. He had a special interest in the management of bleeding peptic ulcer and was advocating the Meulengracht regime in which such patients, instead of being starved, were liberally fed. The teaching on this unit was of high quality and Witts's staff included Ronald Bodley Scott, shortly afterwards to become a notable authority on the leukaemias and later the Royal Physician; Francis Avery Jones, who was justly to earn gastroenterological fame at Central Middlesex Hospital; Eric Scowen, ultimately successor to Witts; and Maxwell Telling. The last was the son of the then professor of medicine at Leeds. Each of the first three eventually received the accolade of knighthood, whereas Witts, a gentle, unassertive man, was later appointed to the Nuffield chair of medicine at Oxford and received only a CBE. My fellow clerks on the firm at that time included Charles Fletcher, Maxwell Bull, and George Lumb. I have already mentioned the first two, who were Cambridge men. Lumb was a London man and later became histopathologist at Westminster Hospital before emigrating to the United States. Fletcher at that time was regularly armed with his Leica camera and took entertaining pictures of senior staff in amusing and sometimes compromising situations. Many of these were published in the hospital journal, with appropriate captions. Fletcher developed diabetes in 1940 and was precluded from war service. After directing the Medical Research Council pneumoconiosis research unit at Cardiff he was an unsuccessful candidate for the chair of medicine at Barts. Scowen was eventually appointed to the chair after several years on trial as the "director."

We had plenty of talent for our Christmas 1938 ward show. George Lumb had become well known as a producer of polished shows. Some years later he teamed up with Professor

Norman Ashton, a distinguished ophthalmic pathologist, to produce a succession of outstanding Christmas pantomimes at the Westminster Hospital. We lacked a good pianist but managed to borrow John Beeston, who had been the musician in my first ward show. In our opening number we each had a characteristic verse to introduce ourselves to the audience. Charles Fletcher wrote mine and I can remember it to this very day:

How d'you do everybody. I am Reggie, Reggie M,
And of all this party you'll agree that I'm the gem,
Though my voice is rather bare, for music I've a flair,
And I know every single bar . . . from here to Leicester Square.

CHORUS: How d'you do, everybody. How d'you do?

The number that brought the house down that year depicted four staff nurses – "blue-belts" as they were called at Barts – seated around the stone edge of the fountain in the hospital square. Its title was "Four Faded Blue-belts" and the chorus between each verse concluded: "We are four faded blue-belts/ And though we look half dead/We're ever so fresh and blooming when we're planted in a bed." All four – Charles Fletcher, Max Bull, George Lumb, and one other (whose name I have forgotten) – looked convincing in their borrowed uniforms, even though the nurses' home sister had been hard pressed to find fitting costumes.

During that December I took the final conjoint examination and then moved to my last appointment as a senior dresser on the surgical firm of Reginald Vick and John Hosford. Although I had not completed my clinical attachments, I managed to trick the final examining boards on the question of my eligibility by giving the date of my second MB examination. The three months I missed while taking the primary FRCS were conveniently overlooked. Even though I was now armed with the MRCS, LRCP conjoint diploma, however, I felt constrained to keep quiet about this, fearing that my chiefs might expect me to be that much more knowledgeable. I doubt that they ever found out. Indeed, John Hosford, whose surgical chief assistant I became some seven years later, cannot even remember me as one of his dressers.

At the beginning of April a number of us began pathology clerkships on the surgical or medical firms of our choice, providing we had been elected in preference to other applicants. These appointments no longer exist, but they gave excellent experience in carrying out basic blood counts and urinary and bacteriological examinations under supervision of the house staff and, when necessary, the professors of pathology and bacteriology. The subsequent house physicians and surgeons were appointed from the ranks of the pathology clerks. I started my clerkship on the surgical professorial unit in April 1939 and my opposite number on the medical unit was Peter Candler, onetime Cambridge rugby blue and former England centre three quarter. I can recall one occasion when we tried to relieve one of my migraine attacks by dissolving a tablet of ergotamine tartrate in saline which he then injected subcutaneously.

Although shortly after arriving at Barts I had joined the London University Officers' Training Corps medical unit, in which I served as a private, I was not an enthusiastic trooper. That medical unit was the biggest element of the corps and was commanded for many years by the ever popular Colonel Philip Mitchener, a St Thomas's surgeon. But he relinquished command the year before I enrolled. I only attended two annual camps, at which "Mitchener's Army," as it was still called, was somewhat lively and ill disciplined. Our new commanding officer, Colonel Hope-Carlton, affectionately known as "Hopeless," was a worthy man but he lacked the charisma of his predecessor and was more easily upset when his troops got up to mischief. I recall the occasion when two Barts men at Shorncliffe had managed to "borrow" a boat, to the extreme ire of its owner. One of those responsible, seriously led astray on this occasion, was always a perfect gentleman who subsequently became a distinguished pathologist. At another camp one of our nocturnal raiding parties had brought back a large and varied collection of road signs which were found next morning arranged around and on top of the latrines. After a telephone inquiry from the local police one of our officers, Alistair Frazer, hastily collected the spoil together and dropped it in a nearby canal. After two years I lost my enthusiasm for the Officers' Training Corps. But with the rapidly changing scene when we began our pathology clerkships Peter Candler and I, together with Richard Terry and Oliver Garrod (both later consultant physicians), decided to join the Territorial Army. We regarded war and early call up as inevitable and decided that it would be better to volunteer. Each of us was commissioned the following month into London units based at either Chelsea or City Road barracks.

During my pathology clerkship I graduated with the London MB, BS honours degree in May and at the end of the pathology job I spent a few weeks as a locum in general practice in Norfolk. This was a two man partnership based on Northwold and Stoke Ferry. The Northwold doctor had been under treatment for tuberculosis at Mundesley sanatorium for nearly a year and I succeeded a locum who had been in the practice for six months. There were a number of satellite surgeries in surrounding villages; one of these was held in a scout hut without an examination couch and it was there that I was immensely pleased to diagnose a case of diabetes. A youngish man had been attending for some time with a septic toe and he was annoyed when I asked him for a urine sample. Having retired behind a screen he produced his specimen and I can still vividly remember my sense of triumph when I found it heavily loaded with sugar. At least that was something vital I had learnt from John Hunt on George Graham's firm – in cases of unexplained sepsis to think of the possibility of diabetes mellitus. It may well have been the only good thing I did in that rural practice, for I still feel guilty about my dispensing. There was nothing available which was pharmacologically active, however, and I am sure that my mixtures did no harm.

A few weeks after starting as casualty house surgeon I spent one of the wettest fortnights of my life in Territorial camp at Beaulieu, Hampshire. I had only just returned to Barts when I received a notice that I was to be "embodied" forthwith. On Friday 24 August I reported to the 168 City of London Cavalry Field Ambulance at City Road barracks. My father drove me there, and I remember the momentary tears in his eyes as we set off for the City. I never mentioned the matter later but he must have been thinking that I might never return from the war. It was a shock to be suddenly whisked out of civilian life in this way. On Friday the German panzer divisions swept into Poland and at 1100 on Sunday 3 September we heard Chamberlain announce on the radio that we were now at war with the Axis powers. That broadcast was immediately followed by the air raid sirens and all the London barrage balloons went up; but there was to be no bombing for almost a year.

The day that war was declared one of our field ambulance non-commissioned officers, Corporal Cattermole, told me that he had been listening to a German radio propaganda broadcast in which he had heard a familiar voice. He told me that he believed it to be that of William Joyce, who had been friendly with his sister but who had gone to Germany shortly before the war. I thereupon wrote a letter to MI6 (which I did not send through "the usual channels") to inform them of Cattermole's suspicions. A few days later I received an acknowledgment from MI6 confirming that the voice was indeed that of Joyce – later to be known as "Lord Haw-Haw" – and thanking Cattermole for his help. I only heard that characteristic drawl on the radio once or twice and little did I then think that I would be meeting Lord Haw-Haw at the end of the war.

I fancy that most of us settled down rather uncomfortably to face up to our new situation. We had to continue the training of our troops that we had already started at our weekly sessions before the war. A number of the men of the 168 City of London Cavalry Field Ambulance were educated and well trained city clerks, several of whom were soon promoted to higher rank as their important clerical skills were more widely appreciated. Our commanding officer, James Melvin, was an overkeen amateur soldier who had been in general practice in Streatham with his wife. Hubert Dunn, our second in command, was a stylish and monocled Ulsterman with a fashionable practice in Grosvenor Square. Of our three captains (who were Scottish, like the commanding officer),

McKay Robb was a radiotherapist, Mackay a general practitioner in Balham, and Macmillan a medical officer of health. Lieutenant Murley was junior officer and to him fell many of the training and teaching chores. We shared a mess with the officers of the 140 City of London Cavalry Field Ambulance, commanded by Lieutenant Colonel Crosby. The most junior officer, who had qualified and joined the Territorial Army at the same time as me, was John Nabarro (later a distinguished endocrinologist at the Middlesex). I became friendly with a Captain Neville Oswald of that unit who had just returned from the United States on completion of a Rockefeller scholarship.

In our off duty time there were parties with contemporaries, some of whom had been pleased to see us called up in the hope that their own promotion might be more certain. One afternoon I walked with Neville Oswald to Barts. As we passed through the Henry VIII gate there, and on into the fine square, Neville turned to me and said, "What an extraordinary place, Reggie, here in the City." He had graduated from Cambridge and Charing Cross Hospital. The next time he walked into that square was as assistant physician at Barts after the war. He became interested in one of the FANY ambulance drivers at City Road barracks, and I later learnt that he had married her.

One day I chanced to see that the Rev Dr Donald Soper would be preaching on the following Sunday at the Methodist chapel, a short way from my barracks. His wife was a sister of Joe Dean, with whom I had shared a study at Dulwich, and I had known the Sopers for a few years. Donald's father-in-law always referred to him somewhat irreverently as "more of a politician than a priest." When that Sunday came I decided to waylay Donald outside the chapel. I was in uniform and there I was talking to a militant pacifist in a clerical habit. He greeted me cordially and we talked for a few minutes about the implications and likely effects of the war. Having referred to its various evils he suddenly remarked, "As for this blackout, Reg, just think of all its awful effects on sexual morality." I was startled by this remark and promptly rejoined, "Donald, you mustn't put such thoughts into a young man's head!"

Luckily we did not spend long in London, since that period of "phoney" war proved unsettling for many people when German air raids did not materialise and various peace feelers were rumoured. In October we moved to Binbrook in Lincolnshire, where we joined other units of the 1st Cavalry Division; there were more units of that division in Yorkshire and Nottinghamshire. I was billeted in the house of Dr Wilkinson, a charming old local general practitioner. In London our RAMC personnel had been joined by a fine group of RASC drivers, in the command of Second Lieutenant Tony Brooks, all of whom came from the United Dairies. With the eventual arrival of our ambulances, lorries, and trucks we were renamed the 168 City of London Light Field Ambulance, but unbelievable as it may seem we were to be attached to old fashioned cavalry units. Indeed, scattered all around us in the fair countryside of those three counties were yeomanry units from a wide area of England.

It was while we were there that Tony received worrying news from a girlfriend in London who reported that she had missed a period. At breakfast I watched Tony's normally cheerful face cloud over. He cornered me immediately afterwards and asked my advice. When he had earlier consulted me in London it transpired that he and the girl were dependent upon Volpargel without any barrier contraception. Ignorant though most young doctors then were about such matters, I had learnt enough to advise him that they were taking unnecessary risks. It seemed that they might now be faced with the consequences of their imprudence. As I was shortly going on embarkation leave I arranged that Tony should get his girlfriend to send a urine specimen to Dr Bill Brewer at Barts for an Ascheim–Zondek test. I had been out a few days later and when I returned home my mother reported that there had been two telephone calls from a friend of mine at Binbrook and that he seemed anxious. When I called him he said that the result of the test had not come through. I thereupon called Dr Brewer; in his high pitched Cornish brogue he said, "Don't worry, Murley, the test is negative." I explained that the test was being done for "my friend" and Bill cheerfully responded, "That's what they all say!"

5 Cavalry crusade

On returning to Binbrook shortly after Christmas the field ambulance officers and other ranks were sent to various units of the 1st Cavalry Division in preparation for going overseas, in a particularly cold winter. I joined some of the Yorkshire Dragoons at Girsby Manor in north Yorkshire. This yeomanry unit included many of the Yorkshire hunting folk in what was an unfamiliar milieu for me. A few days later, on 9 January, we entrained at Darlington station and travelled to Dover. Arriving there in the afternoon, we embarked on the SS *Shepperton Ferry* for Dunkirk, where we were met by the Duke of Gloucester in general's uniform. He joined the officers for their evening meal in one of the dockside buildings, where opened bottles of wine were arranged along the middle of a wide trestle table. The Duke was sitting almost opposite me and, alas, in reaching forward to a bottle I knocked it over in his direction. A stream of red wine spread across the cloth and a few drops spilled on his trousers. I apologised profusely but he dismissed the incident as though it were a regular event.

By the time our meal was finished the horses had been re-entrained in the boxes, "huit chevaux ou quarante hommes," as our gallant allies so succinctly put it. The weather was bitterly cold and we travelled in unheated non-corridor coaches. Calls of nature either had to be answered through the windows or during the periodic stops to water and muck out the horses. In the course of the night we found that more and more of the grooms had found it warmer to move into the horse boxes and sleep between the centrally facing horses' heads "huit chevaux et quelques hommes." When morning came Peter, a yeomanry second lieutenant, leaned out of the window and summoned his batman in the next compartment. That faithful servant then brought his master's riding breeches along the outside footboard, opened our door, and proceeded to help Peter on with his breeches and boots. The process was carried out in reverse order in the evening and was repeated on the following morning.

For good reasons, which will emerge later, I shall not mention Peter's surname, but his interests were confined to hunting and four letter words. As we passed through pleasant stretches of rolling French countryside he would say, "Bloody marvellous hunting country, but fucking French don't hunt." This litany was repeated throughout the day. We carried some rations in each compartment and the engine driver periodically provided boiling water for our tea. We bought wine at some of the stations where we stopped to attend to the horses. Many of the compartments were so cold that both water and wine froze in the night.

On 11 January, after two nights on that miserable train, we reached Aubagne, which is not far from Marseilles. There we joined other units and were accommodated in an old chateau. It was bitingly cold inside and even worse outside and several chargers froze to death in the horse lines. My records show that we spent 12 days there, during which we made several trips to Marseilles. On 16 January, with Macmillan from my field ambulance, I had a pleasant walk in bright sunshine to the village of Cassis; there we drank wine in a little cafe overlooking the sea. A week later the cavalry division and its horses were moved to Marseilles for embarkation on two troopships, the SS *Devonshire* and the SS *Lancashire*, and three horse ships, the SS *Dilwara*, the SS *Rhona*, and the SS *Talamba*, which were converted British India liners. In the afternoon of 23 January our ships were gathered outside Marseilles harbour; they formed up in convoy with two destroyer escorts. We were reminded of the three musketeers as we passed chateau d'Yf and started a rough voyage through the Mediterranean.

I travelled on the SS *Talamba* with a few other officers and some 400 horses with supporting personnel. The senior army officer aboard, Major "Flash" Kellett of the Notts Yeomanry, was OC ship. There was a ship's adjutant, a veterinary officer, and a second lieutenant, Lord Ronaldshay, the heir to the Marquess of Zetland. Kellett was a smart and handsome man and a member of parliament. He was killed in the western desert a year or so later. I used to accompany him each day on inspections of the ship and quickly came to admire him. I only remember one of the ship's officers well, and that was the (inevitably) Scots engineer. I recall one day when he stopped me on deck and said, "You know, Doctor, that Ronaldshay says we are going to see great changes after the war; he's a real socialist." Many years later, when he had succeeded to his father's title, I met the Marquess of Zetland at a surgical dinner in the Cleveland Hills. He was amused when I told him what the Scots engineer had said and gently protested that he had never been a socialist.

As we proceeded through the Mediterranean the weather became more windy and the sea much rougher. Our horses were housed in boxes both above and below decks and the holds were left uncovered to ensure adequate ventilation. Conditions for these creatures soon became atrocious. The journey took six days and we lost 13 horses. Several developed pneumonia and had to be put down, as did others that had suffered fractures. The corpses were hoisted by crane from the deck or the holds and then dropped overboard. Although Italy was not yet in the war we kept our two destroyers until we had passed Pantellaria, continuing with one escort to Haifa, where we arrived in the early morning of 29 January.

The personnel of 168 Light Field Ambulance gathered together again in a pleasant hutted camp at the seaside town of Nathanya, then a centre for the local diamond trade. The accommodation was good and all our men had metal bedsteads. Unfortunately we had not reckoned with *Cimex lectularius*, the common bed bug. Within a day or two most of our men had been repeatedly bitten and we found an increasing number of blood engorged bugs on them and the bedclothes. But hot formalin treatment for the blankets and linen and the application of blowlamps to the metal beds finally got rid of the bugs. The unit remained at Nathanya for several months, but until 6 April I was there only intermittently. My first detachment with my field ambulance section was to Gedera, further south, where we ran a small camp hospital for the Yorkshire Hussars and Essex Yeomanry (gunners). I started to mess with the Hussars, but their charges were high and they expected me to wear blue patrols (formal dress) for dinner. It had not occurred to me to bring such clothing away to a war; but on the advice of an old campaigner from the first world war I had brought Wellington boots and an umbrella. Partly for economy and partly because the company seemed more fitting to my humble status I went to mess with the gunners, where I felt more at home.

There was not a lot of work for my men so I passed the time by giving them lectures on various interesting tropical and other diseases, for which my copy of Letheby Tidy's *Synopsis of Medicine* proved invaluable. Tidy had written that book when serving in Mesopotamia during the first world war, allegedly a precis of Price's *Medicine*, in preparation for his MRCP examination. I had managed to nip up to Jerusalem in my small Austin staff car. There I bought much reading matter for myself, including a book on Palestinian Arabic. My library of small books, mainly in the Everyman series, thereafter accompanied me to many foreign regions. My early education had been sadly lacking and now I had the opportunity to make good by a belated study of novels by Dickens, Thackeray, and Jane Austen, as well as a number of historical books. At that early stage of the war the bookshops in Jerusalem were still well stocked.

Having no previous experience of riding, I thought it opportune in such a large cavalry camp to seek instruction. Through the Yorkshire Hussars doctor I was put in touch with one of the regiment's sergeants. He took me to the horse lines one morning and quickly picked out a charger which he described as "a nice little filly." I was offered no supervision and thought it prudent not to advertise my riding virginity. Mounted on my steed I gently trotted out of the horse lines; but the trot soon developed into a canter. Then my "nice little filly" spotted a squadron of the Scots Greys galloping off in the distance. She rapidly accelerated; I hung on for dear life. I am not clear why she shortly turned about and decided to make for the camp. She went straight for the dhobi lines, with all the washing hanging out, and there I was swept off her back right in front of Private Shipp, my batman. He stood there roaring with cockney mirth and said, "That's the funniest fing Oi've seen in a long time, sir." I am of a nervous disposition and have rarely sat on a horse since.

After I had been at Gedera for just over a month I was sent to relieve the medical officer of the 1st Battalion of the Beds and Herts Regiment at Nablus, one of the towns in the so called terror triangle. It was an interesting and purely Arab town, which featured Jacob's well in the valley and a Samaritan temple on the top of nearby Mount Gerizim. I got on well with the "beds and farts," as they were vulgarly called, and I especially liked their Lieutenant Colonel Mills. Within a few days of returning to Nathanya I was once again off on detachment.

My next posting, to relieve a regimental medical officer who had gone on leave, was not so good. This was in Hebron with the 2nd Battalion of the Hampshire Regiment. I did not establish rapport with any of them and I am sure that the feeling was mutual. The battalion had been in India for quite a few years and was not a happy unit. I was mystified when they reprimanded me for not having dropped "cards." I had no visiting cards but if I had I would certainly not have taken them to war with me. The weather was wet, and as we were living in stone buildings which were fairly scattered I carried an umbrella between the mess and the medical inspection room whenever it rained. The adjutant ticked me off and said that an umbrella was against army regulations. Alas, at that time I had not heard of the only things I had in common with the Duke of Wellington, who always kept a library of books with him and who also declared that a brolly was quite in order so long as it was not used on the battlefield. The adjutant had also taken a dislike to me because I refused to take an armed escort when I visited outlying detachments. But in talking to both Jews and Arabs it was clear that "the troubles" were over for the duration of the war. In these circumstances it seemed absurd to go around armed to the teeth; indeed there were no further terrorist incidents in Palestine until peace was declared.

But, whatever my relationship with the officers was, in Corporal Seale I had a shrewd and experienced medical inspection room orderly. On one occasion a soldier attended the morning sick parade with a streaming dose of gonorrhoea. I inquired when he was last with a woman and he denied any such contact. I regarded this as a typical old soldier's story and sent him off to the VD unit in Jerusalem for treatment. At the end of the morning Seale looked at me knowingly and said, "By the way, sir, I wouldn't be surprised if that chap with the clap wasn't speaking the truth." I expressed my incredulity and rather sarcastically asked Seale if he supposed that the man had acquired the disease from a lavatory seat, or simply caught a cold while peeing against a strong breeze. Seale was undeterred and asked me if I had seen the small Arab boy who sold newspapers in the camp. I replied that I had. He then firmly concluded, "Well, sir, them papers ain't the only thing he sells in this camp!" I was slowly being educated in those facts of life which had largely escaped me at Barts.

While still at Hebron, having been commissioned for one year, I was promoted captain early in May. The war in Europe hotted up and the great German breakthrough began. Holland was overcome and when the Belgian king capitulated I was wise or foolish enough to predict that the Germans would soon be through to the French coast. "Defeatist talk" was a much advertised offence in those days and, unknown to me, it seems that the adjutant had assembled a file of Murley's more imprudent utterances. On the morning of 31 May 1940 I found myself under open arrest and the Hampshire Commanding Officer said that I would be taken before General Giffard, the GOC in C Palestine. I was driven to the King David Hotel in Jerusalem and duly brought before Giffard in a large room full of top brass as well as the Hampshire adjutant and commanding officer. Accusations of "defeatism" were duly made against me. I replied defiantly that what I had predicted had already occurred (indeed some 80 000 British troops had been awaiting evacuation from Dunkirk on the previous day).

General Giffard struck me as a kindly man. After listening

to the charges against me, and my own response, he gently pointed out to his fellow officers that here was a young and newly qualified doctor, a Territorial volunteer, who was unfamiliar with the habits of the services and whose whole education and background were quite different from theirs. He could not find me guilty of any serious offence; but having said that he then turned to me and said that any further suspicions of this kind might well lead to court martial. Colonel Large, Army Medical Service, the director of medical services, Palestine, who had been present, took me down to his office and told me that I was to receive a final ticking off from the one eyed brigade commander who had been with us upstairs. The colonel added, "Now be a good chap, Murley, just stand to attention and salute him smartly." The brigadier arrived and repeated the admonition about possible court martial. When he had gone Colonel Large told me that I could now go back to the 168 Light Field Ambulance. But, awkward to the very last, I said that I did not really get on with the overenthusiastic Colonel Melvin. The director of medical services sighed and said, "You are hard to please," but he then willingly posted me to the 170 Light Field Ambulance, a Birkenhead unit with the 1st Cavalry Division, which was stationed at Hadera, a coastal town some way south of Nathanya.

I arrived at Hadera as the evacuation of Dunkirk was being completed and the future of France lay in the balance. The commanding officer, Lieutenant Colonel Stewart, was a Manchester anatomist and his second in command, Major Cameron Armstrong, was an Australian orthopaedic surgeon from Liverpool. Two general practitoners in the unit, both captains, were Robert Pearson of Birkenhead and Tom Seager from Heswall in the Wirral. I settled down very well with my fellow officers and I liked the men of the unit, most of whom had been employed in the Leverhulme factory at Port Sunlight. I had a splendid batman, Brown, who emanated from the Potteries and had a rich Staffordshire brogue.

A week or so after my arrival at Hadera I was warned that my section of the field ambulance might shortly be needed for a secret mission. This sounded very exciting. A few nights later I was awakened in the small hours by batman Brown, who planted a large mug of hot tea beside me and cried, "Wakey, wakey, sir, the secret mission." When we had dressed and loaded our transport we were told to drive to a map reference which proved to be a crossroads near the south end of Lake Tiberias. It was shortly after dawn and a military policeman directed us to a nearby station of the Transjordan Frontier Force, situated at Samakh on the lakeside. I was told to report to Lieutenant Colonel Dugdale of the Yorkshire Hussars, who was to be my commanding officer.

On arrival I introduced myself to Thomas Dugdale, a pleasant dark haired man from north Yorkshire who was a member of parliament. He acquitted himself admirably after the war when as Minister of Agriculture he resigned over the Crichel Down scandal for which he was in no way directly responsible. He was almost the last minister to resign on a point of honour and later moved to the upper house as Lord Crathorne. I did not realise that he and his camp adjutant had each been promoted by one rank that very morning. The adjutant was now a captain and there was nothing irregular about his appearance. On meeting Dugdale, however, I was puzzled to see his pip mounted above the crown on each epaulet. I tactfully told him that his badges of rank were upside down. He screwed his head round sideways to inspect each shoulder in turn. He then said, "Oh, surely that's all right, isn't it?" I told him that a lieutenant colonel's crown had to go above the pip. He still persisted that all was well. I next told the adjutant, a regular officer, but to my astonishment he said that Dugdale was right. Shortly afterwards I saw that they had followed my advice. Only later did I learn that Major Dugdale's yeomanry batman had added the extra pips in the most accessible position immediately above the existing crowns.

Before Dugdale had adjusted his dress he told me that Marshal Petain had just capitulated in France and that some 10 000 Poles in French Syria might wish to join us later that day. All we had was a large grass airfield next to the Transjordan Frontier Force camp and a supply of tents. "Of course, Doctor, you will be reponsible for the latrines and camp hygiene," said Dugdale. Good Heavens, I thought, how many latrines are needed for 10 000 men? I said that I needed a working party and was introduced to a squadron sergeant with some 60 strapping Wiltshire yeomanrymen. I instructed them to dig shallow trench latrines, in triplicate; 20 yards of trench with 10 yards of open ground in between, and to repeat this several times. Meantime I had another party working on more permanent latrines. In the event, later that day, between two and three thousand Poles arrived by train at the nearby station. This was part of a division of reservists which had managed to get away to the south after the invasion of Poland. Many of the officers were university dons and professional men. I asked one what he did in civilian life: he sadly replied, "I am professor of international law at Lwow. Alas, there is no international law now." None of these men had the remotest idea what had happened to their families at home, and even those who survived would be lucky to meet their loved ones again. We all felt depressed by their plight. Most of them were anything but downhearted, however, in marked contrast to a few French officers and other ranks who had decided to accompany them from Syria and who, shortly after their arrival, sat dejectedly at the edge of the lake.

The detachment of the Transjordan Frontier Force at Samakh was commanded by Major John Hackett, who was seconded from the 8th Hussars. He was always known as "Shan" and was supported by two more British officers, Captain Tony Widdrington and Lieutenant John Hay. The troopers were mainly Arabs and Circassians and were fine horsemen. I shared a bungalow with Hay and Widdrington and Hackett lived next door. On visiting Hackett's bungalow I was astonished to see his fine collection of books and to learn that he was an Oxford graduate. I had often been dismissive of those in the regular services and tended to assume that the profession of arms was no place for clever and intelligent men. But I was quickly learning how wrong I had been, and in writing to my father in New York I remarked on the many interesting people I was meeting. I added that one of the regular officers could equally well have been a don and that if he survived the war I felt sure that he would go right to the top. Shan did just that, ultimately becoming deputy chief of the Imperial General Staff and commander of NATO forces in Europe before being appointed principal of King's College, London, on leaving the army.

Shan had brought out from England a small high wing, dual control monoplane, which he kept on the airfield. He occasionally took me for a trip to a frontier force station in Transjordan (now Jordan), on arrival swooping down over large boulders before picking a smoother place for landing. As we were flying back one day he invited me to operate my controls and continue on level flight. After a while he told me to circle gently; this I did. I was next told to read the altimeter, cut the engine back, and glide in circles. Concentrating hard to maintain a correct attitude, I managed that too. After a few minutes he chuckled and told me to look at the altimeter. To my astonishment I found that I had climbed 2000 feet or so. Unknown to me, the cunning chap had set me up over one of the rapidly rising thermal currents coming up from the Jordan valley.

But at that time Shan was not interested solely in military matters. Late one evening, as I was taking a nightcap with Widdrington and Hay, I was surprised to hear half a dozen shots being fired near the end of the lake. The others reassured me, "Don't worry, it's only Shan returning from a visit to his lady love. As his car approaches the camp he always discharges his revolver to warn the guard to open the gates." He was indeed courting a young Austrian widow with two little girls; she ran the Tiberias Hotel. Some months after I had left Samakh he married the beautiful Margaret and I am pleased to report that they are still very happily together some 47 years later.

I have one more tale to tell about the Poles at Samakh. Despite all our preparations, many of the Polish troops were defaecating all over the airfield. Dugdale and I had a regular morning meeting with the Polish general and an interpreter. In desperation I gave my report on the unsatisfactory state of camp hygiene and ended by asking the interpreter to explain to the general that his troops were crapping all over the airfield. The general listened quietly, smiled gently, and back came the interpreted reply: "The general says that most of his men are simple peasants: they crap on their own fields and will certainly crap on your airfield too!"

All too soon these brave men moved off to a new camp near Latrun and I returned to the 170 Light Field Ambulance, which was now at Haifa. It was early July and the Germans were facing Britain across the channel while we in the Middle East were basking in the summer sunshine. We sometimes wondered whether we would ever see our homes again; but despite all the setbacks morale remained high. Some of the wives and camp followers of our yeomanry units in the 1st Cavalry Division, however, had been foolish enough to join their menfolk in the Middle East before Italy entered the war and the Mediterranean became closed to through shipping. It was a trifle redolent of that old campaign in the Crimea when there were fair numbers of camp followers. Moreover, the news that some of us were occasionally to be seen disporting ourselves on the sandy beaches of Palestine had clearly got back to Lady Astor. In a speech in the House of Commons she suggested that we had an idle army in the Middle East, addicted to sunbathing and poodle faking. She added that if and when we eventually returned home we would be sheer menaces to all respectable young women and that we should therefore be compelled to wear yellow armbands so that they might be plainly warned.

Well, it was not quite as Nancy Astor had said. I returned to my unit at the Italian hospital, on the lower slopes of Mount Carmel, on the day Italy declared war. That very morning there was an air raid warning and from the window of our mess in the hospital I watched a squadron of Savoia bombers fly in over the harbour, disturbed only by sparse antiaircraft fire, to bomb the oil refinery just to the north. They scored direct hits on a number of the oil containers; then they turned away and flew back whence they had come, probably to airfields in Tripolitania. A few minutes later I drove over to the refinery and took some photographs of the conflagration. But it was now time to move to places further south and distinctly warmer in more ways than one.

6 The grim and gaunt Sudan

There is a rather unfair little ditty which goes: "In the grim and gaunt Sudan,/Home of prehistoric man,/Where the Dinkas' doodles dangle all the day." In fact this largest of all African countries is where I had an interesting and challenging time during the war and where I later had much enjoyment – first as an examiner in the primary FRCS and then as a university visitor. That the country now has considerable internal political and religious problems is undeniable, but it is surely not unique in that respect. I am saddened, however, by the present economic plight of the country I first knew and loved in 1940.

As soon as Italy entered the war it was clear that an overall strategic plan had come into operation with the object of driving her out of her African colonies. In view of the fluctuating state of the campaign in the western desert, and the problems which would shortly arise in Greece and Crete, it was remarkable that now, virtually alone in the war, Britain had the enterprise and determination to open a fresh front in East Africa. I was lucky enough to take part in that first completely successful operation of the war and was never thereafter involved in an unsuccessful action. But I must confess that things often looked different in the course of some of these campaigns.

In August 1940 our field ambulance left Hadera in its own transport and moved south through Palestine and the Sinai desert, crossing the Suez Canal at Ismailia en route for Cairo. There we entrained late at night for a long journey up the Nile valley to Aswan. I was fortunately awake at dawn and raised the curtains of my compartment to look upon the richly irrigated land beside the river and the many villages and small towns through which we were passing. It was a wonderful time to see Upper Egypt as the villages came to life and the women fetched water from the wells. After arriving at Aswan we were joined by a squadron of the 6th Royal Tank Regiment for a trip up the Nile on a Thomas Cook river boat. I do not know how long this approximately 250 mile river trip would have taken in peacetime, but we travelled slowly with large lighters carrying 15 medium and light tanks, lashed on each side of the boat. Our speed was no more than two or three knots upstream on what, with the building of the new high dam, has now become Lake Nasser. We were reasonably well accommodated and fed aboard that boat for three days before reaching Wadi Halfa on the north Sudan border. Early in the morning of the last day we passed the temple of Abu Simbel in all its splendour. Later it was dismantled and rebuilt high up on the west side of Lake Nasser. At the time I was so ignorant about Egyptian monuments that I did not appreciate my good fortune in going on such a splendid journey at the expense of His Majesty's taxpayers.

After disembarking at Wadi Halfa we had a comfortable journey on the Sudan railway to Khartoum, where we camped on the edge of the airfield. It was there, in a much delayed batch of mail, that one of our sergeants received the disturbing news that his wife was pregnant: the news was distressing because he had been abroad for almost a year. Until then few of us had any experience of marital infidelity as a common but less publicised consequence of war. A few days later we moved into barracks by the Blue Nile and found that one of our neighbours was the Emperor Haile Selassie, awaiting his opportunity to return to Addis Ababa. Our friends from the 6th Royal Tank Regiment were in the same barracks and Tom Seager and I became especially friendly with their squadron commander, Major Milner. We were then informed that our two sections of the 170 Light Field Ambulance were to become part of a mobile strike force, together with Ken Milner's squadron of tanks. Faced with the likelihood of imminent engagement with the enemy I thought it was time for me to make a will. So I visited a Greek lawyer and arranged to leave all my worldly goods to my mother and father, duly informing my mother in London and my father in New York of my action. I had taken out a life assurance policy for £1000 just before leaving England with the intention that this should repay my parents for the sum of £1000 I had received at the age of 21, itself derived from a policy my father had taken out when I was very young. As I look back I find all this rather comical; and I am still paying an annual premium of £12.39 for that policy.

Shortly afterwards we moved to Atbara, which was the headquarters of Sudan railways. The workshops there provided us with two special trains which were to carry personnel, transport, and tanks so that they could be off loaded at any point on the long loop line which ran at varying distance from the Eritrean border down to Kassala. This "Gazelle force," as it was called, was a small mobile group to strike at vulnerable points along that frontier before the full invasion of Italian East Africa, which would take place when enough troops were available. Soon after declaring war the Italians crossed the Eritrean/Sudan border for a short distance and occupied Kassala, but it was not long before they were driven out again. Indeed, Skinner's Horse, then a motorised unit of the 5th Indian Division, managed successfully to hoodwink the Italians by a simple expedient. At night, with their vehicle sidelights on, a single battalion of Skinner's Horse had driven round and round one of the stony jebels near Kassala, thereby giving the impression that a much larger force was moving into position for the attack. The Italians thought that we had two or three divisions there rather than one brigade and shortly returned to their side of the Eritrean frontier.

In the meantime Tom Seager and I accompanied the light and medium tanks further south to Gallabat, in preparation for an attack on Fort Metemma just over the Abyssinian border. The tanks were both old and outdated and did not take kindly to their long journey. At Gallabat we were joined by a brigade of the 5th Indian Division, which included the 1st Battalion of the Essex Regiment and some attached troops of the Sudan Defence Force. Our air support consisted of a few Gladiator biplanes of the South African Air Force and a Vicker's Virginia transport plane which was to be used as a bomber. After a few running repairs had been done to the tanks we reached Gallabat in the late afternoon and put up our dressing station tents in an open glade. We then laid up in a deep wadi with the tanks for the night. Shortly before dawn we were woken by the tank crews making ready and they soon moved off. The Vickers Virginia flew over us and we later heard that the bombs for Fort Metemma had been rolled out of the doors of that transport plane, as we had no bombers. We were excited to see our fighter planes weaving about in the sky above us, but they were completely outmanoeuvred by the faster and livelier Fiat fighters and we later learnt that our entire Gladiator flight had been shot down. A steady stream of casualties began to arrive, including an extensively burnt South African fighter pilot whose injuries were so extreme that he died later that day. Tom Seager and I were much concerned to hear that most of our tanks were disabled and out of action owing to land mines and other problems. The squadron sergeant major and several other troopers were killed. When Ken Milner, the squadron commander, climbed out of his damaged tank it was found that he had sustained a through and through soft tissue wound of one buttock.

By midday our advanced dressing station was full of casualties. I was attending to Ken's buttock when we heard the drone of approaching planes. On Ken's advice I went to the door of our operating tent and looked up. I called out, "Three white three engined planes with bomb traps open." He promptly rolled off the stretcher on to the ground and shouted, "They'll be Savoias. Get down." I was still looking up at the planes no more than two or three thousand feet above us when I saw the bombs released and spinning earthwards. I lay on my back and screamed; the three sticks of bombs fell right across our dressing station site and not a single person was hit. It was quite miraculous as there were large craters within 15 feet of each end of our operating tent and I had seen the walls of the tent rock back and forth with the blast. Our main tents were plainly marked with red crosses; but it is just possible that, approaching at low level, the crews might have had difficulty in spotting these in time. We were badly shaken by this first experience of aerial bombardment in open country. Thereafter I always felt sure that the next bombs or missiles were bound to hit me. But with the collection and evacuation of still more casualties we had no time for such idle speculation.

Our next disturbance was not by Italian aircraft. A little later, in the heat of the afternoon, troops of the Essex Regiment started to run through our dressing station shouting, "Retreat, retreat!" With stretcher casualties lying all about us it required no act of courage for Tom Seager and me to remain where we were. A few minutes later my general practitioner companion, Tom, with his thick spectacles and looking, as always, like a wise old owl, made a simple proposition: that we should don our red cross brassards. Until then we had not worn these on active service, although we had used them in prewar Territorial Army exercises. Tom pulled his own from his pocket: "Reggie, there's a good chap. Just tie this on for me and I'll tie on yours. They say that these Abyssinians go for your goolies [an Arab slang word for testicles]." If the red crosses on our tents had afforded us no protection from the Italian airmen we at least hoped that their native troops – if they had any fighting for them – might have heard of the Geneva Convention.

Our work continued until nightfall with no signs of a general withdrawal. Only later did we learn that the Italians had more or less simultaneously evacuated Fort Metemma. Tom and I cursed ourselves for not having strolled down the road and occupied the fort to record the first RAMC victory in East Africa. The explanation of the hasty retreat – for which the Essex battalion was subsequently disgraced and its commanding officer relieved of his command – was that those troops had seen a number of black soldiers moving alongside them. They mistook these members of the friendly Sudan Defence Force for Italian colonial troops who had somehow outflanked them.

By this time General Platt, our GOC East African forces, decided that Gazelle force had no future role. With the arrival of both the 4th and 5th Indian divisions all was ready for more effective action. We remained for some time detached from the rest of the field ambulance and joined the 5th Indian

Division at Kassala before moving to Tessenei behind the fast retreating Italians. At Tessenei I had my first meeting with Major Dick Handley, then attached to an Indian field hospital as surgical specialist. After the war he would be a surgical colleague at St Albans and we later served together on the council of the Royal College of Surgeons. At Tessenei too I was compelled to act as an ersatz Catholic priest when a severely wounded British soldier died shortly after arriving in my dressing station. Our cockney cook, the astute Alfie Hammond, reported that the dead man was a fellow Roman Catholic and that I must give him an appropriate burial. Thereupon, while some of my RAMC orderlies and RASC drivers dug a grave, dear Alfie composed a suitable form of words for the burial. I explained that as I was a sadly lapsed protestant it might be better if I authorised Private Hammond to officiate. But Alfie would have none of it: when I had done my stuff, and the body was lowered into the grave and duly covered, he warmly commended me by saying, "Yer dun 'im proud, sir, wiv' a proper caffolic send off!"

From Tessenei we went on rapidly into Eritrea, with but a brief delay at Agordat before moving up to the formidable fortress of Keren. Lieutenant General Sir Geoffrey Evans, a postwar GOC Northern Command, who commanded one of our Indian brigades at Keren, subsequently described this as his stiffest battle of the war. As Winston Churchill writes in volume III of his *Second World War*:

> The flanks of this position could not be turned: only direct frontal attack was possible. To build up his resources for this effort and to deploy both his divisions Platt had but a single road, which lay in full view of the enemy. Railhead was 150 miles away, so that not only did his preparations take several weeks, but surprise was out of the question.

While those preparations were under way I had time to make friends with a Sikh doctor, Captain Alawalia, whose smartness, meticulous cleanliness, and gentlemanly style deeply impressed me. I recall that he invited me to breakfast early one morning and that I arrived before he had dressed and completed his toilet. I was astonished to see the care with which he prepared his long hair and powdered his body before putting on his uniform. I also briefly met the English surgeon, Major Edward Muir, who had not long before been elected to the staff of King's College Hospital at the tender age of 30. I would much later serve under him on the college council and be next but one to succeed him as president of the Royal College of Surgeons. What surprising things life held in store for those of us who were lucky enough to survive.

How well I recall that "single road . . . in full view of the enemy" which Churchill describes. When Driver Bailey drove us in our solitary 8 hundredweight truck on a sunny day early in January 1941 at first all was deceptively peaceful. We turned off the road into a deep wadi to make a reconnaissance of the site where my dressing station would be located next day. It was late morning and we had brought our luncheon rations with us, so we walked along the wadi and climbed its east bank, from which we had a splendid view of the formidable granite heights of Keren. There we sat down to eat our sandwiches, with the warm sun on our backs. After a few minutes I noticed a stone suddenly spin away from between Bailey and me; a moment later it happened again, but Bailey still had not noticed anything and continued to make short work of his Spam rolls. It was only when stones on the other side of me were scattered that I finally realised that we were the targets of rifle fire. Just as I told Bailey that we must take shelter, we saw Major Cameron Armstrong, our second in command, walking towards us in the wadi as several mortar bombs exploded in between. We all took cover under the steep bank and shortly returned to our unit, duly impressed by our proximity to an unseen enemy

The following morning my field ambulance section joined a huge convoy of lorries on the same road that we had taken the day before. But on this occasion we saw puffs of smoke all along the mountain ridges on both sides. At first I naively assumed that those puffs must be our own shells hitting the Italian positions, but the regular whistle of shells and explosions along the road soon reminded me that our convoy was the target. We were relieved to turn off into our wadi and set up the dressing station. Initially all was fairly quiet there, apart from our own 25 pounder guns just behind. We had been told to dig slit trenches for shelter, but the ground was so stony that we only managed a number of short trenches no more than 2 feet deep, in which I later spent a number of uncomfortable nights. Casualties soon began to arrive. If the dressing station was visible to the enemy we hoped that the red crosses on our ambulances would signify our non-combatant status. But it was not long before we were subjected to intermittent bombardment by mortars and shells. One of my RAMC men, about to load a casualty into an ambulance, became so scared that he abandoned the stretcher and did a bunk for a slit trench. I hounded him out of this and back to duty, but there was no bravery on my part. I am sure that I was just as scared as him, but I was the officer in charge and had to set an example. In the next few weeks I was to learn how tenuous was the boundary between relative composure and breaking point in battle.

I cannot remember how many days I was in that wadi; but there were many casualties and after the first few days there was a pause for regrouping. At that time my section was withdrawn to Agordat and then moved to the north side of Keren where we joined a Free French force composed of Foreign Legion men and huge black troops from French colonial Chad. In that force we became part of a Free French field hospital whose commanding officer was Commandant Fruchot, a veteran of the first world war and recently professor of surgery in Tripoli, Syria. Fruchot had the reputation of doing much of his operating at a table in the open air – which was true. There chanced also to be a young Lieutenant Schick in that unit whose name I mentioned in a letter to my father in New York. Several weeks later I learnt that Schick was the son of a Jewish fur trader in Paris, a business friend of my father's in occupied France to whom he somehow found means of sending news of the son.

A lull in the battle during our first few days there gave us the opportunity of hunting kudu and gazelle with which to supplement our rations. Late one evening, armed with two service rifles, I had been out looking for game with a French captain. In the gathering gloom I spotted some gazelle several hundred yards away. Poised on the top of our 8 hundredweight truck I took careful aim at a white mark on the rump of one animal and fired. My companion leapt from the truck, shouting, "Bon chasseur." I had not realised that I had hit the creature, but he dashed off and returned breathless with a fine young animal. We returned to the unit for our evening meal, and the chef prepared our gazelle for later consumption. In the course of the meal the chef entered, with the gazelle's heart cupped in his hands. "Bon tireur, monsieur le capitaine Anglais," he said. To my utter astonishment there was my .303 bullet lodged in the heart and pericardium. The fact that I had managed to hit the creature in that fading evening light was certainly a complete fluke, but I basked in this undeserved applause.

A few days later I had fallen ill with a fever just when we were due for a visit from General de Gaulle. I lay on my camp bed in an unoccupied reed hut where I recorded my high remittent fever on army graph paper. I still have that chart on which I also recorded my symptoms. After a few days I thought I could feel my spleen, but I am so ticklish when others lay a hand on my abdomen that none of my colleagues could confirm this. We had not been on suppressive quinine (the only antimalarial then available) as this had not been ordered. I suspected that I might have malaria, but there was a view prevalent then that "blunderbuss" treatment without a confirmatory blood smear was undesirable. I doubt whether that had any validity, but as things later turned out this could have been life saving for me.

Charles de Gaulle arrived while I was still *hors de combat*. After his inspection I heard powerful African voices and soon learnt that the Chad battalion had been singing their theme song: "Les couilles de mon grand père sont pendues sous l'escalier." ("The balls of my grandfather are hanging up under the stairs.") Many years later in Philadelphia I was to earn the plaudits of some French surgical colleagues when I sang this stirring song to them. On a much sadder note I have to record that one afternoon a British sapper officer friend of ours came to visit me. He entered my hut and said, "Reggie, can you take a shock?" I thought he must be joking and said, "Of course I can." But he asked me the same question again and then added that he had the remains of our transport officer, Tony Brooks, and his driver in an ambulance outside. I staggered to my feet and one glance in the ambulance at the jumbled mass of trunks and limbs was enough for me to see that they were both dead and disintegrated. Poor Tony! He was a delightful man, but had always had a great interest in explosives. All along the roads to the north of Keren there were many mines, dug out by our sappers, still lying awaiting collection or disposal. One common Italian vehicle mine was improvised by placing two fairly large shells nose-to-nose with a detonator mounted in between. The whole thing was then enclosed in a long wooden box, rather like a small coffin. In many places we had seen these boxes dug up and piled three or four deep. The attraction for Tony proved fatal; the sapper officer had warned him only the day before that the mechanism was "light on the trigger." Tony's truck was found nearby with the two bodies blown apart by a stack of four mines consisting of eight high explosive shells.

Keren fell on 27 February and my fever had burnt itself out by 6 March. Some days later we returned to Keren to climb the granite hills which had been occupied by the Italians. We were astonished to find how visible the site of our original dressing station in the wadi was, and how obvious was the bank where Bailey and I had eaten our sandwiches. The rest of the Eritrean campaign was soon completed. Asmara, at an altitude of over 8000 feet, fell on 1 April and we moved on down to Massawa on the Red Sea coast. The final battle for Massawa was on 8 April. I awoke early that day with a splitting headache and visual disturbance which I attributed to migraine. I soon recovered. The Italians surrendered outside the town by midday and we took 10 000 prisoners. By late afternoon I was instructed to go into Massawa and take over the naval hospital by the harbour. Bailey took me there in the 8 hundredweight truck. I reported to the colonel in charge and we saluted each other. I told him that we had come to take the hospital over for our use and he said that he had been informed of this. He spoke only a little English but politely invited me to join the Italian doctors' mess for dinner.

Once my luggage had been installed in the doctors' quarters

I returned to the mess for dinner and was seated next to Majore Regio Moise. He spoke excellent English and we were amused at the similarity of our first names. I learnt that he was a malariologist, and he was interested to hear that I had recently dissected anophelene mosquitoes at the malarial research station in the Hule marshes of north Palestine. We had much to talk about during a good dinner accompanied by some excellent Chianti. The officers' mess and the hospital were efficiently airconditioned, but our living quarters were not. The heat and humidity in Massawa was intense, in marked contrast to Asmara, but I was tired and slept soundly. I awoke early, again with a splitting headache, and I felt terribly hot, despite immersing myself in a tepid bath. On taking my temperature I was astonished to find the thermometer recording 106.5. I picked up the bedside telephone; the telephonist answered. "Majore Regio Moise prego," I said in my hesitant Italian. I was put through and said, "Are you the English speaking Major Moise I sat next to last night?" continuing, "I think I have malaria. Could you please do a blood smear?" He was with me within a few minutes, took a thick blood drop on a slide and left for the laboratory. By the time he returned about a quarter of an hour later I felt very ill and confused. He brought a large filled syringe with him. He told me, "I have seen one ring form of the malignant tertian parasite and that is enough." He then sat down beside the bed and gave me a slow intravenous injection of quinine. I felt relieved and deeply grateful. After sleeping for a few hours I awoke with a falling temperature and feeling much better.

The rest of my field ambulance arrived that afternoon, and a few days later I was sent to convalesce at a hotel in Asmara which was used as a headquarters mess. With my post-malarial anaemia I felt quite breathless back at 8000 feet. At lunch on the first day I was seated alone when a pleasant looking captain came into the dining room and asked if he might join me. I welcomed his company and, in rather typically English fashion, we did not exchange names. We quickly fell into animated conversation about the war and a number of the events preceding it. I recall that I was highly critical of Chamberlain, and of Baldwin, and he did not dissent from my views. We went into the lounge for coffee where we joined a number of headquarters officers, including Alec Carmichael, previously in my field ambulance but now a deputy assistant director of medical services. "Who is that officer I was sitting with?" I whispered to Alec. "Oliver Baldwin, Stanley's son," he replied. "Oh God, I've just been criticising his father," said I. "Don't worry," said Alec, "He strongly dislikes his dad!" After Oliver Baldwin had left the table I was told that he was quite a thorn in the flesh for General Platt, and that he had suggested that the main streets of Asmara should be renamed with all manner of anti-fascist labels.

On one or two evenings in Asmara Alec Carmichael and I had dinner at a restaurant where there was a band and a small dance floor. He pointed out one of the headquarters staff officers dining and dancing with an attractive young woman who, so he claimed, had been "bailed out" of the officers' local brothel. It was alleged that the madame had been prepared to release one of her "best girls" for a suitable consideration.

I completed my convalescence at the end of April and returned to work in the Massawa hospital for two or three weeks. During that period I had an Indian sepoy with several chancroid sores who died dramatically of a fulminating haemolytic condition after treatment with sulphanilamide. This became the subject of my first published paper but deserves no further mention now, other than to say that it became an important means of my later translation to surgical training following two and a half years of field service. We had conquered Eritrea. All that was now necessary was to get the Italians dislodged from their last East African stronghold and to pop Haile Selassie back on his throne – though not for long!

7 Won't you come to Abyssinia, won't you come?

I had, of course, been on the Abyssinian border at Gallabat, but had not entered the country. As we left Asmara, bound for Ethiopia on one of the fine roads which the Italians had built, I could not help thinking of one of those prewar Christmas ward shows at Barts just after the Italian invasion of East Africa. The chorus of the opening number went as follows:

Won't you come to Abyssinia, won't you come?
  Bring your own ammunition and your gun,
Mussolini will be there, blowing raspberries in the air,
  Oh, won't you come to Abyssinia, won't you come?

As we followed the road south and crossed the Abyssinian border that song went racing through my head. We paused at Axum to visit the Coptic cathedral where Haile Selassie and all his predecessors had been crowned (Lion of Lions, King of Kings, Emperor of Ethiopia, as each was styled). I entered that small cathedral with my batman and driver to witness an interesting little service in which a number of men, including some Coptic priests, gathered on each side of the altar steps and then danced back and forth across the nave while chanting a canticle. I was able to take some photographs of them outside the building, with Italian film salvaged from a sunken ship at Massawa.

After leaving Axum, our destination much further south was the village of Adi Arcai, situated on a high plateau with stupendous mountain scenery to the east. The highest mountain, Ras Dasian, was over 15 000 feet; although it was only eight degrees north of the equator its peak was often snow covered. Some 20 miles further on, up a steeply winding mountain road was the village of Debivar situated at the foot of the formidable Wolchefit pass, which rose above the village to some 13 000 feet. One of our infantry battalions was occupying a small area there and was intermittently under shell and mortar fire from the heights above. A patriot force with some British officers was operating in the country behind the Wolchefit pass in the hope of discomforting the Italians, who were hardly vulnerable to frontal attack up the steep road. I had reconnoitred Debivar on the first day and decided that there was no point in having our dressing station under fire. For that reason we established a small hospital in a stone building at Adi Arcai, close to a Roman Catholic mission, where the priest and nuns seemed well disposed to us. Indeed it was not long before our men had arranged for all the washing and mending to be done by the nuns.

My selection of that site was, so I thought, soundly based. We could receive sick and wounded from other units such as the Sudan Defence Force as well as from that isolated battalion at Debivar. Moreover, we were able to combine with Captain Townsend-Coles, one of the Sudan Medical Service doctors, and his men, and had an Indian Medical Service surgical team under the command of Major Jack Maud and his anaesthetist, Captain McElvey. Jack made some excellent sketches of the local people as well as an amusing drawing of one of our many spirited mealtime arguments in the mess. He also had a collection of interesting drawings from his earlier spell in the Western Desert of Egypt. Every Abyssinian male in those days seemed to carry a rifle and they were liable to shoot one another, either in argument or inadvertently. I recall one man who was shot through the chest by his "friend" when he was bending over to pour coffee. He was shocked and had clearly lost a fair amount of blood. Jack decided to give him a transfusion before anything else was done, and a blood compatible relative was found. Then, using an Italian direct transfusion syringe, of which we had all seen pictures but never used, the shot man was given a blood transfusion from his relative, with a discreet screen arranged between them. The donor repeatedly asked about the recipient's progress and was duly reassured; but, alas, the patient rapidly deteriorated and died. I was much impressed at the way Maud and McElvey, with Townsend-Coles as interpreter, managed to complete this procedure without telling the donor of the patient's death until some time after he had been disconnected from the two way syringe.

But trouble shortly reared its ugly head in the form of a visit from the GOC, General Platt, usually known as the *Kaid* (chief) in those parts. He angrily confronted me to ask why my dressing station was not at Debivar. I explained that I had visited Debivar several times and was convinced that it was a totally unsuitable place for a field hospital. But the general didn't like this. After further exchanges with me, he shouted, "Stand to attention, man!" I dutifully shuffled my feet and he added, "*Go* to Debivar." I calmly – but perhaps, somewhat impertinently – replied that I was under the command of the deputy director of medical services. The *Kaid* was practically apoplectic and stormed off. Oh dear, I thought, this time it will surely mean a court martial. I heard nothing further; but from time to time I had to drive about 180 miles north to Asmara. On my next visit there I called on the deputy director of medical services, Colonel William Russell (MC with bar from the first world war), who had previously commanded my field ambulance for a short time. I mentioned my little fracas with the *Kaid*. Willie just chuckled and said, "Oh, so it was you, Murley. The *Kaid* couldn't remember your name but said that you were an undisciplined captain with red hair." My hair was, in fact, always fair until I went bald. The only red headed captain happened to be with the patriots behind the Wolchefit pass, though he made occasional trips to our side down one of the donkey tracks. Willie told me that he had mollified the *Kaid* by telling him that he would deal with that officer when he next saw him.

I made frequent trips to Debivar and loved driving my 8 hundredweight Morris truck up that impressively winding road with the many startling hairpin bends that I knew so well. One day we were visited at Adi Arcai by Brigadier Mills, whom I had known when he commanded a Beds and Herts infantry battalion in Palestine. He asked if I could take him to Debivar, which I did. He thoroughly enjoyed the trip and had the battalion commander there explain all the details of the Italian position before I took him back to Adi Arcai. Only later did I hear from Willie Russell that Brigadier Mills had told the *Kaid* of his trip to Debivar, and what a marvellous mountain road driver Captain Murley was. However, the *Kaid* did not realise that this was the same truculent captain he had met.

The men of my field ambulance section greatly enjoyed their spell at Adi Arcai, where we mainly looked after the sick since there were then few casualties. There were a number of soccer matches against local units of the Sudan Defence Force. On these occasions it was amusing to see that whereas our own troops put on their boots before taking to the field the Sudanese took theirs off and left them beyond the touchline. The feet of the Sudanese were not only remarkably tough but they were usually much more shapely and beautiful than those of the average European.

All of us had been greatly impressed by conditions in Sudan, that largest of all African countries, before we moved into Eritrea and Abyssinia. Although officially governed by a condominium between Britain and Egypt, the latter had had virtually nothing to do with the running of Sudan for many years past. The civil administration was of a high standard; all the district commissioners were Oxford or Cambridge graduates and had often been sports blues too – "a nation of blacks, governed by whites, with blues," as was often said. It was clear that they had been well selected by the Foreign and Colonial Office. I especially remember W G R M Laurie, a former Cambridge rowing blue, whom I met in Abyssinia with the Sudanese Defence Force. When the administration was "Sudanised" after the war and Laurie received his golden handshake he had gone back to Cambridge and the London Hospital to graduate in medicine. Moreover, he and another former Sudan administrator, J H T Wilson, after assiduous retraining won the Olympic coxless pairs event in 1948.

Apart from Townsend-Coles I only knew one other Sudan Medical Service doctor really well and that was Louis Brown, a South African graduate from Guy's, who worked at Atbara, where he had occasionally invited me to breakfast – a common form of hospitality in Sudan. We were impressed by the British doctors we met and by the high standards of competence of those Sudanese who had trained for four years at Kitchener College, Khartoum (later to become the medical school of the new university in 1955) and who then served as "assistant surgeons." Many of those Sudanese looked after dispensaries and small hospitals in the more remote areas, where they certainly maintained a very satisfactory rural service. Moreover, they were capable of recognising when sick patients required referral to the more fully staffed main hospitals. Whatever may now be said by critics of the *ancien régime*, I would regard that old British administration as having been both just and enlightened.

When we were at Adi Arcai Haile Selassie was returned to his capital by camel train, arriving there on 5 May 1941 duly escorted by Major Last, an Australian officer in the RAMC, who later became a highly successful and popular teacher of anatomy at the Royal College of Surgeons, where he was also the first warden of the Nuffield residential college. I cannot remember when those Italian troops surrendered at the top of the Wolchefit pass; but with a South African army moving up rapidly from the south under General Cunningham's command several isolated pockets of Italian troops were left to their own devices while we moved most of ours back via Egypt to help finish off the Vichy French forces in Lebanon and Syria. Having so recently been associated with General de Gaulle's Free French in Eritrea I was sad to be fighting enemy French in their formerly mandated territory from which we had previously received those brave Poles.

8 Back to the Holy Land and beyond

The 170 Light Field Ambulance had now been separated from the 1st Cavalry Division (later the 10th Armoured Division) for almost a year. It must have been in early July that we returned to Palestine, though this time we journeyed up the Red Sea from Port Sudan to Suez. I had been at Massawa in April, but when we arrived in Port Sudan some three months later it was even more hot and humid there. One afternoon a large number of British and Indian troops boarded an aging ship hoping to be at sea within an hour or two. Alas, after going aboard we heard that one propeller shaft was in need of repair and that a group of South African army engineers had gone into the tunnel to do some welding. The heat there must have been unbearable. By the time these men came up and the ship set sail they were in a bad condition. Two of them were suffering from heat stroke and both died within 24 hours. In view of all that they had done to make our ship seaworthy it was a melancholy moment when we buried them at sea. We reached Suez two days later and as we approached the docks an Arab dhow just ahead of us was blown out of the water – presumably by a delayed action mine.

I have no clear memory of the journey from Suez to northern Palestine, but on this occasion we travelled by train. We were stationed in the far north of the country for a month or so, first at Tiberias and then at Safad. In Tiberias we became friendly with Dr Torrance, who ran the Scottish Mission Hospital. When in Hebron I had known his colleague Dr Elliot Forster and his wife, both of whom had introduced me to some of the local Arabs, shown me the ancient mosque, and taken me down to Jericho and the Dead Sea. Dr Torrance's father had first opened the Tiberias mission hospital when he was an enthusiastic evangelist. His son told us that when his father had been there 10 years and had converted only one Arab to Christianity he decided to confine himself to medicine. The younger Dr Torrance and his wife had kept to that policy.

Once Dr Torrance invited Cameron Armstrong, our Liverpool orthopaedic surgeon, to operate on an Arab child with club foot. When they were scrubbed up in the theatre and the boy was wheeled in under Mrs Torrance's anaesthetic Torrance turned to Armstrong and inquired, "Would you say the prayers?" The agnostic, if not atheistic, Armstrong responded in his strong Australian accent, "Oi think it'd have more meaning if you did it, Torrance." So Torrance obliged. We sometimes had tea with the Torrances; and they were kind people. I still had many of my books with me in the tin trunk which I had kept in store in Palestine; these I left at the mission hospital, with the exception of one on the natural history of Palestine which I gave to Denis Glass, my prewar dental friend, who happened to meet me on my return to Tiberias. Like the Iron Duke I had a travelling library and a brolly. It was my brolly that had so upset the Hampshires' adjutant. Later, when using it as a sunshade, I had inadvertently left it under a thorn tree in Eritrea.

During a trip further south to Jerusalem, where I sought some help with the paper I was preparing, I chanced to call at a hospital in Rehovot and found that Neville Oswald, formerly with the 167 Cavalry Field Ambulance in London, was now a medical specialist there. It was good to see him again after almost two years. When we had exchanged news Neville said, "You must meet my opposite number, Rodney Smith. He's the surgical specialist here." Rodney was a St Thomas's graduate who, after house appointments there, had taken his final FRCS and the London mastership before working as a registrar at Middlesex Hospital with, I think, Gordon Gordon-Taylor. He had only recently been called up and until then I had not heard of him. On this occasion Neville took me to visit him in the theatre, where I watched him remove a kidney and do another operation. I remember that I was impressed by his neat technique. After the war he was appointed surgeon at St George's Hospital and I was eventually to succeed him as president of the college of surgeons. It is interesting that I had also so recently met Edward Muir with his surgical unit at Cheren, for he it was who preceded Rodney as president. Possibly one of the greatest bonuses of wartime medical work is the remarkable range and variety of doctors that one meets. As a Londoner I especially appreciated meeting so many from provincial cities and from Scotland.

I was three times in Palestine during the war and spent a total of about 18 months there. Having seen many different parts of the country I came to know it well. Just before the war "the troubles" had been much in evidence. But when the war began it soon became clear that neither Jews nor Arabs wished to fight the British. Officers of our field ambulance who were entertained in Arab villages or Jewish kibutzim were often amused by the remarks of their hosts. For they all confirmed that everyone would lie low "for the duration," but that there would be real trouble once the war was over. There was commonly some allusion to the arms they had stacked away in the basement "to shoot all those bloody Arabs/Jews [strike out what does not apply] when you people have gone," as they so clearly put it. I became fascinated by the recent and ancient history of the country and was lucky enough to have time for extensive reading when I was there.

I think that I can fairly claim to have had genuine sympathy with both sides. To me it seemed clear that the early Jewish settlers in places such as Degania in the Jordan valley presented little problem to the indigenous Semitic population, whether Jewish or Arab. By 1914 there were nearly 100 000 mainly Russian and Rumanian Jews in the country, but that number was considerably reduced by 1918 during the demise of the Ottoman Empire. I have always felt unhappy about the circumstances in which the Balfour declaration was made in 1917 "to facilitate the establishment . . . of a Jewish national home." This was partly by way of a reward for Chaim Weizmann's valuable work during the first world war. At the same time, for equally good reasons, we were courting the Arabs too and perhaps "El Laurens" (as the Arabs called Lawrence of Arabia) encouraged some of them to expect too much. The brief honeymoon of genuine Arab–Zionist friendship came to an end shortly after that war, mainly due to general disappointment of Arab hopes in the peace settlement. Had it not been for Hitler I doubt that there would ever have been pressure for massive Jewish entry to the country. Indeed several times in the past 80 years the number of emigrant Jews has exceeded those immigrating. Once that pressure built up, as it did so excessively during the Nazi regime, the situation became unbalanced. And so, as with many other highly sensitive racial and religious situations, we find that the problem is largely man made. Now, as a result of Jewish developments in the so called west bank – an area I knew so well in wartime – I must confess that I have considerable sympathy with the Palestinian Arabs.

During this period I also spent a short time in Jordan (then Transjordan). Its capital, Amman (the biblical Raboth Ammon), then had quite a small population but this has since grown dramatically. Before the war I had been fascinated by T E Lawrence's description of the Arab revolt and, at my own suggestion, I had been given a fine edition of his *Seven Pillars of Wisdom* for a birthday present. I asked my mother to send the book to me; the bulky volume happily arrived undamaged in my wartime post. Indeed I can remember sitting on a hard bench at a deserted station on the Hejaz railway rereading Lawrence's description of an action which had taken place nearby.

By way of confirming what we had been told of the certain exacerbation of trouble once the war was over I am reminded of a conversation I had with the wife of one of my house surgeons. He was a Jewish graduate from Guy's who later emigrated to Israel and became a surgeon. While still in England he visited us at home with his young Israeli wife. When she learnt that I had been in Palestine she eagerly asked whether I knew the King David Hotel in Jerusalem. I replied that I certainly did and that I had once been taken there under open arrest to be reprimanded by the GOC. She then said, "Well, my grandmother put the bomb there which blew it up!"

When we reached Palestine from the Sudan we were,

perhaps fortunately, too late for the battle with the Vichy French, who surrendered on 12 July. I would certainly have been sorry to fight against the troops of a nation we had not fought since the battle of Waterloo. Not long afterwards I was stationed near Tyre and Sidon, where I met Philip Lever of the Cheshire Yeomanry, whom I would later know much better when he had succeeded to the Leverhulme viscountcy and was chairman of our fund raising committee at the Royal College of Surgeons. I then spent some time in Damascus where I had a tiresome attack of Dengue fever. One of the compensations, however, was a few days' sick leave in Beirut, where I stayed at the St George Hotel by the sea. It was at about this time that I was trying to write the paper on fulminating haemolytic anaemia in relation to sulphanilamide, so I seized the opportunity of visiting Dr Sayoun, the professor of pathology at the American University there. He was most helpful: he cut further sections of the tissues I had preserved, provided photomicrographs for publication, and gave me his expert opinion.

Beirut was then an attractive town. When I was walking near the hotel one evening I noticed a slightly familiar figure just ahead of me, a lieutenant colonel with dark hair hanging over his collar. Sure enough it was Edward Cullinan, the Barts physician on whose firm I had once worked. He greeted me like a long lost friend and we had dinner together. As Edward had some interest in liver diseases he came to the university with me the next day to meet Dr Sayoun and discuss my case with him. When preparing that paper for publication I used to borrow one of the unit typewriters and tediously bang the whole thing out with one or two fingers. I remembered this only when a typescript of that paper turned up recently in one of my old files.

Not long after returning to the 170 Light Field Ambulance in Palestine I was sent to Cairo on an officers' gas course. This lasted two weeks; the teaching was excellent, and we had officers from nearly every Dominion and Allied force. My brain had been so starved of challenges of this kind that I found myself effortlessly soaking up everything that I heard and read. We all had to sit an examination at the end of the course. To my surprise I came top and a month or two later I was offered the post of medical adviser in chemical warfare at Middle East Command. This meant promotion to lieutenant colonel, a flat in Cairo, and – who knows? – perhaps a dusky mistress there as well. I had no hesitation in declining this invitation because I was becoming more and more anxious about getting back into clinical medicine. By now it was clear that the war was likely to last for four or five years – or even more, as it did – and I feared that I might miss the chance to take up surgery.

There was an amusing side to this chemical warfare offer. Some time after I had returned to the field ambulance at Safad the unit had a gas exercise, of which I took a number of photographs. As had been my custom in Palestine I had the pictures developed and enlarged at Gompert's photographic shop in Haifa. The Dutch Jew who owned the shop when I first went there in 1940 had left some time before, bound for the Dutch East Indies. He had, alas, arrived in Sumatra at just about the time when the Japanese invaded. Some weeks after those pictures were processed we were informed that the medical adviser, chemical warfare, Middle East, would be coming to visit us. He was about my age and dolled up with "pips and crowns," whereas I was still a captain (I began to think that I might have been unwise to miss the promotion I was offered). He saw my photographs and asked if he might have copies. These I duly supplied at my own expense. It was only by chance about a year later that I was told of the excellent photographs of field ambulance gas exercises that had been taken by Lieutenant Colonel X and which were much appreciated at Middle East headquarters.

During that second period in Palestine, in 1941, I had two interesting experiences which increased my scepticism about psychiatry. The first concerns one of the RASC drivers with the 170 Light Field Ambulance. This lugubrious looking man, in peacetime a miner from Blythe, Northumberland, came to my sick parade complaining of hearing strange voices. I spent some time talking with him on several different occasions and concluded that he was suffering from a genuine psychosis. On referring him to a psychiatrist, however, I was assured that there was nothing wrong with him. Though somewhat incredulous at this decision I assumed that it merely confirmed how inadequate my psychiatric training had been. Not long afterwards, when I was no longer with that unit, I heard that the man had committed suicide. I realise that this may not mean that I was right and the psychiatrist wrong, but I suggest that the balance of dubiety was distinctly in my favour.

The second incident concerned one of my fellow RAMC officers, a handsome and elegant middle aged doctor who had been in general practice in the north of England. We had both been on detachment in Damascus, where we shared a small apartment and the services of a single batman – the delightful Brown from the Potteries. Bill, as I shall call him, came into breakfast one morning and, after fixing me with a steely glare, accused me of having hit him the night before and then rushed at me with arms raised. I seized his arms and fought him off, and eventually quietened him. He made a few more odd remarks and then lapsed into silence. A week or two later, back in Palestine, Brown came to me one morning and told me that he was worried because Bill had a number of phenobarbitone tablets in a container beside his bed. He thought that Bill might do himself harm but was reluctant to say more. It was at about that time that Bill had fallen off a horse while out riding with one of the cavalry units. The accompanying squadron sergeant major had remarked, "I've never seen a man come off a horse like that in all my 25 years." A few days later Bill was admitted to the officers' ward at the Italian hospital in Haifa, where we had formerly been stationed. Shortly afterwards it was reported that after making three attempts to throw himself out of a third floor window Bill had been evacuated to a psychiatric hospital in southern Palestine, strapped on a Neill Robertson stretcher. At that stage the ever sagacious Tom Seager remarked to me, "I wonder if Bill is putting it all on in order to work his passage home?" I was astonished, but Tom went on to emphasise how remarkable it was that (a) Bill had not taken an overdose of phenobarbitone, despite keeping a large quantity beside his bed; (b) an experienced sergeant major had commented on his unusual fall from a horse; and (c) he had made no fewer than three unsuccessful attempts to get out of a third floor window, each time being held by the legs.

I conceded that Tom might have a point or two, but I just could not believe that a fellow doctor would do this. Tom remarked that Bill had a charming wife at home and four lovely children, all of whom he desperately missed after two years abroad. To satisfy my curiosity I set out for that psychiatric hospital and visited Bill. I gave him the good wishes of the unit, but he appeared remote and uncommunicative. I then saw an RAMC captain, the graded psychiatrist (junior specialist) in charge. He told me that they had decided to send Bill back to England. I brightly remarked, "Perhaps he'll be much better when he is back with his family." The captain somewhat sententiously replied, "Manic depressive psychosis is *quite* uninfluenced by environment." Thoroughly put in my place, I thought, oh dear, why did I not pay more attention to psychiatry in my student days? Well, I am not sure that it would have made any difference, excepting that I might have been wrong on both occasions. Bill *was* sent home; he *did* make a complete recovery and he returned to his practice. Following the war, during a visit to a northern university town, my wife and I met Bill at a medical dinner. Neither of us referred to the Damascus and Palestine affairs and he seemed perfectly sane to me. But then, of course, I am not a psychiatrist!

ORTHOPAEDICS FOR BEGINNERS

Towards the end of 1941, about the time of the episode just referred to, I wrote to Jock Monro, the regular army consultant surgeon at Middle East headquarters, Cairo, asking if there was any chance of a surgical traineeship. Early in 1942 I was posted to 2 Orthopaedic Unit at 12 General Hospital, situated at Sarafand, somewhere between Tel Aviv and Jerusalem. This was a great opportunity. The officer in command of the surgical division was H A Brittan, a distinguished Norwich orthopaedic surgeon. The senior orthopaedist, later to become a general surgeon at Liverpool Royal Infirmary, was Major

Clifford Brewer, who was an excellent surgeon with a brilliantly sharp brain. He was about four years older than I and had James Tulloch, an Edinburgh lad, as his trainee. I was attached to another Liverpool graduate, Captain Bickerton, who practised orthopaedics in Durban after the war. In addition to my orthopaedic duties I ran the hospital blood bank and was responsible for bleeding all the donors. Lastly our commanding officer, Colonel Mackie, a dour but charming general practitioner Territorial from Scotland, persuaded me to organise the occupational therapy department – a special activity in which I certainly did not shine.

We were very busy at Sarafand, where we acted as a base hospital for casualties from Egypt as well as dealing with orthopaedic problems in Palestine. I was eager to learn and I hope that I did not do too much harm to any of my patients. As spring and summer approached we often managed to visit the Jaffa Club in the afternoon, where, rather surprisingly, we enjoyed good surfing at the eastern end of the Mediterranean. On one such visit I recognised another senior officer; he was stark naked and combing his hair in the changing room. That was Clifford Naunton Morgan with whom I had worked on the professorial unit at Barts. Just like Edward Cullinan, Clifford greeted me like a long lost friend and breathed fire about all those young doctors back home who were "hard of hearing" – this was a reference to those who had managed to avoid enrolling in the services. We talked about prospects after the war but that postwar world still seemed far away, as indeed it was.

My paper on fulminating haemolytic anaemia had been completed at Sarafand and was now on its way through "the usual channels" en route to the *Lancet* and the *RAMC Journal*. Luckily it had attracted the attention of Colonel J S K Boyd, the consultant pathologist in Cairo, and we exchanged four letters on the subject. I was impressed by the way that he, a regular and senior RAMC man, addressed me in friendly fashion – "Dear Murley," without the "Captain." Of course some might say that he would have to have written "Dear Reggie" to achieve the equivalent friendliness today. His comments were most helpful. Many years later, when he had become Sir John Boyd and been elected to fellowship of the Royal Society, I discovered that he was living in Northwood. He was then in his 80s and nearly blind. Not surprisingly, he did not remember our correspondence of many years ago, but I reminded him that he had discussed me with Jock Monro who, I strongly suspect, had selected me for my next move only on the basis of that conversation. John Boyd has since died, but I was so glad to have visited him and given him a bottle of his favourite blended whisky.

It was about September 1942 when right out of the blue my commanding officer, Colonel Mackie, told me that a posting order had been received for me to proceed to 1 Maxillofacial Unit at 8 General Hospital, Alexandria, as "assistant surgeon." Delighted though I was by this news I was mystified why I had been selected. Only later did I hear that the two Australian surgeons at that unit had decided that they needed a young man to train and take on the donkeywork. One of them, Randall Champion, had approached Jock Monro at the very time when Boyd and he had been discussing my most amateur first paper, on which I had been working for many months. Serendipity and luck can certainly play an important part in our lives.

9 Plastic and maxillofacial challenge

I believe it was in September 1942 that I moved from Palestine to Alexandria. This was shortly after the Axis forces had driven the Eighth Army back to Alamein, greatly stretching their own lines of communication and conveniently shortening ours just when we were achieving air superiority. It was an exciting time to arrive, and Alexandria was a pleasant city almost undamaged by the war. Number 8 General Hospital was in the relatively new buildings of an Italian school, which had adapted well as an 800 bed military hospital. Number 1 Maxillofacial Unit was commanded by Major Randall Champion, a pleasant but reserved Gillies trained Australian; later he became consultant plastic surgeon in Manchester. The senior dental officer was Major E J Dalling and he was assisted by Captain B V Janes. They had the back up of a good dental laboratory with two or three dental technicians. We also had some facilities for clinical photography. Our anaesthetist, Captain John Taylor from the London Hospital, was good to work with in the theatre. Because there was an Australian division in the Eighth Army we also had an attached Australian Army Medical Corps plastic surgeon, Major David Officer Brown, who had also been Gillies trained. Champion had graduated in Sydney; Brown in Melbourne – though he practised in Sydney after the war.

I could not have arrived at a better unit or at a more opportune time. There was a volume of interesting work, mainly faciomaxillary but also related plastic problems and severe burns. Even between battles we had enough to keep us busy. I covered the plastic unit whole time but I also took my turn on general surgery emergency duty under the officer in command of our surgical division, Lieutenant Colonel R K

Debenham of Birmingham. I had had little civilian surgical training but I was keen as mustard and had excellent guidance and tuition from my senior colleagues. Our unit records were well organised and we had an efficient secretary, the half French, half English daughter of a wealthy Alexandrian family. The unit had between 60 and 100 beds pleasantly situated on the first floor, with facilities for expansion, and we had our own operation room which could take two tables. The officers' mess was in a large mansion about five minutes' walk from the hospital. My companions were splendid, with the exception of one overtly homosexual doctor who made passes at several of the younger officers, but fortunately he never showed any such interest in me.

The officer in command of our medical division was Ronald Bodley Scott, who had taught me on the medical professorial unit at Barts. He was an excellent physician, slightly reserved but a good friend and a good humoured companion once one knew him better. He was friendly with our ophthalmic specialist, the Hon Geoffrey Bridgeman, from St George's Hospital. The general surgical specialist was Briant Evans, a relatively recently appointed gynaecologist at Westminster Hospital. It would have been difficult to find better colleagues or a better ambience in which to work. I count myself fortunate to have fallen on my feet in that hospital. In our sparse leisure time we used to visit the elegant Union Club or the Alexandria Yacht Club. My companions were invariably male and I always maintained a strictly professional relationship with our nursing sisters. Moreover, I had firmly resolved that I would concentrate on my medical work and avoid the possibility of any serious female attachment until after the war. With that general philosophy it was easier to concentrate on the work, and I never had any doubts on this score. Of course, things were different for combatants, many of whom had a strong incentive to sow their wild oats lest they should perish in the next battle. Sadly too there was liberal opportunity overseas for many married men to seek pastures new. Having had little chance of observing marital infidelity in my sheltered prewar life I tended to be a trifle censorious about those individuals who lapsed from grace.

If I was lucky in my surgical chiefs I hope that they felt pleased to have me with them. What I lacked in experience was certainly made up in energy and enthusiasm. In one sense I was contravening all the established conventions of surgical training through having started in the specialties of orthopaedics and plastic surgery. But later I realised how lucky I had been to enjoy this exposure to two such important specialties before settling into the generality of surgery. There was so much, especially in plastic surgery, which had vital application in general surgery and, indeed, in other specialties. The close collaboration with dental surgeons and anaesthetists, which is vital in head and neck work, taught me much which was to be of lasting value later, not only in my own work but also in the training of young surgeons. Moreover, when I was on duty for general surgical emergencies I realised how lacking I was in those diagnostic and judgmental skills which tend to be more slowly acquired in that wide field. But it might ultimately have turned out rather differently had I not later been determined to give myself as wide a general training as possible. That early experience in plastic surgery taught me a great deal about neat suturing, the gentle handling of tissues, and the principles of skin and tissue replacement, which I was able to apply in my general work. It gave me, too, a keener grasp of the breadth of experience which we should aim to provide for our surgical trainees.

With British, Australian, New Zealand, South African, Polish, Free French, and Greek units in our own force, as well as Italian and German prisoners of war, the clientele of our plastic and maxillofacial wards was multiracial and multilingual. It was fascinating to compare the style and habits of these different elements. At one end of the spectrum the Australians were, at any rate by conventional British standards, outspoken and somewhat ill disciplined and contrasted sharply with the Germans. Our hospital was reasonably close to the bars and night life of Alexandria, and the Australians loved their "tinnies" of Foster's – when they could get them – or of Egyptian "Stella" when their own brew was not available. It was impossible to keep the Aussie "up" patients out of the town, and once they were mobile it was useless to try to keep them under control. Empty bottles and cans of beer were commonly kept beneath the beds, to the consternation of one of our more strictly disciplinarian sisters from Paisley. Moreover, even some of those with serious facial injuries, whose broken jaws were immobilised by intermaxillary wire fixation or cast metal cap splints, seemed to have no difficulty in imbibing vast quantities of liquor. It was not unknown for the occasional drunkard, possibly returning from a binge in the town, to get into serious trouble when vomiting ensued. I can remember one or two who had to have the tie wires which held the jaws together cut by the dental surgeon so that the airway could be cleared.

We generally made a point of putting our allied and enemy casualties in separate wards. Although the general level of discipline of the New Zealand and foreign troops was similar to that of the British, there was a stark contrast when one entered a predominantly Aussie ward. We all – Champion and Brown included – found this more entertaining than exasperating, especially if one's next visit was to a German ward. Immediately we appeared at the door of a ward full of Germans the senior non-commissioned officer would usually call the ambulant patients to attention. Those confined to bed might have their arms – if uninjured – outside on the counterpane, palms downwards. We always made a point of maintaining a formal and strictly professional relationship with the prisoners; only a few of them spoke English and my school German was distinctly rusty.

During the steady build up of our forces before the battle of Alamein there was the opportunity to clear beds by sending some of the more seriously wounded British and Dominion troops to South Africa and the prisoners and allied wounded to Michael Oldfield's 2 Maxillofacial Unit in Cairo. One afternoon in early October 1942 I had a truck trip towards the front at Alamein. After leaving Alexandria I was astonished by the almost continuous encampments and signs of activity along the road, on both sides of which transport, tanks, and service personnel were amassed in great numbers. I had watched the build up of two divisions before Keren, and that was small beer when compared with the seven infantry and three armoured divisions here. The fact that in contrast to the enemy we had short lines of communication and mastery in the air meant that our troops were almost immune to attack by Axis aircraft.

I cannot forget the moonlit night of 23 October when we heard a thousand of our guns open up more than 50 miles away at Alamein and continue their bombardment for several hours. Our first facial casualties arrived early the next morning and we remained intensely active for the next two weeks, until the final breakthrough on 4 November. Our policy was to cope with every patient as fully as possible but to rely on ultimate evacuation to South Africa for the longer term reconstructive work. There was little chance of sending long term cases home round the Cape, so many of these patients went to Jack Penn's unit in Johannesburg.

About the third day of the Alamein battle we admitted a German *Feldwebel* (staff sergeant) named Beick, from a Panzer division, with loss of his lower jaw and overlying soft tissue from angle to angle. He had been given a blood transfusion during his evacuation but reached us in a shocked state. I set up a fresh transfusion and shortly discovered that despite his severe wound, with tongue more or less "floating," he spoke good English. When I visited him again a few hours later he looked up at the bottle of blood suspended above his head and said, "Is that the fourth bottle, sir?" "No, Beick, that is the fifth," I replied. He sighed deeply and said, "Oh dear, by the time this transfusion is over I shall not know whether to say Heil Hitler or God save the King!" The drollery of the response caused me immense amusement and I dined out on that story for a long time.

While I was in Alexandria I was smitten by a sharp attack of bacillary dysentery. This happened during an operation which I had started in perfectly good health. Just after its completion I fainted; shortly after recovering consciousness there was an urgent call to stool and I passed almost pure blood. I was admitted to the officers' ward under the care of Bodley Scott and he, being a good physician, wanted a stool culture done so that I would not receive blunderbuss treatment with an unsuitable drug. All was well for some hours after I arrived in the ward. At about 11 pm that night, however, I felt a powerful urge developing. Anxious that my "specimen" should be promptly tested so that I could quickly get back to work, I sent for the orderly officer – a captain from the VD department – and we mobilised the duty laboratory technician so that my specimen could be taken down to him in a warm bedpan. The venereologist obligingly connived in the deception of Bodley Scott by promptly prescribing a sulpha drug, to which my organism was subsequently shown to be sensitive. Perhaps it was lucky that the VD doctor was on duty because he was used to starting his "clap" patients on treatment before the sensitivity of the gonococcus had been reported. That is the only time I have ever been treated by a venereologist.

While on casualty duty a few days later I was called to see a sick brigadier who had recently arrived from England by air via West Africa. He gave his history in somewhat confused fashion, and had a slight pyrexia. My own experience in Eritrea promptly alerted me to the possibilities. I made a blood smear and took it to the laboratory after sending my patient to the officers' ward. In a few minutes we found that the specimen was teeming with ring forms of the malignant tertian malarial parasite. By the time I arrived at the ward the brigadier was confused and drowsy: I concluded that he had cerebral malaria so I gave him a slow injection of intravenous quinine, such as Regio Moise had given me on that fateful morning in Massawa. Bodley Scott had been enjoying an afternoon off at the yacht club. When he arrived for the evening round he asked Kathie McShane, the ward sister, if there were any new patients. "Yes, sir, a brigadier with cerebral malaria," she replied. Bodley was startled and said, "Good Heavens, where is he?" Kathie calmly replied, "Oh, he's all right; he was diagnosed and treated by Captain Murley." Bodley responded, "You surely don't mean him; he works with the maxillofacial unit." Kathie confirmed my identity and warmly commended her recent dysentery patient. My stock certainly rose sharply; but Bodley had not appreciated how easy it was for me after my personal experience in Massawa.

When I first arrived at 8 General Hospital I heard an amusing story about Kathie McShane. A few months earlier a Major Randolph Churchill had been admitted to her ward one night after a road accident west of Alexandria. He had broken a few ribs and suffered a slight crush fracture of a thoracic vertebra (which was not spotted for several weeks, but no harm was done). When Kathie came on duty the next morning the night staff notified her of the new admissions and she shortly set off on her round. On opening the door of Churchill's room she saw a dark skinned half naked man sitting up in bed. He promptly said, "Sister, I expect you know that I am the Prime Minister's son," to which Kathie naively responded, "Oh. Nahas Pasha?" Randolph snorted and shouted, "*No, Winston Churchill!*" I subsequently asked Kathie about this event and she assured me that, far from trying to score off him, her thoughts at that moment were far away. Although she had seen the name Churchill in the admissions book, when she opened the door of the room she thought that the bronzed patient was Egyptian and therefore had named the Egyptian rather than the British Prime Minister.

On 23 January, three months after Alamein, our troops had captured Tripoli. Within a short time it was decided to send maxillofacial and neurosurgical units to the British hospital there. As Mortimer Shaw, who was at Michael Oldfield's unit in Cairo, was more experienced than I – and possibly seeking a little change from Michael – it was decided to send him to a forward section of 1 Maxillofacial Unit in Tripoli, and I moved to 2 Maxillofacial Unit as Oldfield's assistant. This was certainly good for all of us. So in February 1943 Shaw went to Tripoli as I joined Oldfield's unit at 9 General Hospital in the Heliopolis Palace Hotel. Lieutenant Colonel Robert Keller, an Edinburgh gynaecologist, was in command of the surgical division and George Matthew of Edinburgh, another gynaecologist, was the general surgical specialist; there was yet another Edinburgh surgeon in charge of the thoracic unit.

Michael Oldfield was exceedingly industrious and single minded, but he had a reputation as a tough task master who many people found difficult to work with. This applied to both doctors and nursing staff, as I was soon to learn. He had two splendid dental surgeons, Major Wilfred Roberts and Captain Ronald Pook, and an excellent anaesthetist, Alfie Raffan of Aberdeen. Pook and Raffan became my lifelong friends, the former being my postwar dentist until his retirement. Oldfield's unit had a dental laboratory and staff similar to that in Alexandria, but he had a more highly organised photographic department. He also had two special RAMC orderlies as "dressers" and these men did many of the daily wound and graft dressings under our supervision. I was also struck by the fact that he was undertaking a lot of longer term reconstructive work, much of which I thought inappropriate to wartime circumstances in Egypt. For example, he was raising a large number of tube pedicle grafts, shifting skin and subcutaneous fat from the abdomen and chest region by a method that was time consuming as it needed several staged operations. Indeed, several of his patients developed urinary tract stones, partly because they were confined to bed for so long.

It will be appreciated that the Cairo unit contrasted sharply with what I had become used to in Alexandria, but it provided me with excellent experience. We did quite a lot of homografting of burns and we generally stored any "spare" donor skin in the refrigerator so that it might be available for the more severe burns cases. We had one burnt soldier who had skin applied from donors of no less than seven different nationalities. Until then I had not been familiar with homograft rejection but now I saw its regular occurrence. Oldfield would emphasise that the later a graft was applied the more quickly it would be rejected. At that time Medawar and Gibson's work on the antigenicity of skin had not yet been published. It was an extension of that study which was eventually to bring Peter Medawar the award of a Nobel prize.

I was unprepared for Michael's extraordinary and intermittent irascibility. He was slimly built and always used rather shrunken cotton operating suits. His assistants had to squeeze themselves into similarly tight garb. One morning as we were scrubbing up I remarked on the extreme tightness of my trousers. Michael responded, "Well, you can go then." I took no notice of this seemingly disconnected remark so he glared at me and shouted, "*You can go!*" Apparently his mind was made up, so I promptly disappeared to the wards. When I next met him he seemed perfectly cordial and made no mention of the incident. But I learnt that the nursing staff suffered in similar fashion. He had two excellent theatre sisters, one in her early 30s and Miss White, who was grey haired and possibly in her 50s. They were both proud products of the Edinburgh Royal Infirmary. A few weeks before my arrival Michael had been doing a nephrectomy on one of his longstanding patients who had a huge staghorn calculus in one kidney. He indicated that he would like a drainage tube and Miss White duly placed one on the theatre trolley. Now Michael had a habit of peering sideways and speedily picking on any practice of which he could possibly disapprove. On this occasion he said, "From where did that drainage tube come?" "Out of the emergency drainage tube jar, sir," replied Miss White. "And how was it sterilised?" asked Michael. "In carbolic solution, Major Oldfield," said Miss White. Without another word Oldfield turned to the trolley, grasped the towel on which the instruments lay, and pulled everything on to the floor. He then calmly sat on a theatre stool, "And now, Miss White," he said, "just boil those up for 20 minutes." That was done. After the operation Miss White waylaid Michael to have a private word with him. They retired to the anaesthetic room where she said, "Major Oldfield, I have worked with some of the finest surgeons in Edinburgh and I have *never* been treated like that. If this happens again I shall resign." Michael blandly replied "Well, go now, Miss White!"

Michael had an obsession about boiling everything as this, apparently, had been the routine in his native Leeds. All our surgical gloves had to be boiled and then put on wet. Now there is little worse than having water slopping about under one's gloves while operating, and wetness certainly tends to promote wound contamination. But he would not accept gloves sterilised in the autoclave and manufacturer packaged presterilised gloves were, of course, not then available.

Sadly, Michael could be his own worst enemy. On the

several occasions when I went to the Heliopolis sporting club with him, or when we met after the war, he was always charming and friendly. But he still had much the same reputation among those who worked with him. He died of a myocardial infarct in his early 50s. Whatever my own feelings were about him in wartime I greatly enjoyed my five months in Cairo. We lived in a pleasant little hotel just across the road from the hospital and our regular army commanding officer was the delightful Colonel Oram. He was a perfect gentleman and had been a radiologist in the army in peacetime. Although we all lived in that small hotel the officers had a dining room in the hospital, and the American bar – still with its illuminated outside signs – was immediately adjacent. Oram usually reached that bar first for his preprandial lunch-time drink and one morning a group of American other ranks walked in through the outside door. They ordered four whiskies and the barman looked a little dismayed. But Oram turned to them and said, "Gentlemen, you must have these drinks on me." The Americans were agreeably surprised and started an animated conversation with the colonel. Gradually the bar began to fill up with other RAMC officers. The Americans noticed the maroon tabs on Oram's lapels, and on learning that he was a colonel one of them exclaimed, "Gee, Colonel, are we in an officers' mess? We must beat it." Oram reassuringly replied, "Oh, do please finish your drinks first."

After dinner one evening Colonel Oram brought out a photograph album and told us the fantastic story of a successful prewar hoax. A new military hospital in Haifa was due to be opened by Lady Hood, the wife of the director general of Army Medical Services, but she was taken ill. Shortly afterwards it became known at the hospital that the opening would be performed by an Arab sheikh. The great day came when the Sheikh of Hokes was said to be arriving from Transjordan. An aeroplane – by kind cooperation with the RAF – flew over and landed at a nearby airfield. Shortly afterwards the sheikh and his entourage appeared in two large limousines. A pair of huge Sudanese with coloured sunshades (all hired from a local restaurant in Haifa) climbed out of the leading vehicle and provided cover for the sheikh as he got out of his car. A guard of honour greeted the distinguished visitor and Major Oram (as he then was) drew his sword at the wrong moment. That distracted attention from the sheikh, who then proceeded up the steps (with QAIMNS sisters on each side) to the red ribbon across the entrance: this he cut with "scissors, stretcher-bearer nine inch," gold plated for the occasion. After a full tour of the hospital the entourage ended up in the sisters' mess for tea. At that stage the identity of the sheikh – by now sitting crosslegged on the floor – was strongly suspected by one elderly and wily RAMC officer. He kept his suspicions to himself and, as tea and cakes were served, he whispered to matron, "Don't feed the sheikh, it's Ramadan" (indeed it *was* the time of that Muslim fast and the sheikh got nothing to eat). It was only as the visitors left to enter their cars that a sister at an upstairs window remarked, "How like Captain Watts that sheikh walks". He *did*, for he *was*; and John Watts was on short leave of absence for the event.

Colonel Oram told this story with puckish glee as he turned the pages of his album and showed us pictures illustrating every stage of the hoax, including the elaborate make up of Captain Watts at an Arab barber's shop. After the event the hospital personnel divided into two camps, the first firmly declaring that it had been a hoax and the others equally firmly declaring that they could not possibly have been deceived in this way. That, said Oram, is the real test of a successful hoax for if nobody finds out it is not nearly so much fun. Perhaps the more diligent of the sceptics were convinced only when they failed to find Hokes on the map. It was regulars like Oram in Cairo, Large, the deputy director of medical services in Palestine, and Willie Russell in Abyssinia who convinced me that I must not categorise people according to my misconceived notions.

After I had spent a few months with Oldfield it was suddenly realised that I was not an officially graded specialist, so I was given welcome and belated recognition on the recommendation of Robert Kellar, the officer in command of our surgical division. Not long after this, in June 1943, I replaced Shaw in Tripoli and he rejoined Oldfield in Cairo. Number 1 Maxillofacial Unit closed down in Alexandria; its dental officers and other personnel and equipment were moved to Tripoli, and David Officer Brown returned to Australia and Randall Champion to England. The Axis armies in Tunisia were finally defeated on 13 May and there was a lull before the invasion of Sicily and Italy. During that short lull we were attached to 41 General Hospital. We were awaiting the arrival from England of our new commanding officer, Richard Battle. Those few weeks I spent in Tripoli were especially interesting because of a penicillin conference which was attended by representatives of both the Eighth and Second armies and the consultant surgeons of the British, American, and New Zealand forces.

Only during the last stages of the North African campaign did a small supply of relatively crude penicillin become available. Unlike the later, much purer, crystalline preparations our initial supplies were rather brown in colour. Moreover, as so little was available it was customary after wound excision and toilet to insert small tubes through which a solution of penicillin could be injected. Although the dosage was low by modern standards the initial results were impressive and the object of our one day conference was to facilitate fuller reporting and exchange of ideas. After the morning session and lunch we reassembled under the chairmanship of Howard Florey. He quickly observed that our recent lunch and the hot afternoon had made some people a little sleepy. "Is there a beach to which we could adjourn?" he asked. There certainly was, and transport was soon organised to take us all to the sisters' bathing beach. We travelled in open trucks in the middle of a passing convoy, and the troops were astonished to see a number of top brass of the American and British armies travelling in this fashion. We included colonels Churchill and Naffziger of the American army; Stout, the New Zealander; and Heneage Ogilvie, our own consultant surgeon, then a major general. As it arrived at the beach the truck in which I was travelling stuck in the soft sand, and I shall never forget the sight of Howard Florey helping to push the vehicle free. Once we were on that beach the conference continued in relaxed style.

The invasion of Sicily was due to begin on 3 July in a

campaign which lasted 38 days, and until our own unit moved over to the island during August we continued to work at 41 General Hospital. There we were teamed up with 4 Neurosurgical Unit, with which we would continue to work in Sicily and Italy in the ensuing 14 months. Whereas 1 Maxillofacial Unit had just one theatre sister – Mary Beardall, who had been with us in Alexandria – the neurosurgical unit had two special ward sisters and two theatre sisters. That unit had earlier lost one theatre sister in the desert in strange circumstances, which are worth relating. While she was working in the western desert with the unit, a few months after arriving from England, that sister began to get fat. There was much good natured joking about this, in which she happily joined. They had come out around the Cape, and about eight months after sailing from England she went back to Cairo on leave. It was shortly after this that Kenneth Eden, the neurosurgeon in charge, had gone to Cairo to see the patients he had evacuated to Peter Ascroft's neurosurgical unit there. While in Cairo he was asked to call on the matron-in-chief. "What *have* you been doing to sister D?" said matron as Eden entered her office. He was completely mystified and asked, "What do you mean?" To which matron rejoined, "Mean, Major Eden? Mean? I mean she's pregnant." Kenneth Eden slapped his head and said, "Oh, *that's* why she's been getting so fat!" It seems that the sister herself thought that her missing periods were due to life in the desert and did not suspect her true condition until she went to Cairo. That is why she had so cheerfully accepted chaffing by the team. Even the matron-in-chief was more philosophical once she realised that the baby had been fathered by one of the ship's officers on the way out and not by the neurosurgical team.

The two neurosurgical ward sisters, Mary Turner and Mary Bailey, were both splendid "nightingales" from St Thomas's: highly competent, full of good humour, and most industrious. It was usual for the neurosurgical team, having dealt with a penetrating brain wound, to apply a plaster of Paris headcap with dates and details inscribed thereon with a blue pencil. One hot afternoon a patient of theirs went berserk and rushed stark naked out of the ward into a small copse alongside the hospital. Mary Bailey duly went off in search of him while many of her other patients, at the windows of the ward, gave her instructions as to where the patient had gone. Within a minute or so Mary Bailey, in her immaculate white uniform, emerged from the wood arm-in-arm with the now compliant soldier, who was wearing nothing but a plaster headcap. There were great shouts of applause from the assembled company and it was certainly a performance of which Florence Nightingale herself would have been proud.

10 An unholy trinity in Italy

It was about the end of the first week of August when we prepared to move to Sicily. Richard Battle had still not arrived from home. He had been in the army at the start of the war, serving in France; but after Dunkirk he returned to England and was attached to Professor Pomfret Kilner's unit at Stoke Mandeville. We boarded the hospital ship *Maine* one evening for a comfortable voyage in warm summer weather. All the ship's lights were aglow. What a welcome contrast to the usual blackout. On going below in the almost empty ship I found some extra luggage near mine; and on a bedside table there was a silver cigarette lighter engraved "RJVB." I knew that Dick Battle had arrived and I soon found him up on deck. I felt immediately that there would be no problems with him in charge. We had much to talk about as we exchanged news from England and North Africa. The following evening we entered Augusta harbour in Sicily, where I met one of my near contemporaries from Barts, Charles Foster Cooper, with Rowan Nicks, a New Zealander. Both were surgeon lieutenants in the navy. I would next meet Rowan in the final FRCS examination. He has remained a lifelong friend.

We did very little surgery in Sicily because the fighting there soon ceased. After a day or two in Syracuse we moved up to Catania and then to Taormina, where Monty had addressed his troops in the Roman theatre a few days before. While in Catania I met Kenneth Eden, who was in charge of the neurosurgical unit. A few days later he became ill with a sore throat. He was admitted to hospital, where it was thought that there was little wrong with him. With the aid of a mirror, however, he observed that he had some paralysis of his palate. This he demonstrated to his graded surgeon, John Gillingham, who had only just returned from Cairo, where he had been sent for special investigation after developing a peculiar paralysis of his jaw muscles. Kenneth Eden died of polioencephalitis a day or two later and there can be little doubt that Gillingham had had a similar but milder infection. Indeed, John's jaw muscles were restored to normal strength only many months later. A second graded surgeon with the neurosurgical unit was Hal Slemon, a Canadian from Toronto who had joined the RAMC soon after the war began. There was also a graded neurologist, Llewellyn Smith. Hugh Cairns had had all these young men with him for training at the Head Injuries Hospital, in St Hugh's College, Oxford.

We had little time to mourn the loss of Eden before the neurosurgical and maxillofacial units were moved by landing craft across the straits of Messina into the toe of Italy. This was in late July. We had our own transport and, having disembarked at Reggio di Calabria, spent the next two days in relatively wild country, moving via Loeri and Catanzaro to Taranto. We reached Taranto a day or two after a British parachute brigade landed there from a naval cruiser. I was fascinated to hear that Shan Hackett, no longer with the cavalry, was in command of that brigade. I was sorry not to see him there and I was not to meet him again until some years after the war. In Taranto we were joined by 1 Mobile Ophthalmic Unit under the command of Major Edward Zorab, who had recently been with the Second Army. Thereafter, on the Adriatic coast of Italy, our neurosurgical, maxillofacial, and ophthalmic units would remain together. The first two were subsequently split into forward and base sections, the eye unit staying with the advanced sections. Edward, always known as "Z," was a charming companion and a highly competent eye surgeon. He came of a large medical family and had four brothers; three of them were doctors and one was a dental surgeon. Their father had been an eye surgeon in Southampton. Father and sons were all trained at Guy's. Edward was a keen poker player and during lulls in the fighting could often be seen having a round or two in the mess. He almost invariably had a cigarette in his mouth. It was at about this time that Charles Donald, then our consultant surgeon in Italy, playfully dubbed us "the unholy trinity." That name stuck for the rest of the campaign and meanwhile a similar group of units, formerly with the Second Army in North Africa, provided the service on the west side of Italy.

This was the first time in the war that a comprehensive "head and neck" service had been provided and that such units had functioned with casualty clearing stations well forward. Strategically placed in this way, we were normally able to collect our casualties within a few hours of their being wounded. If there were multiple wounds elsewhere on the trunk and limbs the general surgical teams would collaborate with us. This arrangement set the pattern for all subsequent campaigns in the war and I do not think that we could have provided a more efficient service for these patients. Suffice it to say that even under peacetime conditions there are few parts of the country where a similar concentration of specialist services is provided at a single hospital. We were privileged to be able to work in this way and to gain unrivalled experience.

Our units first opened up in Bari, but the advanced sections soon moved to Barletta further up the Adriatic coast, where we were attached to 48 General Hospital and located in a school. At that time the neurosurgical unit was joined by a new graded surgeon, Campbell Connolly, from the Head Injuries Hospital at Oxford. In addition to our own and enemy casualties we soon started to receive Yugoslav partisans who were flown across the Adriatic. Such was our ignorance of Yugoslav affairs that we still believed Mihailovic to be in charge there. But the mention of his name rarely produced any positive response; these men constantly spoke of Tito, of whom we had not previously heard. The Yugoslavs were in all age groups from young boys to elderly men. Typical of some of the latter was a man in his 70s who had never before been far from his native village; he had sustained a nasty face and jaw wound when hit by a fragment of an American bomb. A few hours later he was astonished to find himself in a British Army hospital in Italy. We also had quite a large number of burns casualties in Barletta; they were nursed in wards protected by insect screens, for flies were in abundance. We made extensive use of Bunyan–Stannard envelopes for many of the limb burns as these gave further protection.

The Italians had surrendered on 3 September, shortly after the invasion of Italy, so our early advance was swift. It took the Germans a while to move in, but they were able to contain the Salerno landing, south of Naples, for some time. On the Adriatic side the advanced sections of the "trinity" moved on to San Severo from mid-September to mid-October and then to Foggia for a week. By mid-November we moved to Termoli for a month, by which time the important airfields at Foggia could be brought into use. It was then that bombers would set out from England and land at Foggia after bombing German targets en route. Further raids could then be made on the return flight. But we were now at the beginning of winter. The ground became steadily more boggy and German resistance strengthened, aided by the many rivers which ran from the Appenines down to the coast. The winter in Italy in 1943 was cold and miserable and, after four years, we had begun to think that the war was interminable. It was clear too that the Germans were putting up a much stiffer fight than had the Italians. During a quieter spell at San Severo General Montgomery came to visit our casualty clearing station, which was in a school building. He wandered into my operation room wearing his beret with the two badges. He was clearly intrigued, and not a little pleased, to see the neat and cheerful Mary Beardall and promptly said, "Whatever are you doing here?" She replied, "I work here, sir. I'm the theatre sister and I'm a regular just like you." Not to be outdone he retorted, "But how do you get on with all these terrible men?" Mary replied, "They're not terrible, sir, they look after me very well." On that same visit to our clearing station Monty delivered many books and magazines which had been sent to him by well wishers, including a copy of a Johannesburg newspaper for 1 January 1900, printed in gold to celebrate the beginning of the century.

Notwithstanding the sometimes discouraging conditions, we in the unholy trinity were usually very busy and were learning a lot from each other. When facial or cranial casualties were many the units would help each other out. And so I gained considerable experience in dealing with penetrating brain wounds and compound skull fractures. In collaboration with our neurosurgical colleagues we were able to achieve early and efficient treatment of some of the serious craniofacial injuries. Moreover, even in the lulls between battles a steady stream of road casualties would arrive. We worked in close concert with our surgical, dental, and anaesthetic colleagues and our task was a fulfilling one. There was little time for depression about the many severe injuries which passed through our hands. All parts of the trinity continued to keep good and careful records, and if any of the men with graver facial injuries died I did a necropsy examination whenever possible. From those necropsies I learnt that many of these patients had aspirated a considerable amount of blood into the lungs. This aspiration of blood often gave rise to serious trouble later; and we began largely to solve the problem by early tracheostomy to allow better toilet of the trachea and bronchial tree.

At Termoli there was one November day when we admitted a number of New Zealand casualties from north of the Sangro River. One of these was a young officer with a wound of the face caused by a shell fragment which had passed through the upper jaw, below one eye, and lodged high in the neck. Despite fairly heavy loss of blood, he arrived in good condition from a New Zealand dressing station where he had been briskly and efficiently transfused, as was the custom. On examining him in the preoperative unit I noticed that his skin was rather warm; the thermometer showed a high fever, and a blood smear confirmed the ring forms of malignant tertian malaria. There had been many such cases from the Sicilian campaign but few fresh ones in Italy. We postponed operation and in collaboration with the medical specialist, Philip Evans, we treated him with quinine. While he was sitting up in bed on the sixth day his breathing became increasingly laboured and bubbly and he rapidly died. I did a necropsy in our tented morgue and found that his heart was filled with bubbled blood. The shell fragment was lodged in a partly divided jugular vein and air had passed down the wound track into that vein, and so to the right side of the heart. Philip and I thought the case important enough to warrant publication; I later wrote it up and sent my script to him when we were at separate units. Philip greatly improved my paper and I was grateful to him for embellishing my earlier humble effort before publication in the *British Journal of Surgery*. As he succinctly pointed out, had this officer been lying down, rather than sitting up in bed, he might well have had a secondary haemorrhage instead of suffering the much more serious hazard of air embolism. Had it not been for the malignant tertian malaria the wound would have been fully dealt with, the shell fragment removed, and the jugular vein repaired on the day of admission. The outcome was sad; but, once again, a battlefield necropsy had prevented us from overlooking an otherwise unsuspected complication.

We in the unholy trinity moved up to a British casualty clearing station at Vasto in December and it was there that we spent Christmas. We dealt with a lot of casualties on Christmas Day and Boxing Day, but things soon became a little quieter. There was also a Canadian clearing station in that small town and, with fewer mid-winter casualties in the New Year, a number of lively parties were held. At one of these Arnold Gourevitch of Birmingham, and Dalling, our dental surgeon, managed to pour a huge quantity of fruit salad and tinned cream over each other. I shudder to think what some of those civilians back home might have said, living on fairly tight rations, had they been able to see us. But this horseplay did provide opportunity for harmlessly letting off steam. On a more serious and romantic note, a Canadian RAMC officer with our clearing station began to court one of the sisters from the nearby Canadian unit. They were married a few months later and I found myself wondering whether this wartime marriage would last. Alas, it did not. They had two children and the wife later developed poliomyelitis. By the time I visited him in Toronto in 1955 there was a new spouse and then, unbelievably, no fewer than three more.

During that period our neurosurgical unit dealt with one patient with a middle meningeal artery haemorrhage. A Canadian medical officer, quite drunk, was found on the side of the road, presumably having been hit by a passing vehicle.

He had been missing for several hours and was found in a deep coma with dilatation of the pupils on both sides. No anaesthetic was needed, but the anaesthetist intubated him to secure the airway. A huge extradural clot was found on the left side; as this was evacuated the patient began to recover consciousness and later made a remarkably good recovery. That experience was to prove immensely valuable to me because I had a number of similar patients after the war.

It was at this quiet time at the beginning of the year, following the heavy casualties around Christmas 1943, that General Montgomery visited the three casualty clearing stations. I vaguely recall a conversation at luncheon with one of Monty's staff when I was somewhat critical of the recent fruitless engagement during a particularly muddy Italian winter. But my old friend Alan Birt, then working with a field surgical unit at the nearby Indian casualty clearing station, later told me that he had heard that I had protested directly to Monty, telling him that next time he decided to start a battle in such unfavourable conditions he should first consult his surgeons for their advice about the likely casualty list. It is possible that the general may have been sitting not far from those to whom I directed my criticisms at the luncheon table – or his staff officer may have passed on my remarks; but it is certain that Alan Birt received an apocryphal version of what really happened.

Shortly after this the time came for Mary Beardall to return home on what was known as "python." After four and a half years overseas we were eligible for home leave. Mary had been in Egypt with the regular QAIMNS before the war and so qualified for python earlier than the rest of us. Before her departure we had a splendid "TPU" (trinity piss-up) – which was not such a drunken event as the name might imply – in which the personnel of all three units took part. Eric Dalling, the senior officer, climbed on a chair to make an appropriate farewell speech. He concluded, "Unholy trinity, raise your glasses on high as I give you the toast to our Mary, our virgin Mary, and there can't be many units which could say that after nearly four years overseas!" Mary was a cheerful and hardworking woman who got on well with all ranks. She had a fine sense of humour and could always touch on the risqué without becoming vulgar. She would often laugh about an event which had occurred shortly before my arrival in Alexandria. On that occasion two or three naval officers were at a brothel called "Mary's House" when they suffered injuries during a bombing raid. Mary claimed that their record cards were appropriately inscribed "Wounded in action."

On another occasion in our postoperative ward at Vasto I had mislaid my pen when writing up some case notes. I called over to Mary Turner, the neurosurgical ward sister, "Mary, could you please lend me a pen." She put her hand in the pocket of her gown and pulled out a pen, together with a French letter. Quite undismayed, she said, "Gosh, that looks bad doesn't it?" Condoms, teat ended with a rubber tube tied on, were extensively used in preference to indwelling urethral catheters for many of our more serious cranial cases with incontinence. Indeed they could be a godsend in keeping the beds dry. In these more promiscuous times which so many people now suffer, rather than enjoy, I often look back on those days in sheer wonder. Our womenfolk were treated with chivalry and we enjoyed the best of professional relationships with some quite outstanding nurses.

As spring approached fighting on both sides of Italy steadily increased and our trinity moved up to Porto San Giorgio, where we were attached to a Polish hospital in a good building. These Poles were not those we had met in Palestine in 1940 but were part of a Polish corps under General Anders which had been allowed out of Russia via Iran. Most of us enjoyed excellent relations with the Poles, partly because we appeared to have a somewhat similar sense of humour. I recall that one of my Scots anaesthetists had asked a Polish radiologist how he would translate that English vulgarity, "Get up them stairs." The Pole thought for a moment and said, "Well I suppose that 'Hotch me spatch rasim' [speaking phonetically] is as near as one can get." The anaesthetist practised this for a few moments and then went to the wards to order some preoperative medication. Having signed up the drugs, he then said "Hotch me spatch rasim?" to the pretty Polish sister. She looked a trifle surprised and then said,

"Tak." The anaesthetist did not recognise that she had said "Yes," and only later learnt that the radiologist had given him the rather free, if not loose, translation of "Would you come to bed with me?"

The weather was steadily becoming warmer and we were able to brave the Adriatic for regular early morning swims. One sunny day, around 0700, we sighted an American cruiser steaming south. Suddenly her guns fired briskly at a couple of motor torpedo boats. So far as we could tell neither of them was hit; which was fortunate since we learnt later that these were friendly craft, not enemy ones. But the time came for us to part from our new Polish friends and, as had been the case since leaving San Severo, each new move took us across one or more of the many rivers which proved so helpful to the Germans in their slow and tenacious retreat. The Italian campaign used many of our valuable resources, but it also stretched the enemy at a time when he was under severe pressure on the Russian front.

We had crossed the Chienti and Potenza rivers during this move to Loreto and were then attached to a British general hospital at a superb site. We were housed in a fairly new Italian orphanage on a steep hillside, overlooking the Adriatic. On the top floor of this building the trinity had a magnificent combined operation theatre which comfortably accommodated four operation tables. The tables were not rigidly allocated but were used in various combinations by the three teams according to the flow of casualties. During our time there we had many casualties from British, New Zealand, and Polish units, with a fair number of wounded prisoners as the Germans fell back to what were to be their main winter defences on the Gothic line. A sad event one morning was the arrival on stretchers of two magnificently built military policemen, both casualties from the front seat of a jeep. Each of them had an identical mid-cervical spinal injury with paralysis of all four limbs. The vertebral displacement was such that it is most unlikely that there would be any significant recovery later. These were two extreme examples of the steady stream of road accident victims which the trinity received even during the height of battle.

We had many Canadians with craniofacial wounds at that time. Among the apparently more severe was one soldier whose facial skeleton was totally bared from the chin to the top of the forehead. His eyes were intact; some teeth were damaged, and there was loss of much of the nasal supporting structures. Happily, tucked away under a huge shell dressing which had been applied over his ghoulish visage there was a flap of facial soft tissue, hinged at the forehead. Brief inspection proved that this was viable with an adequate blood supply from the scalp. After the patient had been resuscitated our dental surgeon tidied up the teeth and I repaired the rest of the face, leaving restoration of the nasal skeleton for Dick Battle's subsequent skilful attention at our base section. A number of our colleagues were impressed by the result of the primary operation; in fact, it was among one of my easier pieces of forward repair work.

Mention of Canadian casualties reminds me that Hal Slemon became a casualty to holy matrimony while we were in Vasto. After a wedding and honeymoon on the other side of Italy he was replaced in the unholy trinity by John Gillingham, who had been with the base section. We missed the outspoken Hal, the son of a family doctor from Bowmanasville, Ontario, for he had an entertaining turn of phrase. Once, on entering a lavatory and finding the seat missing, he had cried out loudly, "Hi there, who's pinched the frame?" After a heavy party with a neighbouring Canadian casualty clearing station during a lull in the campaign he had greeted the ever pale faced and dark eyed Llewellyn Smith (even darker eyed with a serious hangover) on the following morning with the epic remark, "Good God, Smiddy, your eyes look jes' like two piss holes in the snow."

At about the same time we were all appalled, despite our long experience, to receive a German prisoner of war who had either lain unseen or been left for dead. He had suffered terrible facial wounds from a land mine. Both eyes were totally destroyed and the sockets were full of maggots; and both upper and lower jaws were severely damaged. When we had resuscitated him we examined him under anaesthetic, removing the maggots, the metal and wood splinters, and the many detached teeth and bone fragments. I do not know whether I was especially tired, but I was shattered by this man's condition. I went quietly to a side table in the theatre, picked up a syringe, drew up no less than three grains of morphine, and injected this intravenously. I thought it would be enough to put him out of his present plight and save him future misery. He returned to the ward with respirations falling to between five and two per minute. Several times in the night it was thought that he was on the point of death; but by the morning his respiration rate slowly increased. A few hours later – I think it was in the early afternoon of the next day – with his face completely enveloped in dressings he sat up in bed, raised his right arm on high, and shouted "Heil Hitler." It was with some difficulty that the RAMC orderlies prevented him from being attacked by the New Zealanders on each side of him. I did not see any of these last events myself, but they were reliably reported to me by the sister in charge. This was to be the first of only two occasions in my professional life when I deliberately attempted to end the life of a patient. Both attempts failed.

On a lighter note there is the story of a Canadian patient who had suffered a relatively minor soft tissue wound of the face. As one of our anaesthetists, Major Jock Harbord, sometimes arrived a little late for the morning list, I decided to anaesthetise this patient with a local injection. Because when pressure of work was particularly heavy it was our practice occasionally to put a patient to sleep and ourselves pass the endotracheal tube to continue anaesthesia from the standard Oxford vapouriser, I took the opportunity to pull Jock's leg. The Canadian was a willing collaborator, so I towelled him up with the connecting tube from the vapouriser tucked in under the towels while I got on with the surgery. The other three tables were already in use with patients under the care of John Wyman, our second anaesthetist. A few minutes later Jock looked in through the door and asked, "Everything OK, Reggie?" I had just said "Yes, Jock" when he spotted the immobile anaesthetic bellows on the top of the Oxford vapouriser. He hurried to my table, saying, "He's not breathing." Just as he arrived at the table I tapped the patient on his right shoulder; at that prearranged signal he raised his right arm and called out, "Hiya, Dr Harbord!" Everyone, Jock included, joined in the fun.

Jock Harbord left us a little while later to join a surgical shock research team on the west side of Italy: this presaged his later inclination to a more academic life. Our other anaesthetist at Loreto, later consultant anaesthetist at the Westminster and dean of the medical school there, was John Wyman. He was highly skilled and thought nothing of running three tables simultaneously while, just occasionally, quietly excising and suturing a scalp wound at yet another table. Lest this should sound horrifying to those accustomed to more leisurely peacetime practice, I shall explain. Firstly, every one of our patients was run at a light level of anaesthesia; secondly, they all had the airway secured by an endotracheal tube; thirdly, the Oxford vapouriser, properly used, was an ideal machine for this type of work; and, lastly, I never saw a patient put at risk in John's safe hands.

Next we moved with the Poles to Ancona. This must have been at the beginning of August because the Poles had a celebratory lunch on the cliffs to commemorate "Soldiers Day" (15 August), when the Russians were defeated at the gates of Warsaw. Foolishly, I did not attend the lunch because I had been told that this anniversary had strong political connotations. Indeed, I learnt later that a Polish journalist had spoken to the British troops, in excellent English, and had concluded his speech: "Officially the Russians are our gallant allies; but we Poles know only too well that they are, in fact, our bitterest enemies." He was loudly cheered by the Poles but coolly received by the British. But most of us, fed for so long on the official propaganda about "dear old Uncle Joe" (Stalin), regarded that Pole as being needlessly offensive. It did not take me long to learn how wrong we were. At about this time news came from Dickie Battle, at our base section, that I was to become a surgical specialist with the rank of major. It was an unexpected and welcome surprise as I had had no chance to sit for the final FRCS examination. Brigadier Harold Edwards of King's College Hospital, who had replaced Charles Donald as our consultant surgeon, kindly made this recommendation, for which I was extremely grateful.

We were not long in Ancona for the Germans had now fallen back to their strongly prepared positions on the Gothic line, which they were to hold through another cold winter. During that autumn they started to shower our troops with propaganda leaflets, often disguised as match packets. One of those leaflets depicted about 20 ways of "going sick" by simulating a number of different types of illness or injury. Apart from such simple ideas as putting pepper in the eyes and beating the knee with a wet towel to produce a joint effusion, it included a cunning way of simulating pulmonary tuberculosis. For this ingenious simulation you had to report with chronic cough. Then, before a chest *x* ray was done, you had to rub lead ointment into a small area of the skin, no larger than a 6d piece, below one clavicle. It was suggested that the doctors were unlikely to take a lateral view of the chest, but that eventuality was also catered for. The *pièce de résistance* was the sputum test. A little blood was to be introduced from the gums, plus a spot of smegma from under the foreskin, with the intention of the acid fast *Bacillus smegmatis* being confused with the acid/alcohol fast tubercle bacillus. I am not aware of any men who made use of these 20 ways of going sick, but it would be remarkable if one or two had not tried some of them on during a long, cold winter.

Later in September we, the unholy trinity, moved to a hospital by the beach in Rimini. It is normally a lovely beach, and so it was when I visited it again after the war. But it was heavily mined when our units arrived there and so bathing was forbidden. Our unit's anaesthetist at that time was Frank Logan Turner, unofficially known either as "Happy" or "Lightning." He had been with us before but had spent more time with Dick Battle at the base section. He was an excellent anaesthetist. Of his two sobriquets he earned the first by virtue of his often lugubrious countenance and the second from his slowness in getting out of bed in the morning. Indeed, when sharing a tent with Dick Battle and two others at Bari he had become notorious for slow rising. In Bari Dickie would often greet Frank with a cheerful "Good morning, Happy." Frank would respond with a grunt, "What's bloody *good* about it?" He would then add, "Give us a few bars, Dickie." At that, Dickie would pull his trumpet out from under the bed and say, "What would you like, Happy?" Frank might reply, "Give us a few bars of Purcell's Trumpet Voluntary, now attributable to Jeremiah Clark." Dick would oblige and his trumpet would be heard all over the camp. In fact he was a first class musician and also played the French horn and saxophone. While at Cambridge, to the dismay of his father, a surgeon at St Thomas's, Dickie had spent a little too much time running a successful jazz band. But he subsequently made good with some very hard work.

In late autumn we once again became exceedingly busy at Rimini. When my replacement, Captain Raoul Sandon, arrived towards the end of October I knew that my python movement order could not be far away. A few days later I received a posting to Naples transit camp en route for home. By then I had been overseas for four years and nine months. Looking back I realised how lucky I was to have survived the bombs at Gallabat and the shot and shell at Keren, not to speak of the malignant tertian parasites in Massawa; how lucky too I was to have enjoyed such a rich experience of surgery and the acquaintanceship of many fine men, most of whom had had to suffer far greater discomforts and dangers than a mere RAMC doctor. Only later did I fully appreciate how privileged I had been to graduate from that great university of life – the army in wartime.

Throughout the campaign in Sicily and Italy I had had a Geordie batman, Jack Love, a coalminer from Ashington, Northumberland. He was almost totally bald and was affectionately known as "Curly"; I cannot remember any of us, officers or other ranks, ever calling him anything else. Curly was a splendid man, immensely loyal and hard working, with a soft Northumbrian accent. He once hesitantly confessed that he had been a "bed wetter" well into adult life. I reassured him that this was nothing to be ashamed of and that it was far more common than many were prepared to admit. That information may be relevant to something I learnt about him 25 years on, to which I shall return later. Curly's opposite number in the neurosurgical unit was George Cook, a cockney who had been a night porter at the Hans Crescent Hotel, Knightsbridge. He kept us all in good humour, and often in fits of laughter, with his rich stream of cockney jargon and stories about the hotel. Of course both these batmen had far more important medical tasks in the trinity than merely looking after their officers. They were especially useful in nursing and during operations. Our unit's operating room attendant was Corporal Dakin. He was a regular soldier, as was our senior dental mechanic, Sergeant Wheatley. They had both given us first class service and I wrote a rousing citation for them, for which each was awarded the BEM. In this connection I should mention that nearly all the officers in the trinity ended up with the pink ribbon of the MBE. I became so concerned about this when the first award was made that I forbade Dick Battle to enter my name for "a pink ribbon." My reasons were simple: firstly, I was doing a most interesting job in my own profession; secondly, I was at less risk than many civilians in Britain; thirdly, many doctors had been in the forward areas for far longer than I and many had served under worse conditions than I had suffered even in Eritrea. It may be asked why I was so inconsistent in recommending awards for the two non-commissioned officers. A good question. Quite simply, I felt that these men were much more deserving than I. After the war, when I again met Tony Jackson (an ex-prisoner of war in Japan – after capture in Hong Kong) and Raymond Ramsay (a former Chindit who had been captured in Burma), both of whom had deservedly been awarded the MBE, I was relieved that I had avoided the same award for doing a satisfying job in relative comfort.

Before going on python I bade farewell to my unit and the rest of the trinity and set off to cross the Appenines in a truck, a journey of some 250 miles which took me through Arezzo, Orvieto, and Rome on my way to Naples. We were in the transit camp for two days and then boarded an ocean liner, a "dry" ship, as were all transports after the Americans came into the war, but one on which we were sumptuously fed as we sailed home to a strictly rationed Britain. But that "dry" ship was the undoing of one young officer who had been drunk for most of his time in the transit camp. We were at sea for little more than 24 hours when this officer developed delirium tremens. An escorting destroyer came alongside and our patient was lowered overboard, strapped in a Neill Robertson stretcher. Though we were aboard a 30 000 ton liner, she heeled over at quite an angle as all the troops gathered at the starboard side to watch the transfer. It was left to us to conjecture whether the patient would receive treatment ashore or whether he would merely be "resuscitated" with a few tots of gin from the wardroom or rum from the seamen's rations.

I have only one more story to relate about that voyage. We had about 3000 troops aboard, including many of those who had first gone abroad with me in January 1939. Among the officers was one whom I had met before. I found him in the lounge surrounded by an admiring group of nursing sisters, WRNS, and other lady officers, plus a few of his friends. He had been promoted to captain, and I was startled to see that he was wearing the ribbon of the Military Cross with two bars. He was telling his admiring audience some spicy stories of war in the desert and weekends in Alexandria. At one point he said, "By Jove, how well I remember when I caught my third dose of clap!" Though well used to his foul language on the French train, I was astonished to hear him talking like this to a mixed audience. But I was left with the sobering thought that he had done no more than precisely match up the number of bravery awards with his doses of clap. Although I had heard of the occasional purple heart being inadvertently pinned on the breast of a stretcher borne American VD casualty, I cannot believe that there has ever been an award of the Military Cross only for a brave encounter with the gonococcus!

11 Python and back to war

Early in November 1944 we disembarked at Liverpool and travelled to London by train. In my compartment there were two New Zealanders, recent prisoners of war in Italy now enjoying a first visit to Britain. They were delighted by the verdant countryside through which we passed. After nearly five years abroad even I had forgotten how green England could be. When I had been at home for two weeks I managed, through a little low cunning, to persuade the War Office to post me to Shenley military hospital with secondment to the Barts sector hospital at Hill End, St Albans. Although I was officially attached to Rainsford Mowlem's plastic unit, with his connivance I in fact attended the general surgical units for about six weeks. I knew that I would only be in England for three months and that it was essential for me to be better prepared to take on general surgery. Furthermore, I was anxious to sit the final FRCS examination as soon as I was properly prepared.

I lived in the mess at Shenley. One of my fellow officers there was Geoffrey Brooks, who had been regimental medical officer to the Notts Hussars with the 1st Cavalry Division. When this later became an armoured unit in the western desert he had been severely wounded in one arm and shoulder and had been awarded the MC. During his evacuation from around Tobruk, back to Cairo, he had developed infective parotitis first on one side and then on the other. The first infection had been left to take its course; but on the second occasion, at a New Zealand unit, the gland on the right side was promptly drained. He had no more trouble on that side but suffered profuse gustatory sweating on the left whenever he took hot soup or spicy foods. He returned to his family practice at East Bridgford, Nottinghamshire, after the war. The bothersome sweating continues to the present time, though rather less severely.

I used to bicycle from Shenley to Hill End every morning, returning there at night – a journey of four miles each way. I occasionally sped down Shenley Hill into Radlett; but I never suspected that I would later live there for more than 40 years. Each day at Hill End I tried to learn as much as I could from the various surgical firms, working mainly with John Hosford. But James Paterson Ross was kind in setting and then discussing a number of specimen examination questions with me. He was an excellent coach in the little spare time he had; and I used those same exercises when I began to teach fellowship candidates a year or two later. The Barts surgeons had minimal assistance in wartime and I remember how annoyed Ross was after a visit to James Learmonth's unit in Edinburgh. Ross and Learmonth were each in charge of a university surgical unit; but in contrast to Ross Learmonth had a complete staff with most of the amenities that one would expect under peacetime conditions. After the war both these men were to cooperate in the surgical care of King George VI when he developed arterial obstruction in one leg. At Hill End I also attended some of the other units to broaden my knowledge. I was especially glad to have gained experience in thoracic work for in north west Europe I was soon to deal with patients with chest and thoracoabdominal wounds.

After several weeks at Hill End I was posted to the Cambridge Hospital, Aldershot, as a general surgical specialist. A pleasant Australian, Keith Moore, who had been a prisoner of war in Italy until a few months before was also posted there. The officer in charge of our surgical division was Gordon Bryan from St Mary's Hospital. He was a sullen and uncommunicative man who sometimes snooped in the theatre when I was operating – perhaps to make sure that I had not picked up too many bad habits with the plastic surgeons. I watched him operating once or twice and was appalled to see him close a nephrectomy incision with half a dozen huge silkworm gut sutures passing through all layers. I had never seen anything quite so primitive as this. Our orthopaedic specialist was Lloyd Griffith from Manchester. He was one of the most voluble and entertaining people I have ever met and there was rarely a dull moment with him in the mess. During the month I was at the Cambridge Hospital there was an amusing incident each week when Colonel O'Riordan, a regular, did his official round of Griffith's ward. On arriving at the bed of a certain Cypriot – whose sole reason for being in hospital was that he was awaiting the supply of some special boots – Griffith would stand sharply to attention and say, "Colonel O'Riordan, sir, this is Private Nicolaides of the Cypriot Pioneer Corps now in his eighth (ninth, tenth, etc) week of waiting for the supply of special boots." I had left by the time those boots arrived and although Lloyd Griffith later told me the final weekly score I cannot now remember what it was.

One afternoon in the outpatient department at the Cambridge I encountered a near contemporary at Barts. He had been a year junior to me and was just a little "hard of hearing." He had passed his MD and MRCP examinations and worked as a wartime chief assistant. Now, recruited in late 1944, he was resplendent in the uniform of a lieutenant and told me that he had been visiting the medical specialist. I assumed he was to be a new graded physician. "Oh no," he said, "I have been to see the physician about my hay fever and he has certified me unfit for the Far East." I was flabbergasted and briskly rejoined, "Jimmy, you never had any serious trouble when I knew you." I continued to castigate him and ended, quite inadvertently, on my trump card: "If you've any guts at all you'll tear that certificate up and go to the Far East. Just think of all the wonderful experience of tropical diseases you will get." I did not meet him again until a year or two after the war. He then told me that he had torn the certificate up and gone to the Far East, where, as a physician, he thought that he had had the most marvellous experience. He said how grateful he was to me, but I sometimes wondered whether he deserved such good advice.

The Cambridge Hospital officers' mess enjoyed – or suffered, according to your taste – almost total silence at breakfast. The food was good and the catering was in the hands of the capable Miss Cuffy. She was the only non-military female allowed in that mess and I recall one day when Dr Edith Summerskill, the Labour MP, came to visit her husband, then a major. Edith breezed in at teatime and was briskly escorted from the dining room by Miss Cuffy. The officer in charge of our medical division was John Richardson of St Thomas's. Just after the war he had the misfortune to develop tuberculosis, which he had almost certainly picked up from the many displaced persons with phthisis he had attended after VE Day. During the war John struck up a close friendship with Harold Macmillan, to whom he acted as physician in North Africa (where Macmillan had been Minister of State). When my old chief, Alec Badenoch, did Macmillan's prostatectomy it was John who received the knighthood, and later a baronetcy and a peerage. It will be recalled that Macmillan, although he made a speedy and uneventful recovery to survive well into his nineties, resigned the premiership while still in hospital. Never once did he discuss this matter with Alec, and I doubt whether resignation was ever advised by John Richardson. During my last week at Aldershot, in January 1945, in the gathering dusk we watched huge numbers of Lancaster bombers amassing above us for the thousand bomber raids on Germany. After all we had been through in the previous five years it was a goodly but sobering sight. As I looked up I wondered whether death, when it came to them, was so different from that of our ground troops, especially our tank crews.

All too soon my three months was up and I had a new posting order. The German counteroffensive had been successfully held in December, and in February 1945 I was off to the continent. We landed at Ostend and I spent one night there in a staging camp where I shared a room with two St Thomas's men, both surgical specialists. Bernard Williams went to Portsmouth shortly after demobilisation and Guy Baines became a urologist at the Queen Elizabeth Hospital, Birmingham. Bernard had had considerable experience with a field surgical unit in the western desert. He was a pleasant companion and I remember a significant remark which he made to me after the war. We were seated at a dinner at the College of Surgeons when he said, "Reggie, we surgeons are very fortunate: firstly, we deal with people, and people are always interesting; secondly, we have an intellectually challenging job; thirdly, above all we use our hands, and that is something which many people itch to do." I have often thought that Bernard's sage aphorism was most apt.

After a day in the impressive city of Bruges I was moved back to 13 Field Surgical Unit, which was attached to 25 General Hospital at Amiens. Preparations were then being made for the Rhine crossing and my unit helped that hospital in the interim. An old Barts contemporary, Kenneth Burrow, was a graded surgeon at the hospital and Nigel Compston (trained at the Middlesex and later on the staff of the Royal Free) was a graded physician. The regimental sergeant major of the hospital was a tall, handsome, and well spoken man. On discovering that I was from Barts he inquired whether I knew his brother-in-law, Oliver Garrod. I told him that we had joined the Territorial Army together and that we were good friends and almost contemporaries. I did not then suspect that the regimental sergeant major and Oliver would both be my brothers-in-law less than two years later.

An especially amusing feature of 25 General Hospital was the temporary attachment of a section of an American field hospital. We understood this to comprise one quarter of the hospital and were intrigued to find that the American medical and kitchen equipment was roughly equivalent to that for an entire British hospital. The American section was commanded by Major Burkhardt from Tipton, Indiana, who practised surgery there. Of his fellow officers I can still name Chauncey M Stone Jr, Irwin Weiner, and Foley D Woods, but I forget the names of the others, which may be prudent as I must tell a story about one of them. He had a lady friend in Rouen, some 50 miles away, and he paid frequent nocturnal trips in an ambulance to visit her. She was the French wife of a French civilian husband, who, it appears, always welcomed the captain with open arms. If the captain were to be believed there was a temporary and happy *ménage à trois*. Nor were these nocturnal sexual activities confined to one officer: Kenneth Burrow informed me that there were more exciting goings on in our mess than I could ever have suspected. Major Burkhardt, who was not so involved, used to regard his younger officers with benign amusement.

One morning when I was seated with Burkhardt at breakfast one of the Americans arrived late. As he walked in the others chanted, "Hello, Foley, where's your hat?" There followed much ribald laughter, which mystified me. Burkhardt promised to tell me later. It transpired that our own hospital stretcher bearer officer shared a flat with the American. The Briton returned late from a party and found the door locked. He remembered that there was a high window at the back. So, in bright moonlight, he shinned up the wall. On peeking through the window he saw his American flatmate, *in flagrante delicto* with a young French lady, and still wearing his hat!

Shortly after this, on 23 March, a stream of planes and gliders flew over us as the Rhine crossing started. Within a few days my field surgical unit moved forward through Belgium and southern Holland, crossing the Meuse at Venlo and the Rhine at Xanten, and worked with a clearing station at Munster. I have no detailed record of this period; but, with Captain Pye-Smith as anaesthetist, 13 Field Surgical Unit had to deal with many serious casualties. On moving to Celle, I was ordered to take over 53 Field Surgical Unit at Uchte. That unit was then under the command of Henry Thompson, who was several years my senior and an experienced surgeon who had trained at the London Hospital. He was a superb surgeon who later got on the staff of St Mark's Hospital and became a firm friend of mine. When I first met this charming, reticent, grey haired man I felt overawed. Moreover, I wondered what his men would think of his youthful replacement. But Henry was being posted to the Far East and all went well as the unit promptly moved to 33 Casualty Clearing Station at Luneburg. The war in Europe was nearly over, but we were kept busy throughout those last few weeks. Our anaesthetist was Captain Edward Goldsmith, and my operation record from 53 Field Surgical Unit shows that we dealt with numerous severe

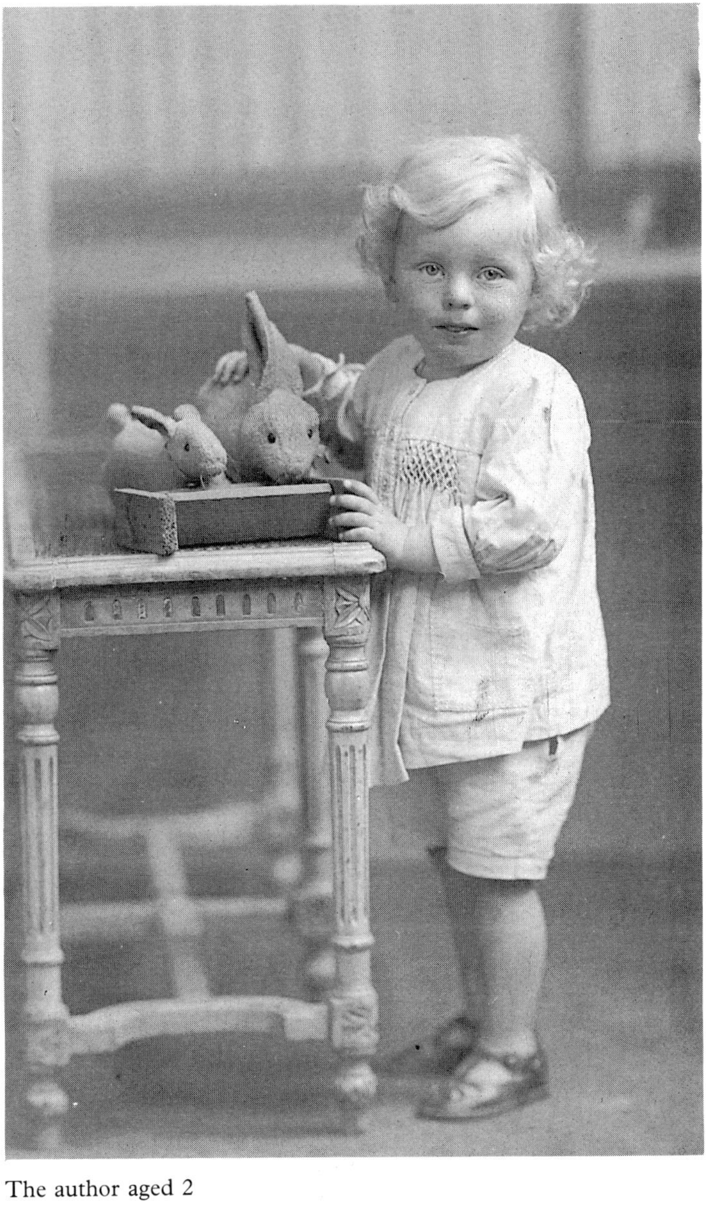
The author aged 2

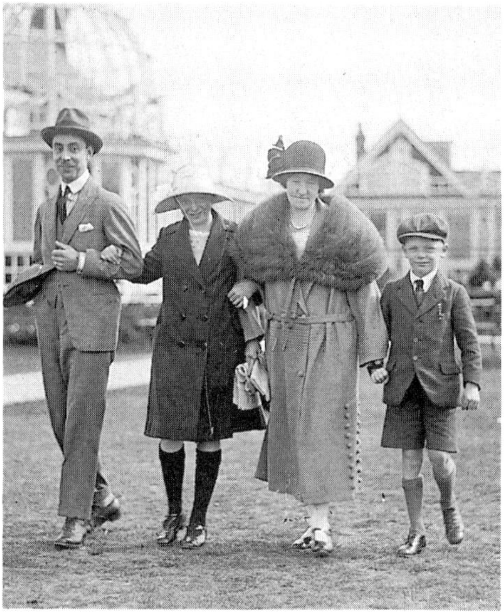

The author (*right*) at Cliftonville with his parents and sister, 1924

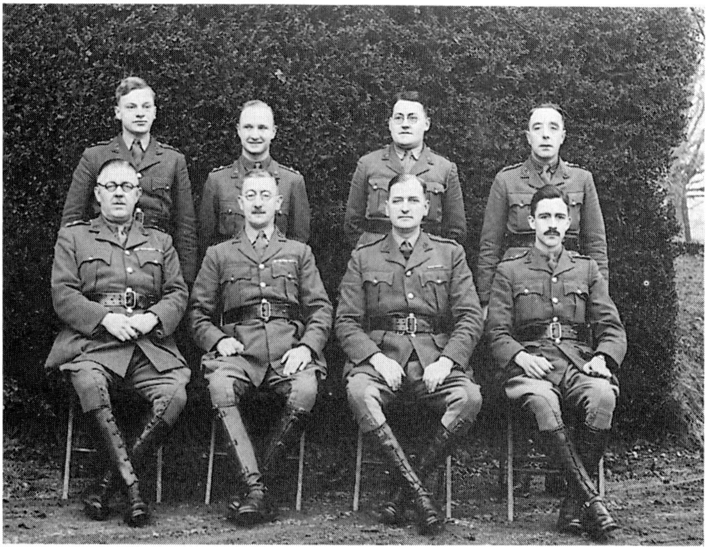

Officers of the 168 City of London Cavalry Field Ambulance, November 1939. *Top left :* the author

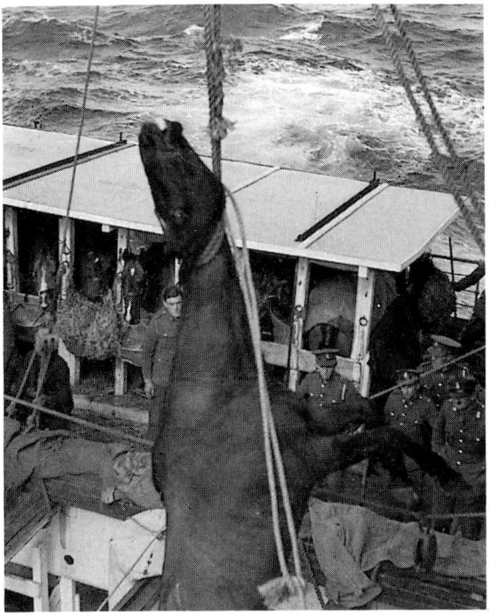

Dead horse being hauled overboard in the Mediterranean, January 1940

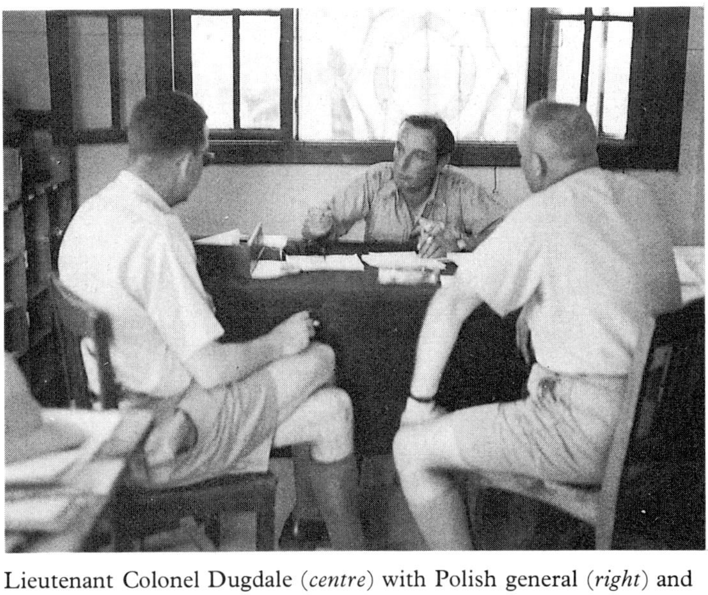

Lieutenant Colonel Dugdale (*centre*) with Polish general (*right*) and interpreter (*left*) at Samakh, Palestine, June 1940

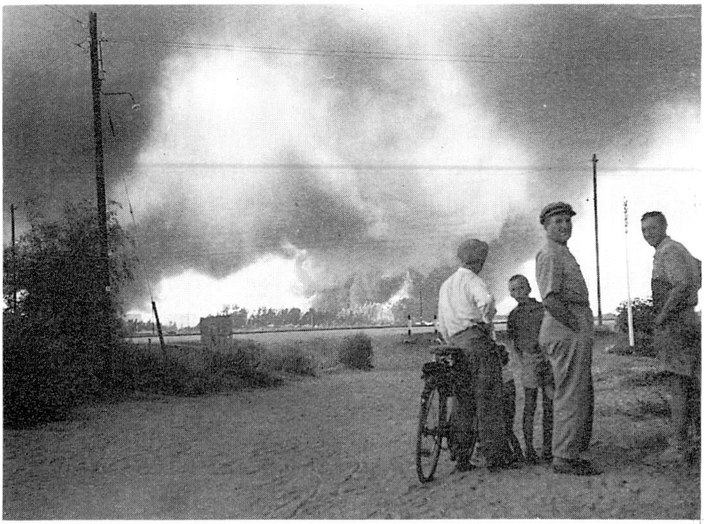

Burning oil refinery at Haifa after first Italian bombing raid, 11 June 1940

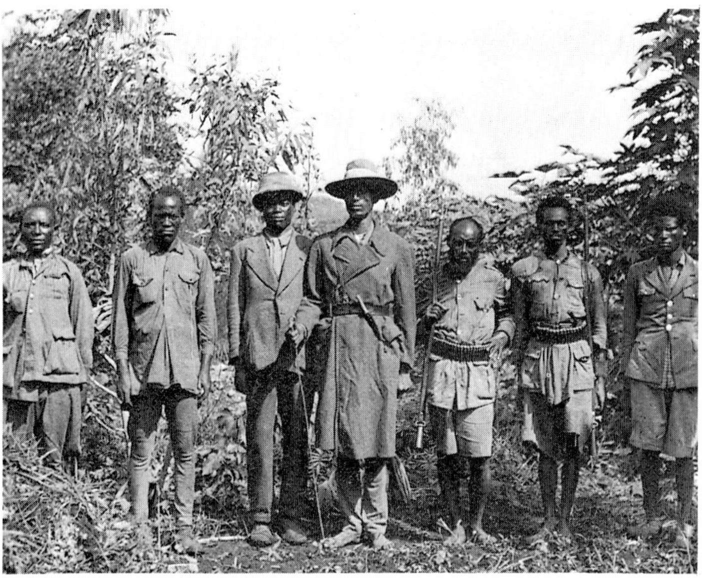

Abyssinian patriot troops, 1941

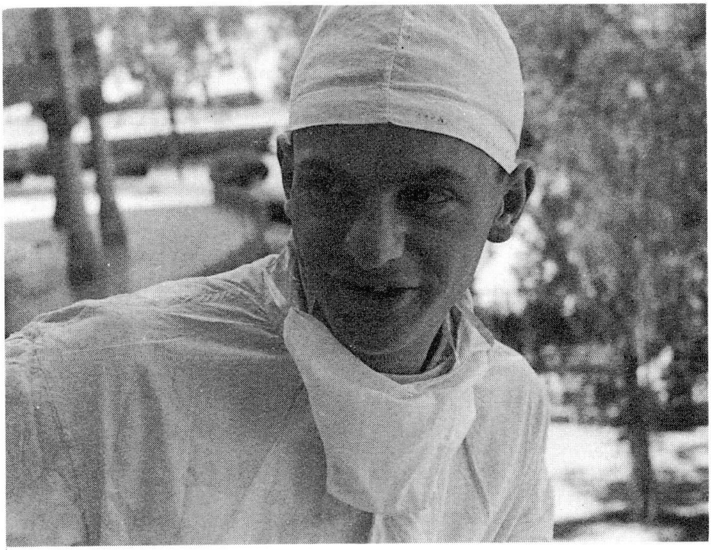

With maxillofacial unit in Cairo, 1943

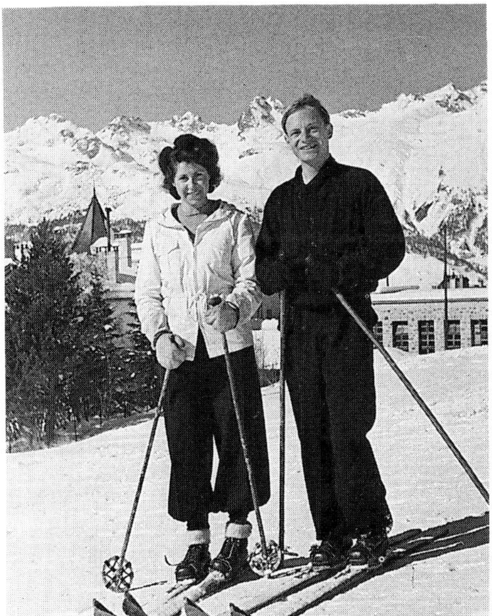

Skiing with Daphne
at Pontresina,
February 1947

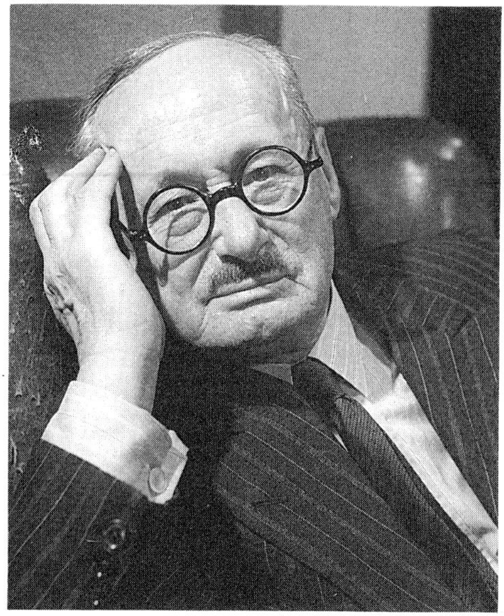

Lord Horder, 1953

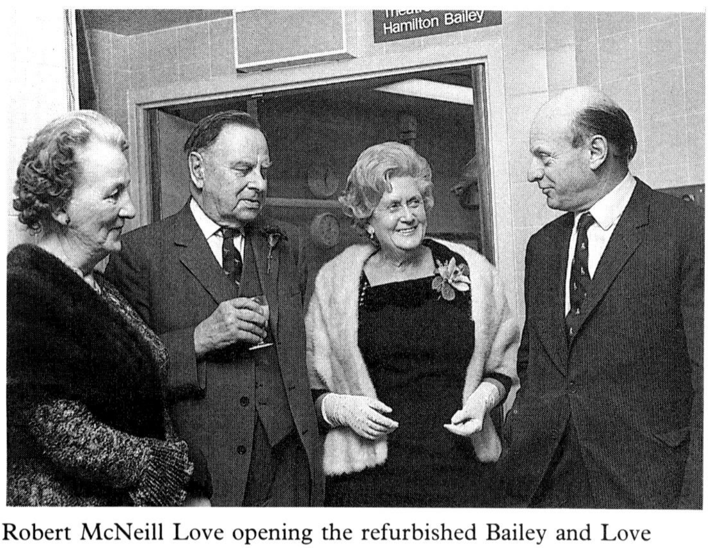

Robert McNeill Love opening the refurbished Bailey and Love theatres at the Royal Northern Hospital, September 1971. *Left to right:* Rhoda and Robert McNeill Love, Vita Hamilton Bailey, the author

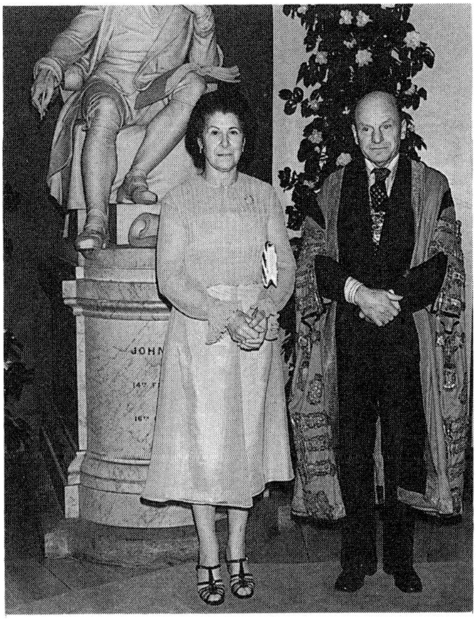

With Daphne at reception at the Royal College of Surgeons to celebrate the 250th Hunterian anniversary, 14 February 1978

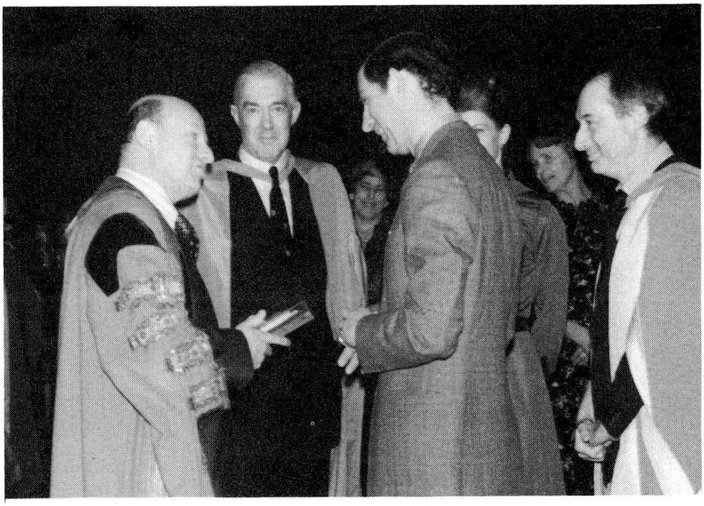

Presenting to the Prince of Wales, on the 250th Hunterian anniversary, a memento for Her Majesty the Queen. *Left to right:* the author, Professor McMinn, HRH the Prince of Wales, Professor Turk

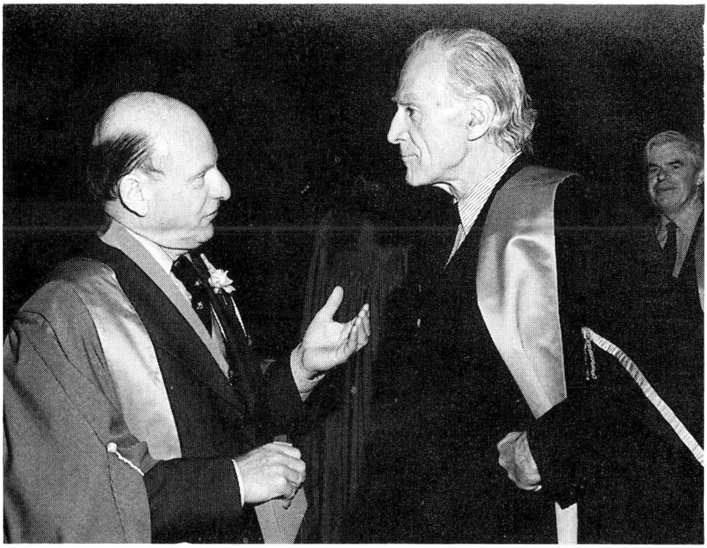

With Professor Kinmouth at the Royal College of Surgeons, June 1981

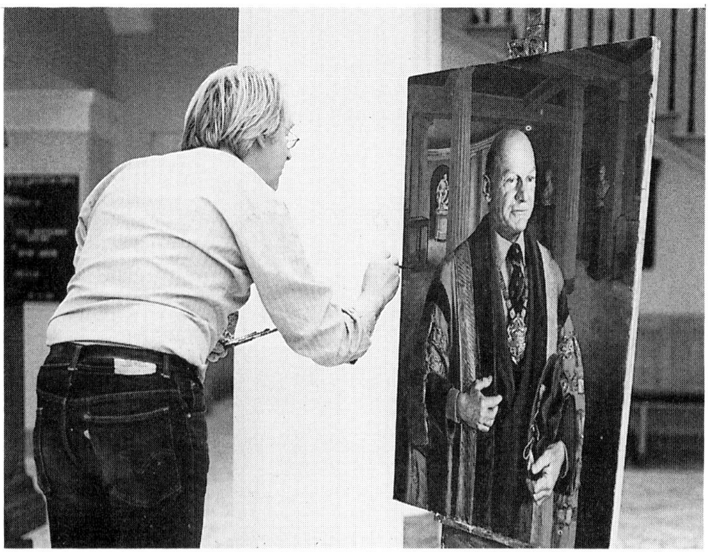

John Walton completing the presidential portrait, 1983

abdominal and thoracic wounds. These patients usually did well and we later regularly received information through the excellent follow up postcard system then in use. By sending one of these self addressed cards with the medical record at the time of evacuation it was possible to ensure that base hospitals overseas or in the United Kingdom would send the necessary follow up information. One could not but be impressed by the efficiency of the army postal system, which had to contend with far greater difficulties than the GPO in peacetime. After all, most of the addressees were frequently on the move and often changing units.

On VE Day, 8 May 1945, my unit was still with 33 Casualty Clearing Station in the SS barracks at Luneburg. Before lunch we had a modest celebration with sparkling German wine ("pink Champagne") taken over from the SS officers. My only operation was the repair of a partly burst abdomen in a soldier whose thoracoabdominal wound I had dealt with some days earlier. All that, and certain other events, have been recorded in "Exciting Times," my contribution to the BMA publication *As You Were*, which appeared in 1984 as a medical retrospect on VE Day and included some 42 contributions. It will bear repetition from "Exciting Times" that I had a disturbing and horrifying visit to Belsen concentration camp on 12 May, just after its liberation.

We moved with 33 Casualty Clearing Station to Schleswig on 18 May and spent nearly a month in that pleasant town. There was not much work for us and we had three surgical teams, so we took turns on duty for the emergencies. The corps commander had the army take over the local yacht club and craft were allocated to various units in the area. Those of us who were off duty had the use of a yacht allocated to the clearing station and there was some good sailing on a stretch of the River Schlei, which opened into the Baltic. With two days off duty I had one enjoyable trip with John Leslie, later a surgeon at Leicester, and his anaesthetist, Greenhalgh. After one long day's sail we moored for the night by a field. The cabin on the craft slept only two so John pitched a tent alongside the craft and Greenhalgh and I stayed aboard. Just in case of any problems in the night we each had our revolvers handy. After a hot meal and a bottle of wine we settled down for the night. Some time later, in the early hours, we were awoken by a succession of revolver shots. We ran out on deck to hear John shouting, "Bloody cow, stuck its head into the tent!" Fortunately the cow was not hit, but the tent was a trifle damaged.

Soon after we returned to the clearing station at Schleswig late in the following afternoon there was great excitement when we heard that Himmler and William Joyce had been spotted in a nearby wood and that when challenged by some British troops Joyce had tried to escape but was then "winged" with a shot in the buttocks. Himmler was taken into custody and bit his cyanide capsule shortly afterwards, but Joyce was admitted to the clearing station when Buckley Hamer, a Lancastrian surgeon, was on duty. John Leslie and I went to the admissions room to see Joyce lying comfortably on a stretcher. Leslie mentioned to Joyce that one of his cousins had known him before the war. The response in that unmistakable "Garmany calling" voice was, "Oh, such a nice girl!" to which John brusquely retorted, "Well, Joyce, I hope they hang you!" The corps commander had sent Buckley a message: "Be sure to preserve this man so that he can be tried for treason." There must have been about 20 people in the theatre when Joyce was brought in under Bill Scriven's anaesthetic. There was a superficial perforating wound through one buttock with a bullet lodged in the other "cheek." The "Haw-Haw" buttocks and the bullet were duly photographed; but, alas, I have since lost my print of the traitor's arse. He was evacuated from the clearing station and was duly hanged on 3 January 1946.

I did my last operation at Schleswig on 13 June. Towards the end of the month 53 Field Surgical Unit was moved to München Gladbach under the control of the deputy director of medical services in Hamburg. Goldsmith and I were given the task of visiting the many German hospitals and *Lazarette* in the area, partly to ascertain their precise condition and partly to assess what could be done with the many thousands of patients, including both military and displaced persons. I find that I still have a copy of my report, dated 21 July 1945, and entitled "A medical appreciation of the situation in the German hospitals and PW cages of the 53 (W) divisional area." The conditions in some of these hospitals were appalling with two tier, and sometimes three tier, bunks where pus could occasionally be seen dripping through the mattresses on to those at the lower levels.

I was for a short time in Hamburg where I was accommodated in the fine Vierjahreszeiten Hotel by Lake Alster. It was one of the few intact buildings adjacent to that lake, on the far side of which there was an endless line of devastation all the way to the docks. A waiter in the hotel told me that during one of the great air raids on Hamburg the whole of the town on the far side of the lake was on fire and hundreds of people rushed off the streets and into the lake to escape the conflagration. Of the thousands that perished, in addition to those who were killed by high explosives many were burnt to death or drowned. I confess that after all the horror and suffering which the Nazis had inflicted on millions of others I did not feel any sympathy for the Germans. But with the object of easing the situation Count Folke Bernadotte, the head of the Swedish Red Cross, and some of his colleagues were also staying at the Vierjahreszeiten Hotel.

With the end of the war in Europe many of those whose demobilisation would not be due for some time were sent to the Far East. But with five and a half years' service I was not to be one of them. Many long serving RAMC officers, however, became frustrated because they felt that their demobilisation was being needlessly delayed, as will emerge shortly. In the course of my report on the military hospitals I seized the opportunity of visiting a large German plastic surgical unit in Hamburg in the hope of tracing my old patient, Feldwebel Beick. I found a friendly and charming elderly surgeon in charge and I explained to him that Beick was an orphan who had lived with an aunt in Hamburg. When I mentioned the name and described the details of his wound the German surgeon's face lit up. "Oh yes," he said, "I remember him well. He was evacuated here from Cairo and I completed his reconstruction work." I told the German that Oldfield had been reluctant to repatriate him and inquired whether he had gone back into the army. "No, he did not rejoin the army," said the surgeon, "but he became leader of the Hitler youth here in Hamburg."

During my time in Hamburg and München Gladbach I was able to visit many places in the predominantly industrial area of Duisburg, Dusseldorf, Essen, and Wuppertal where the bomb damage exceeded anything I had seen in Britain. The remarkable speed and efficiency with which many of these areas were later cleared and rebuilt speaks volumes for the energy and determination of our former enemies. At the same time, had Hitler won the war I doubt that we would have had either the opportunity or the enterprise to rebuild our own towns so quickly. Fortunately we were spared that eventuality, but one can only deplore the slowness with which we tackled the problems of postwar reconstruction in a predominantly socialist society under both Labour and Tory administrations.

Throughout most of the war my father had been working with the Hudson's Bay Company in New York. He had been invited there early in 1940 when fur trading in London had practically ceased. My mother and sister, being reluctant to go to the United States, had remained in England. Not long after VE Day my father visited London on business and I arranged for a short leave at home. I know that it was early in June because the general election was pending. I recall hiring a car and driving my parents to Brighton for Sunday lunch at the Royal Albion Hotel. On our way through Streatham and Mitcham my father was astonished to see all the Labour election posters in what had been a predominantly Tory area before the war. I told him I felt sure that Labour would be elected because there was not a single man in my unit (myself excepted) who intended to vote in any other way. From my regular reading of the service "educational" papers I was in little doubt that they had a powerful doctrinal effect on many people's already confused political judgment. Baldwin and Chamberlain were blamed for many things for which they were not directly responsible, and most people had conveniently forgotten that Labour had consistently voted against rearmament, thereby strongly contributing to our unpreparedness and the inevitable encouragement of Adolf Hitler. The outcome in no way surprised me.

Shortly after my return to the British Army of the Rhine it became known that there would be a series of meetings for doctors on the subject of the postwar civilian medical services. During the war there had from time to time been correspondence in the medical journals on the possibility of nationalised medicine, but few of us abroad had had much opportunity to consider the implications. There were 10 of these meetings under War Office sponsorship and the visiting group included Lord Moran and Dr Harold Boldero from the Royal College of Physicians, an army brigadier, and various officials from the Ministry of Health in Savile Row. It came to be known as "Lord Moran's Circus" or, more irreverently, as "Corkscrew Charlie's Circus." I happened to attend the last of these meetings in Hamburg. It was said to have been one of the largest. Moran did most of the talking from the platform and was anxious to tell us how much the government would be doing for us after the war. He went on to say that those of us who had been away for "two or three years" would be anxious to get updated. As most of the audience had then been in the services for five or six years many were irked by this remark. His lordship was brought to order by a colonel seated just in front of me. We were told of the creation of government paid postwar specialist registrarships, but this was not generally well received. I thought I discerned considerable scepticism in the audience. At the end of the meeting I ran into Arthur Porritt, then our army consultant surgeon in BAOR. I commented that a number of the platform party seemed ill informed on our real problems. Arthur chuckled and agreed, but he went on to say that having attended the first and a few of the other meetings he was fascinated to see the way in which Moran had taken over more and more of the proceedings.

It was in the course of my hospital and other visits that I became aware of the large number of doctors with little or nothing to do in Germany. There had been critical leaders and letters in the medical press, and questions were asked in the Commons, as a result of which the then Minister for War, Sir

James Grigg, had made a statement to the House. In that statement the Minister gave some figures purporting to show that the proportion of doctors to patients in the area of the British Army of the Rhine was similar to that in the United Kingdom. His statement, reported in the *Lancet*, was so manifestly incorrect that I wrote a carefully composed letter to that journal in which I suggested that Sir James's figures must have included all the displaced persons in West Germany, most of whom were not the direct responsibility of service doctors. To show the genuineness of my concern I sent a copy direct to Sir James; both letters were despatched on 16 July. In a letter dated 20 July Dr Theodore Fox, then editor of the *Lancet*, replied that he would be publishing my letter but that as I was a serving officer he had taken the liberty of arranging for it to appear anonymously over the nom de plume "Major, BAOR." I promptly sent him a cheerful reply saying that he was not to worry for a copy had been sent direct to Sir James.

My letter duly appeared in the *Lancet* in July; but, as I already had a posting to 67 General Hospital and was awaiting the necessary movement order, I had put "67 GH" on my letter to the minister. Before I arrived at that hospital, situated at Rendsburg on the Kiel canal (a place I had once visited in my schooldays), the director general of medical services, Sir Alexander Hood, on a visit to Germany, had gone hotfoot there in search of me. On arrival he asked Colonel Bourne if he could interview Major Murley, the surgeon. The colonel replied that there was no such officer on his staff; and how the plot then thickened. I arrived at the hospital in mid-August, a week or so later, and while I was doing a ward round on my second morning one of the office staff sergeants came to ask me to report to the commanding officer "with my hat." Now, I was well known in the service for frequently being hatless and I had brought none with me from the mess. Thereupon I borrowed the staff sergeant's hat and went to the colonel's office. As I entered and saluted him he said, "Murley, I think this may mean a court martial." I cheerfully responded, "Oh, sir, do you think that will get me home more quickly?" "Don't be facetious," said Colonel Bourne. He then asked me why I had not sent my letter through the usual channels. I replied that I had. So he asked, "Who was your commanding officer?" I said, "I was, sir." Bourne snorted and said, "But a field surgical unit is not an independent command." I responded innocently, "Oh, isn't it, sir?" He then inquired, "How long have you been in the army, Murley?" I replied, "Six years, sir, and a damned sight too long." The commanding officer seemed astounded: "What, six years, and you didn't know that?" I firmly pointed out that my unit had been working quite independently without any official attachment. Bourne, a regular soldier, immediately became most friendly and helpful, saying, "Well, I think that should be your best defence." He promptly settled down to help me compose a suitable letter of apology to the director of medical services for having bypassed "the usual channels." I am happy to say this was accepted, but the brigadier himself came to give me a further ticking off – just as had happened in Palestine in 1940.

A little before my arrival at Rendsburg I had started a correspondence course for the final FRCS. It was a good way of stimulating my reading and it gave useful practice in writing answers to papers. I was sadly lacking, however, in normal peacetime experience and felt that this might be a serious handicap. I had time to swot at Rendsburg and I was given study leave for the examination in November, when I flew to Northolt with some sick and injured. But a too friendly New Zealander, rather than the examiners, was an important part of my undoing in that examination. While awaiting the morning paper I met the splendid Rowan Nicks, last seen in Augusta, Sicily, resplendent in the uniform of a surgeon lieutenant commander. At lunchtime he took me to London House, where he had once lived when taking the primary FRCS before the war. We had a good lunch but the two or three pints of beer proved too much for me: I felt rather dopey and unfortunately went to sleep during the afternoon paper. It is difficult to say how long I was "out," but it was somewhere in the region of half an hour. As with the migraine in my first MB, I thought of but once again resisted the temptation to plead a migraine attack. I failed the examination, but I doubt whether my coma during the second paper was the full explanation. In truth I was a trifle puzzled by some of the clinical cases. Rowan Nicks, coming of tougher Kiwi stock, sailed through but remained repentant about me. When I first put up for council of the Royal College of Surgeons in 1968 he wrote saying that he had firmly cast his vote for me, concluding his letter with "I owe this to you, Reg, after all the trouble I caused you in 1945."

After the examination I returned to Rendsburg for a short time. I had enjoyed my four months there with Bill Sillar of Edinburgh and Pat Hardie, a near contemporary of mine at Barts, as graded surgical colleagues. Another more senior Barts man, Hall Drake, was in command of our surgical division. There had been enough to keep us busy and, just after the fellowship, I collected a much neglected French casualty from a small German Hospital. Major Emile Comparot had suffered severe injuries in a road accident and had been somewhat neglected. He had sustained severe "car bumper" open fractures below his right knee, with an extensive soft tissue wound of the right thigh. He also had an open fracture of the left femur and a bad scalp laceration. By the time I found him in the German hospital his right leg was gangrenous and I did a through knee amputation to preserve maximum length. He was embarrassingly grateful, and when I was on holiday in Brittany in August 1948 he insisted on coming to stay at my hotel so that he could express his gratitude. He later emigrated to Mexico to run an estate belonging to one of his aunts.

After six years and four months in the army I did my last operation on 13 December and returned to England the following day. Coming ashore – I think it was at Folkestone – there were troops wheeling prams full of personal belongings and loot, but the customs took no more than a perfunctory look at them. I was demobilised at Regent's Park barracks, in Albert Street, where I collected shoes, socks, underwear, a suit, a soft trilby hat, and a raincoat. I do not remember any medical examination but I am sure that I filled in a form with details of all the diseases I had acquired on His Majesty's service. I had already asked Barts medical college about the possibility of an anatomy demonstratorship and I learnt that one would be available. The preclinical medical school of

Barts had been at Cambridge since the beginning of the war, and it was there I would be going early in the New Year. I had also been in touch with Professor Paterson Ross, who had indicated a readiness to take me into his unit in due course. But more of that later.

12 A don at Cambridge and Charterhouse

Following my demobilisation I spent Christmas at home and then made a brief visit to Cambridge so that I could confirm the arrangements for my appointment and fix up some accommodation. I had been given the name of a Mrs Goodchild, the mother of a Barts nurse. Mrs Goodchild was said to be living in the vicarage of All Saints in Jesus Lane, where, allegedly, there was no present incumbent. After calling at the anatomy school I went to Jesus Lane and knocked on the vicarage door. To my surprise it was opened by a soberly clad, dark haired young man with a dog collar. I explained that I was a doctor from Barts and that I had been told to call on Mrs Goodchild. In a quiet ecclesiastical voice the gentleman introduced himself as Hereward Hard and added, "Oh, I'm afraid that Mrs Goodchild vacated the vicarage quite recently." I apologised for troubling him and was about to leave when he invited me in to tea. It was a large house and there in the lounge was a little old man, also dog collared. I was introduced to Hereward's widowed father and we settled down to an excellent fireside tea provided by their housekeeper. While I was eating dainty cucumber sandwiches and sipping tea in my best vicarage manner, I discerned that I was getting the cautious once over from this brace of vicars. After a short time Hereward said, "Father, do you not think that we might offer Mr Murley a room?" His father responded, "Yes, certainly, we have that spare room at the back," and Hereward added, "And, of course, he could have the downstair room as a study." I said that I had no wish to be a nuisance, but they assured me that this would be no trouble as they already had three other lodgers in their large house. When I asked what they would like me to pay they at first refused to accept any rent. I protested and they eventually agreed to full board at £2 (or was it £2. 10s?) a week. They then took me to look at two quite adequate rooms. I moved in a day or two later. I rarely met one of the others lodgers, an elderly anatomist whose nocturnal coughing occasionally disturbed the house. But Richard de Grey and his wife usually joined us at breakfast and dinner. Richard had been a prisoner of war in Changi gaol, where he taught history in the lively "university" which was set up there. Apart from our mealtimes, and an occasional walk along the river Cam towpath, I rarely saw Richard as we both had plenty to keep us busy.

The Barts students had been resident in Queens' College during the war and our anatomy school was accommodated in Professor Henry Harris's department; our students, however, were confined within a roped off area of the dissecting room. I learnt that Harris had accepted them rather reluctantly. My fellow demonstrator, Tom McKane, had been a year or so senior to me and he too had been in the RAMC throughout the war. He and his wife, a former Barts nurse, rented a house in the town; they had two little girls at that time. Although there was a Barts reader in anatomy the chair was vacant because Professor Hamilton had recently accepted the regius chair at Glasgow. In the meantime, for reasons best known to the Barts dean, Michael Boyd, recently demobilised and now deputy director of Ross's surgical professorial unit at Barts, was acting as part time director of our anatomy department. He spent half the week at Cambridge living in the Temperance Hotel (a source of some amusement to many of his old friends) and the other half in London. This was especially helpful for me since he gave me surgical coaching at the vicarage on two evenings a week. He had been first assistant on the professorial unit before the war and then had been in command of a surgical division in the RAMC, part of the time at Helmiah when I was with Oldfield at Heliopolis.

Cambridge to me was sheer magic. As a London "red brick" undergraduate I had had no idea of the pleasures of collegiate life at one of the older universities. Moreover, the move from the army to the teaching of anatomy was a welcome change. It had always been my intention to return to a demonstratorship after the war and I had made a point of keeping my anatomy up to date. In this I had been greatly aided by always keeping handy a copy of *A Synopsis of Regional Anatomy* by T B Johnston; it was a splendid little book.

A week or two after starting the anatomy appointment I met a former orderly room clerk from 19 Casualty Clearing Station in Italy. Albert was a well spoken and intelligent young man who had always seemed out of place as a private. I was pleased to learn of his belated admission to the university to read for an Arts degree. Albert had not been at all popular with the regimental sergeant major of that casualty clearing station and we recalled with some amusement the occasion in Italy when he had a frightful ticking off for not wearing his service "ribbon." Like many of us, Albert just had not bothered to sew the ribbon on his uniform. The following day, at the morning parade, Albert wore two ribbons: the Africa star with Second Army clasp and the coronation ribbon. The sergeant major moved along the assembled company and when he sighted Albert's chest his eyes almost popped out of his head. "Why are you again improperly dressed?" he asked. "I *am* properly dressed and you *did* tell me to wear my service ribbon, sir." "*I* told you to put up your Africa star: what the hell are you doing with a coronation ribbon?" Albert responded sweetly, "Well you see, sir, I *was* in Westminster school choir for the coronation." Collapse of sergeant major!

With Michael Boyd's coaching I passed the final fellowship in May at my second attempt and continued the anatomy job until the end of the summer term. Much to the relief of Queens' College and Professor Harris, the Barts students then returned to Charterhouse Square in London. The premises of the Merchant Taylor's school had been acquired when the school moved out to Sandy Lodge. Girling Ball, our dean, himself an old Merchant Taylor, had managed to buy those splendid premises for £120 000, just when I became a clinical student. I had never worked in the new departments, but because I realised that many of those returning from the forces would need intensive tuition I decided to set up a course for the primary FRCS. I did this in collaboration with George Cunningham, later professor of pathology at the Royal College of Surgeons; Reggie Shooter, who succeeded Paul Garrod as professor of bacteriology at Barts; and John d'Silva, who shortly took the chair of physiology at the London Hospital before moving to King's. Each of us had responsibility for the new style primary; in my day the only subjects were anatomy and physiology. When the dean, Dr Charles Harris, heard of our course he was contemptuous of it. He wondered what the hell we were doing trying to run a course for postgraduates in an undergraduate teaching hospital.

We had 16 ex-service doctors on the course; according to Reggie Shooter they all got through. But that is not strictly true: one of them failed – but he passed the examination the next time he sat for it. In that class we had John Loewenthal, a future president of the Royal Australasian College of Surgeons; my Barts "twin," Douglas Nicoll, who, like me, had been born on 2 August 1916; and Raymond Ramsay, just two weeks younger than I, who was shortly to be my best man. Before and during this two month course I had been thinking seriously about my professional and personal future. In regard to the first of these, Michael Boyd had told me in Cambridge that I would be returning to the professorial unit as first assistant. I said I could not believe this as I did not think I had enough experience for the post. Following my spell with John Hosford at Hill End a year earlier, I had decided that it would be far better if I were to train with him. Originally I had been attracted to the idea of academic surgery, but I was beginning to have doubts.

Shortly before the course began a surgical chief assistant post was advertised, but, as was then the confusing habit at Barts, the specific unit was not indicated. Somebody said it was John Hosford's post, so I thought it important to clarify matters with Paterson Ross. I called on him and mentioned Michael's firm contention, which of course I had not believed, that I was to be first assistant. Ross seemed taken aback and said that Cedric Longland, two years my senior, would be taking that post as soon as he was demobilised. Thereupon I asked if he would mind if I put in for Hosford's chief assistantship. He surprised me by saying that the one advertised was for John O'Connell's neurosurgical firm; but he told me to talk to Hosford. I did this and Hosford confirmed the nature of the advertisement and then added, "If mine were advertised would you be interested?" I said, "Most certainly," and he replied, "Well, in that case I shall have this done; but I am not promising you the job." I afterwards talked to John O'Connell, who urged me to get the Hosford job, saying, "Reggie, you really cannot do better than that." The Hosford advertisement soon appeared and I was delighted to be able to start that appointment on 1 October 1946. Incidentally, my old friend and contemporary John Gillingham took the neurosurgical job. He was later appointed to a consultant post in Edinburgh and then succeeded Norman Dott in the chair of neurosurgery. He was ultimately elected president of the Edinburgh college of surgeons some six months after I became president of the Royal College of Surgeons of England.

There had also been vital developments in my personal life. In the Easter vacation from Cambridge I had been coaching Oliver Garrod and Robert Macpherson in surgery and anatomy for the London BS; both had failed this part of their final examination at the beginning of the war. This time they were each successful. Garrod had been a student contemporary and his younger brother Tony had been at Dulwich with me. I had met three of their four sisters before the war, but not Daphne. As a reward for my unpaid coaching Oliver gave me Bunnell's *Surgery of the Hand*, which I was keen to have. On a beautiful spring day he and his wife, Barbara, took me to Kew Gardens. When we returned to Hampstead Oliver invited me to tea at his father's house in Church Row. As we entered the hall his widowed sister, Daphne, was coming down the stairs with Susan, a pretty dark haired four year old girl. There were other children in the house because Oliver's youngest sister, Hilary, had just had another baby at St Mary's. She was married to the St Mary's physiologist Alistair Frazer (the officer who had disposed of all those purloined road signs at the Shorncliffe Officers' Training Corps camp many years before). After tea Alistair, Oliver, and I went to a local pub, where we were later joined by Daphne. Good stockings were hard to find in those days: I noticed that one of Daphne's was laddered and repaired and made a mental note to get my father to send some from the States. Just after that I passed the final FRCS and returned to Cambridge for the summer term. One afternoon Richard de Grey and I had been for a walk; as we returned to the vicarage we saw an unfamiliar elderly woman in the front room, inspecting the curtains with Hereward. Richard said, "Are you thinking what I am, Reggie?" I said, "Yes, he must be going to get married; that's his future mother-in-law."

That same evening Hereward rather shyly told us that we would not be able to stay after October as he was just getting engaged. I assured him that all would be well as I was due to return to London with the Barts students. I had spent the whole war determined not to get involved with any woman; but spring was in the air and even young Hereward was preparing to take the fateful step. Daphne was on holiday in Switzerland with her cousin Peter and his wife, and in any case I was determined to think over very thoroughly the notion which had been gradually maturing in my mind since that day at Kew. I had often, to put it vulgarly, told my friends to marry with their brains and not their balls. I was firmly of the opinion that marriage could only have some prospect of success if it resulted from careful thought and preparation. Moreover, there is the old adage about looking at your prospective mother-in-law. That I had done in 1938; but, sadly, Rowena Garrod had died of a meningioma in 1941. But I had known the whole family, with the exception of Daphne. There were two sticking points: first what sort of a stepfather would I make and, much more importantly, would the lady ever accept? After one visit to the theatre with her followed by dinner at the Cafe de Paris I let these thoughts gently simmer in my mind.

By the time the primary FRCS course was completed a new professor of anatomy had been appointed. This was Alexander Cave, a Yorkshireman who came from the Leeds chair and later went on to the Royal College of Surgeons in succession to Wood Jones. We had just heard of the success of our postgraduates when Cave appeared at Charterhouse. I took an immediate liking to him and especially his opening remarks: "Now, Murley, just come and have a cup of coffee and tell me all about these Barts booggers." I was sorry not to have one term with him but we were both due to start our new jobs in the autumn. And I was near to popping the question.

13 Return to Barts and a bride

On 1 October 1946 I moved from the anatomy department to "Barts in Herts" as we called the Hill End sector hospital. Although it was a vast mental hospital occupying a series of two storey buildings, interlinked by long corridors and without any lifts, it was a splendid place in which to work. There were two large general medical and general surgical units and a full range of specialist surgical services – orthopaedic, plastic and maxillofacial, neurosurgery, gynaecology, as well as eye and ear, nose and throat units. The Barts wartime paediatric beds were in the adjacent Cell Barnes Hospital, so there was rich experience for trainee specialists as well as medical students. I took a room in the residents' quarters and was living "over the shop" for the next four months. My original surgical chiefs were John Hosford and Harold Rodgers; the latter had recently returned from the RAMC where he had been in command of a surgical division. John had lived at nearby Bendish during the war and very soon he and his family were sorry to have to return to 58 Harley Street, which had been rented as an American officers' club during the war. Harold lived in St Albans and both he and John were visiting consultants to the Mid Herts Hospital, then a small voluntary hospital of 120 beds. Close to that voluntary hospital was the Herts County Council Osterhills Hospital, a former Poor Law institution of some 220 beds, to which the Elizabeth Garrett Anderson Hospital had been evacuated during the war.

Although I had had considerable operative experience in a wide field during the war I thought it vital that I should assist and work with a master surgeon for two or three years. John Hosford was a superb and gentle operator, onetime deputy director of the Barts surgical professorial unit and Lord

Moynihan's last private assistant in his London practice. Indeed I have only recently recorded John's recollections of assisting Lord Moynihan in London nearly 60 years ago. John had extensive hospital connections at Hitchin, Watford, and Dorking and a deservedly most successful private practice, largely centred on the London Clinic but also at King Edward VII Hospital for Officers. Harold Rodgers worked at Mount Vernon Hospital, Northwood, too.

As I was off duty every other weekend and on alternate weekdays I had some opportunity to further my other absorbing interest. Ralph Garrod had sold his beautiful Queen Anne house in Church Row and moved with Daphne and her daughter, Susan, to a flat in Well Walk. After Rowena's death he had married Helen Payne, a former Barts nurse, whose farming family had been friends of the Garrods for many years. Helen, alas, like many nurses of that generation, had developed pulmonary tuberculosis and was being treated in a sanatorium at Davos. There was a good train service from St Albans to Hampstead and I began to visit Well Walk whenever I was off duty. I had to court both a widow and her child, but this did not prove as difficult as I had expected. Susan, aged four, was a lovely little girl with black hair and dark brown eyes. Her father had been a Canadian pilot; he had been killed in a flying accident over Vancouver Island in October 1942 after surviving two operational spells in Britain. He had died when Daphne was seven months pregnant and when they had been married less than a year. When I met her she was a widow for the second time, for her first husband, a bomber pilot with DFC and two bars, had been killed on returning from a raid in 1940.

It was some time in November 1946 that Daphne and I became engaged, and we planned the wedding for 1 February in the following year. By chance we heard of a Barts professor's house shortly to be rentable in Harpenden. This proved to be the former home of James Paterson Ross's parents and then of one of his brothers who had gone overseas for a while. We clinched the deal, but Ross told me that he felt embarrassed about the rent – £250 per annum when my salary was £600. I assured him that we would regard this as an excellent temporary home while we searched for our own house: my friend Michael Mason (later a distinguished rheumatologist) had rightly warned me that there were broadly two groups of individuals, "landlords" and "suckers," and advised us to buy a house as soon as possible. As my wedding day drew near a number of DC3 aeroplanes (widely used during wartime) had been involved in crashes. While operating one day John Hosford asked, "Would you fly in a DC3 Murley?" I said, "Most certainly, sir: I flew in them during the war and I shall be going to Switzerland aboard one for my honeymoon." In view of the fate of my prospective bride's former spouses, I think that John was somewhat embarrassed about having asked me that question.

My father-in-law had already given away his other three daughters and now he was about to give away the last one for the third time. I felt shy about the possible cost; but if Ralph Garrod was anxious he concealed it well. We were to be married at St Bartholomew-the-Less, the charming old parish church within the ancient precincts of Barts. To satisfy ecclesiastical regulations I was to deposit a suitcase in the flat of Belinda Bartlett, sister in charge of theatres, at the top of the surgical block. It seemed curious that I would be leaving my luggage with one lady in order to marry another. Our wedding day was at the beginning of one of the coldest and longest spells of winter weather on record. My best man, Raymond Ramsay, has already been referred to. With that urbane and kindly ex-Chindit I could not have been in better hands. He premedicated me judiciously with a swig from a flat flask concealed in the tails of his morning suit. As we walked up the aisle together there was a clearly audible stage whisper from Susan: "There goes Daddy." The congregation was amused. One of my contemporaries had led a heavily gravid bride out of church early in the war; but at least nobody assumed that I was belatedly correcting some wartime indiscretion. Now my father-in-law was a stickler for punctuality, tending always to be previous rather than punctual. Before leaving Well Walk he prescribed a small brandy for Daphne, ostensibly to protect her from the bitter weather. They set out in good time; but when they reached the precincts of Smithfield well ahead of schedule he insisted that the bridal car should pause outside the Old Bailey so that they could be sure of arriving at the church "on the dot." Daphne was not certain whether it was the weather or simply their proximity to the Central Criminal Court that brought on a touch of "cold feet" at that moment.

We were married by Canon Francis Donne, the then vicar and hospitaller of Barts. It was all very cosy and intimate with some 200 packed in that small church. For the preliminary "Air on a G string" which Daphne had chosen, but did not hear, Donne had kindly arranged for a violin accompaniment by a Barts nurse concealed in the organ loft. Our reception was at the nearby Apothecaries Hall. We then went to the Savoy for the night, with the intention of flying to Zurich the next day. But bad weather delayed our flight for 24 hours so we spent a second night at the Savoy; there were no vacant rooms so we had to hire a suite for 13 guineas. The next day our DC3 took off from Northolt and landed at Zurich in a heavy snowstorm. As we came in over the pine trees to land I was reminded of John Hosford's remark, but all was well and after one night in the Bau au Lac Hotel we moved to Pontresina for the next three weeks. Neither of us had ski'd before and we enthusiastically joined a class which included at least two other honeymoon couples. Daphne, with a much better sense of balance and with her experience as a prewar instructor in Prunella Stack's Women's League of Health and Beauty, did much better than I. One day we took the train to Davos to visit her stepmother, Helen, in a sanatorium there. This was the last time we saw her alive, for although she looked deceptively well she had extensive pulmonary tuberculosis and died within a year. Streptomycin was only just becoming available and the present effective antibiotic regimes had not then been devised. The cost of our honeymoon, and of a new 1½ litre Riley purchased two months before, was covered by my service gratuity of £850; but I shuddered when I thought of the expense that Ralph had incurred in paying for his wife's medical care as well as our wedding.

When we returned from Switzerland Britain was still in the grip of an icy spell with frozen, and later burst, pipes everywhere. Ralph had been unable to take a bath for almost a month; and our rented house in Harpenden was bitterly cold. There was then no central heating in most houses and fuel was still severely rationed. But our house was only 15 minutes' drive from Hill End Hospital, where I went every day except on Monday mornings, when I worked at the outpatient clinic at Barts itself. Oliver Garrod, my brother-in-law, became chief assistant to Dr A W Spence and Dr Neville Oswald at Hill End later that year, having quickly passed his MD and MRCP examinations after his delayed graduation. In the early spring Jim Ross and his brother Alec called on us at the house in Kirkdale Road, where their parents had lived in retirement. Only a few weeks later we learnt that their other brother would be returning early from abroad and that we had to vacate the house. We were already looking for a house in Radlett, a village conveniently placed between St Albans and Barts. At this stage Professor Lawrence Paul Garrod, a distant cousin of my wife's, offered us the vacant top floor of his Harpenden house as a temporary home, for which we were most grateful. We lived there happily with the Garrods during the summer. After a holiday in the Isle of Wight, spent close to Alistair Frazer's parents in Freshwater Bay, we were able to move into a delightful four bedroom house in Radlett which would be our home for the next five and a half years and where our first three children were born.

This was a period of uncertainty for many doctors as the National Health Service was due to come into effect in July of the following year. It was in anticipation of the inevitable changes that the general practitioner staff of the local St Albans hospitals decided on certain reforms. At the Mid Herts voluntary hospital there were four general practitioner surgeons. One had the English FRCS and had done surgery in the RAMC, but he decided to resign from the hospital staff before the appointed day and stick to general practice. A second, with the FRCS Ed, wanted to continue. Of the other two, neither of whom had a higher surgical qualification, one intended to resign and the other, with the least surgical experience, wished to stay. And so it was that I and one of my contemporaries, Christopher Anthony Jackson (of the pre-

Anschluss Austrian trip), were appointed in September 1947. Tony resigned a year later when he had to commit himself purely to thoracic surgery. From my own point of view, initially with just two sessions a week and with Hosford and Rodgers as senior consultants, it gave a gradual introduction to independent consultant practice. In addition to this John Hosford arranged for me to broaden my horizon by succeeding him as consultant surgeon at Napsbury Hospital, a nearby mental institution in Hertfordshire, then run by Middlesex County Council.

I had excellent experience with Hosford and Rodgers, the latter still being styled as "assistant surgeon," until the inception of the NHS. But within eight months the unit had moved back to Barts at Smithfield and we had changed our assistant surgeon three times owing to staff resignations. The senior of the assistant surgeons, Bill Underwood, was appointed professor of surgery in Johannesburgh; Michael Boyd became professor of surgery in Manchester in succession to John Morley; and then Harold himself was appointed to the chair of surgery in Belfast. As both the full and assistant surgeons were teamed up in order of seniority, and as Hosford was then the most junior of the full staff, our assistant surgeons moved up when each vacancy occurred. Harold Rodgers first moved up in place of Underwood and was himself replaced by Alec Badenoch; Badenoch was succeeded by Alan Hunt, and Hunt by Eddie Tuckwell. I was therefore fortunate to stay with Hosford for three years and to work with four different assistant surgeons. We covered the whole field of general surgery and urology and were lucky enough to draw our patients from a wide catchment area, but much of that was substantially to change in the next few years of the NHS.

John Hosford and Harold Rodgers helped me to get the appointments at St Albans and Napsbury before the NHS came into operation and before our Barts units returned to London. Thus I was able to observe at first hand the changes brought about by the NHS in both an undergraduate teaching hospital and in peripheral hospitals during the crucial early years of the service. Several years later John Hosford was wont to remark that one of the most important early contributions of the NHS was to promote a significant upgrading of standards in many of the regional hospitals. He would often cite St Albans as a good example of this, and I certainly support this view. But it is important to recognise that the chief reason for the improvement was the appointment of those with specialist training in all departments. The days of the general practitioner surgeon and physician were numbered and the early months of the NHS were traumatic for a lot of these men. Thus, although two of the four general practitioner surgeons, including one with the FRCS Eng, had decided to resign, we were left with two general practitioners on the surgical staff. The one with the FRCS Ed was largely self trained; but he could hardly be blamed for this since it had been a common feature of prewar provincial hospital staffing even in places such as Oxford and Cambridge. Moreover, such a competent surgeon as Ronald Reid of Colchester had arrived there from St Thomas's in the 1930s at the age of 26, armed with his mastership and English fellowship, to become the first "pure" surgeon in that town.

Our Edinburgh fellow at St Albans was ultimately appointed as a senior hospital medical officer for five sessions a week and continued with general practice until his retirement. The fourth general practitioner, who had completed a single house surgeon's appointment before entering practice, was quietly eased out by not being given a contract by the regional hospital board. I must confess to being actively involved in that decision since his continued service for emergency surgery and for minor operations seemed quite indefensible. At that stage I was given four surgical sessions. Paul Stringer (trained at Middlesex and Charing Cross) was appointed on a similar basis, with his remaining sessions at Hemel Hempstead Hospital. We still had John Hosford as a "visiting" consultant, and Richard Handley of the Middlesex staff had replaced Harold Rodgers in a similar capacity, with a single session each week. It is important to remember that much of the elective surgery of that area had been done in the Barts (Hill End) and Elizabeth Garrett Anderson (Osterhills) sector hospitals during the war, and that the emergencies had generally gone to the Mid Herts and Osterhills hospitals. As Barts and the Elizabeth Garrett Anderson Hospital returned to London so was the local hospital staffing being progressively changed.

The standard of fracture treatment at the St Albans hospitals left much to be desired. Similar criticism could then be applied even to the fracture work in many of our teaching hospitals. Shortly after the inception of the NHS I had written to the medical staff at St Albans indicating that despite my army orthopaedic experience and higher qualifications (I had passed the London mastership in May 1948) I did not feel properly equipped to take responsibility for all fracture patients. Thereby I hoped to persuade them to shame the general practitioner surgeons into giving up this work. My prewar visit to Böhler's clinic in Vienna had left me in no doubt about what needed to be done. Fortunately, on his return from the Royal Navy Harold Jackson Burrows, in addition to working in the Barts unit at Hill End, was visiting consultant to the Mid Herts Hospital. We were both determined to acquire a young orthopaedic surgeon on a substantial part time basis, and very soon we appointed Arthur Rushforth, then a senior registrar at the Royal National Orthopaedic Hospital. There was a rapid and impressive improvement in the standard of fracture treatment. It is interesting to record that when I began my Barts chief assistantship it was routine for all fractures to be treated on the general surgical units. By the time we returned to London I adopted the practice of calling in the orthopaedic chief assistants to treat all such patients. This practice quickly spread to the other general surgical units and was fully approved by John Hosford, who himself had been an orthopaedic chief assistant before taking a general job and had written a popular student book on fractures.

On the appointed day, 5 July 1948, the Mid Herts Hospital (voluntary) and Osterhills (Herts County Council) were combined under one management committee with the Earl of Verulam as chairman. Most of the management committee members were local people of the old school: public spirited, essentially non-political, and generally devoted to our interests. The North West Metropolitan Regional Hospital Board, then located in Portland Place, was responsible for hospitals – apart from the London undergraduate and postgraduate ones – serving a regional population of some 4.5 million, all the way way out to Bedford in the north and Slough and Windsor in the west. The only saving grace in the early days of this ponderous organisation was the fact that the former chief medical officer of Middlesex County Council, Dr H M C Macaulay, was senior administrative medical officer for the region. He was the one person who saved us from excessive bureaucracy in the first few years of the NHS, but his influence was steadily eroded as lay officialdom and committee management progressively took over.

Before discussing further my work at St Albans and Barts in the early days of the NHS I think it important to describe some interesting medicopolitical turbulence, in which I played a small part. Fortunately there is an accurate contemporary record of this important piece of medical history. How that record came to be made, and eventually inherited by me, will emerge in the next chapter.

14 A tale of turbulent times

For those who were not then qualified it is almost impossible to picture the high tensions and anxiety of the medical profession just before the inception of the National Health Service. Some of the flavour of those times is indicated in the *History of the British Medical Association 1932–1981* by Dr Elston Grey-Turner and Mr F M Sutherland,[1] and in a small booklet, *The Medical Surrender*, which was published by Lord Horder's Fellowship for Freedom in Medicine.[2]

It is sometimes said that most of the opposition to the NHS came from general practitioners rather than hospital doctors, but this is far from true. Most family doctors were strongly opposed to the proposal that the sale of goodwill of their practices would be made illegal under the 1946 Act.* Moreover, compensation for goodwill would only be paid at the time of retirement while, in the mean time, interest on the capital was to be paid at a pretty niggardly annual rate. Aneurin Bevan, the then minister of health, who seldom missed the opportunity for a shrewd blow at the doctors, had emotively referred to the sale of goodwill as "tantamount to the sale and purchase of patients."

In December 1946 a plebiscite of the whole profession had shown a clear majority against entering into negotiations with the minister on the regulations to be made under the Act. And on 8 January 1948 a special representative meeting of the BMA unanimously declared that "the Act in its present form

* There were separate Acts for Scotland and Northern Ireland but the singular is used throughout this chapter.

This chapter was first published as a special article in the Christmas number of the *British Medical Journal* 1984; 289: 1782–94.

is so grossly at variance with the essential principles of the profession that it should be rejected absolutely." A further plebiscite of the whole profession was proposed. In the mean time on 27 January consultants in London decided by 766 votes to 11 that they should not take service under the Act until it had been suitably amended. The forms for that second plebiscite were issued on 31 January, and, in an 84% poll, there was more than a nine to one majority against accepting service under the unamended Act.

RELUCTANCE TO GET EMBROILED

During the ensuing two months a curious lull occurred with little information or leadership from the council of the BMA. It may astonish present day doctors, accustomed to almost annual battles over pay and conditions of service, to learn that hospital doctors had no idea of what their proposed rates of pay or their pensions would be until well after the appointed day, 5 July 1948. Furthermore, family doctors stood to lose all compensation for the goodwill of their practices if they did not sign on the dotted line before that date.

By virtue of their charters the then existing royal colleges (physicians, surgeons, obstetricians and gynaecologists in England, and the physicians and surgeons in Edinburgh) showed some reluctance to get embroiled in the political battle. But Lord Moran, president of the Royal College of Physicians, was rumoured to be engaged in private parleying with the minister. The concern of many specialists was exacerbated when the three English presidents (Lord Moran, Sir Alfred Webb-Johnson, and Mr William Gilliatt) addressed a letter to Mr Aneurin Bevan on 2 January 1947, to which the minister replied on 6 January; both letters were published in the *BMJ* on 11 January 1947.[3 4] Shortly afterwards, at the request of the statutory number of fellows, a special general meeting was held at the Royal College of Surgeons in an attempt to ensure that the president was better acquainted with the views of the fellows. There remained a strong suspicion that their views might be ignored and so, in the following year, only a few months before the appointed day, a group of fellows from London and the provinces duly requested that there should be a further meeting.

THE REBELS

That second meeting at the Royal College of Surgeons was held on 28 April 1948, when some 250 fellows packed into one museum hall which then served as the only available meeting place before the rebuilding after the college's extensive destruction in the 1941 blitz. The "rebel" group, led by Reginald Payne, included several highly respected senior surgeons – A J Gardham of University College Hospital; Basil Hume and John Hosford of Barts; Etherington-Wilson of Torquay; and Eric Lloyd of the Royal National Orthopaedic Hospital. Payne, a Barts man on the staff of the postgraduate hospital at Hammersmith until the inception of the NHS, was a most cultured and civilised person although something of a "loner." An able surgeon and excellent teacher, Payne had been a Hunterian professor of the college on no less than four occasions in the 1930s. The rebels, keen to ensure that the younger fellows' views were taken into account, included in their group a 31 year old Barts chief assistant (the equivalent of a pre-war surgical registrar) – the author of this book. That the group was reasonably representative of the views of the fellows is shown by the support for the three resolutions that they proposed.

The opening speaker, John Gardham, in a telling and restrained contribution that ably expressed the widespread concern of many British surgeons about the virtual nationalisation of medicine, spoke to a resolution: "That this meeting of fellows of the Royal College of Surgeons, being anxious lest the standards of British surgery might be lowered if the NHS is implemented in its present form, urges the council to represent to the minister the views expressed at this meeting." Despite the visible reluctance of the president to submit to anything so democratic as a ballot of the fellows present, the motion, duly seconded by Basil Hume of Barts, was eventually passed *nem con.* There were still deep suspicions that the president might not communicate his fellows' views to the minister.

A second, rather longer, resolution was proposed by Reginald Payne, emphasising that a satisfactory service could be achieved only if free from political control. It may seem naïve to us today that anyone could seriously postulate freedom from political control in a service that would be almost entirely dependent on direct Treasury support. But Payne clearly expounded the dangers of centralised political control, the coercive powers of the minister under what was essentially an enabling Act, the threat to the independence of medical educational institutions, and the problems resulting from dominance by the government actuary and the Treasury. Fortunately, as it now transpires, our medical royal colleges – unlike the universities – have managed to avoid the dangers of governmental financial support.

In the course of a short speech, seconding Payne's resolution, I emphasised the anxieties that so many of my younger colleagues had expressed privately and at their own meetings. I added that "some of these men, through insecurity in their present jobs, have not been keen to express their views in public." I went on to refer to the president's letter of 1947 as a "tactical blunder [which] confused and divided the profession, weakened the position of the BMA and strengthened the hand of the minister." Perhaps I was a trifle ungenerous. My contribution was loudly applauded, though one or two of my colleagues did suggest afterwards that I might find it difficult to secure a senior appointment.

In the ensuing discussion there was a prolonged presidential filibuster in the course of which Sir Alfred rather plaintively asked, "Do you want to put me in the jackpot?" To which inquiry there were "loud cries of 'Yes'." The president tried to persuade the meeting that voting on the second resolution should only take place if the third resolution was withdrawn, but this was rejected by its sponsors. He also suggested that the meeting would be voting, not on the existing Act as published but on a promised amending Bill which had not even been drafted. Despite this attempt to dilute support for the motion I had seconded, it was carried by 153 votes to 73 on a ballot.

Presidential caution about the third resolution was due to its concluding words: "It is not in the best interests of the public, or the profession, that fellows should take service under the present Act." Etherington-Wilson, in proposing the resolution, emphasised the perils of entering a state service on what virtually amounted to a "blind date" with no assurances about professional freedom and the loss of independence of our old established voluntary hospitals. He was seconded by Eric Lloyd, who, in a gently effective speech, emphasised his equal repugnance to control by any of the political parties under an unamended Act. After more than two hours there had been a marked thinning out of the meeting and, on a show of hands, this last resolution was passed by only 67 votes to 58.

MEETING SECRETLY RECORDED

Finally, to satisfy the fellows' consciences and the college's honour, Reginald Payne suggested that a humble petition be sent to His Majesty, but this the president firmly rejected. So ended a historic meeting which the editor of the *BMJ*, Dr Hugh Clegg, was eagerly awaiting to report. The *Lancet* had evinced no special interest in our meeting though it would surely have been different in the days of Thomas Wakley. Alas, we rebels suffered from being too well organised for, anxious to ensure that every detail of the proceedings was accurately recorded, we had spirited an expert parliamentary speedwriter into the meeting from the House of Commons. He sat in the midst of a solid phalanx of our supporters so that none but us could observe him recording every word and incident. Indeed, in the style of *Hansard* he included each round of applause and every spirited interruption. The resultant 49 foolscap pages, double spaced, were to have been made available to the *BMJ* when Payne, a man of unique and rugged integrity, observed that the president was recorded as having said that the proceedings were "secreta collegia." In fact, none of us could remember hearing this though Sir Alfred did sometimes slur his speech or, perhaps, some of us were not as well grounded in the classics as our opposite numbers in Trafalgar Square.* Payne thereupon declared that it would be a breach of honour and of loyalty to his college if he released the record for publication. Clegg was furious, and so were all of us though none could persuade Payne to change his mind. So far as is known, the president did not acquaint the minister with the views of his fellows. The only report in the *BMJ* was a short editorial on 8 May 1948, entitled "Surgeons in Camera."[5]

A few years later I asked Reggie Payne if he would let me have a copy of the record of our meeting. "No," he replied, but added, "I shall bequeath it to you when I die." I enjoyed some years of further friendship with this remarkable man before he died quite suddently at his home of a myocardial infarct on 20 October 1967. He had a happy family life and was survived by his wife and two sons, one of whom is an Anglican clergyman and the other, Dr Richard Payne, a consultant pathologist. True to his father's promise, Richard promptly wrote to me to say that he was sending by registered post certain documents which his father had left me. Thus did I receive the complete and lucid record of that parliamentary reporter whom we had secretly introduced into a vital college meeting. A photocopy of his report now reposes in the library of the Royal College of Surgeons and the college will have the original when I die. It has been read with great interest by several past presidents of the college as well as the present editor of the *BMJ*.

It is a matter for conjecture whether stronger and better leadership might have saved the public and the profession from the viler breezes of nationalised medicine. But it would be wrong to blame the leaders of the royal colleges alone for the unsatisfactory outcome. There were equally strange goings on in the BMA, where a special council meeting was called by

* The Royal College of Physicians' former building was then in Trafalgar Square and was once picturesquely described by a London taxi driver as "the dirty end of Canada House."

telegram and then held on 15 April 1948. That meeting was never reported in the *BMJ* or in the supplementary annual report of the BMA council. Moreover, it is not even mentioned in Grey-Turner's history of the BMA. But it was at that meeting that the chairman of council, Dr Guy Dain, declared that there was no need for a further plebiscite. A wavering minority of the council then requested that the secretary of the BMA be heard. After Dr Charles Hill (now Lord Hill) had spoken a small majority on council voted in favour of holding yet another plebiscite under similar conditions to the second one. Not surprisingly, rumour became rife that the council was divided (which was true). The plebiscite result, reported on 5 May 1948, still showed an overall majority of the profession against accepting service without further safeguards, but the number of opposing general practitioners had not reached the previously agreed majority. Thus did the NHS come into being on the duly appointed day.

Reginald Payne was no blinkered opponent of "progress," but a man of great humanity and wisdom who rightly feared the disappearance of that spirit of service which epitomised the best of the voluntary system. In 1948, in reply to a question about the possible deterioration in standards, he shrewdly predicted, "The NHS will be carried on the broad shoulders of the professions – medical, nursing, and administrative – for a full quarter century; then, and only then, will the real cracks start to appear." That was a truly prophetic remark, for it was in 1973 – just 25 years after its inception – that the NHS first tasted the bitter fruits of so called "industrial action." This was followed by growing evidence of the "closed shop" mentality, the introduction of "statutory holidays" (a device for granting extra overtime payments to ancillary staff while effectively scuppering many regular clinics and operation lists), and of many other measures that seem calculated to promote the comfort of those who work in the service rather than of those they have the privilege of serving.

REFERENCES

1 Grey-Turner E, Sutherland F M. *History of the British Medical Association 1932–1981*. London: British Medical Association, 1982.
2 Fellowship for Freedom in Medicine. *The medical surrender*. London: Fellowship for Freedom in Medicine, 1951.
3 Moran Lord, Webb-Johnson A, Gilliatt W. National Health Service Act: presidents of royal colleges and Mr Bevan. *Br Med J* 1947; **i**: 66.
4 Bevan A. National Health Service Act: Mr Bevan's reply. *Br Med J* 1947; **i**: 66–7.
5 Anonymous. Surgeons in camera. *Br Med J* 1948; **i**: 888.

15 Crossing the Rubicon

The epic meeting described in the last chapter took place just after our surgical firm returned to London. Before our return Reginald Payne and his colleagues had held occasional meetings at Payne's house in Norfolk Road, St John's Wood. It was during 1947 that they had invited me to join them since they wanted some input from young doctors, especially those who had been in the services during the war. Moreover, Selwyn Taylor, who had been in the naval medical service and was later to be appointed surgeon at King's College Hospital and at Hammersmith Hospital and postgraduate medical school, had collected together an informal group of young ex-service specialists to discuss the implications of the new service and related problems in regard to our future. It was from these contacts that I recognised the anxiety and uncertainty which was being experienced by those in my generation, and so I willingly joined Payne and his senior colleagues.

During one of the earlier gatherings at Payne's house we had each agreed to make personal contact with those members of the college council who were best known to us. As Sir Heneage Ogilvie had been my consultant surgeon in the Middle East I was given the task of visiting him. I telephoned his secretary and was asked to call at his flat one Saturday at noon. I arrived in good time and was invited into the lounge, where I joined a large young man, then Heneage's house surgeon, who was about to accompany his chief to Bosham for some weekend sailing. As was not uncommon at that time we did not exchange names and I was shortly invited into Heneage's study, where I explained my business and told him of our concern that the college council should take some concerted action on behalf of its fellows. As I talked I could see that I was not evoking a sympathetic response. After exchanging a few further comments and questions Heneage said, "Well, we shall see." I left his flat feeling rather like a small boy who had not been able to give the headmaster a satisfactory account of his deviant behaviour. A few minutes later Heneage and his houseman left for Bosham. During the journey Heneage said, "Parks, did you see that young man in my lounge?" His houseman replied that we had exchanged a few remarks. Heneage then went on to say, "That chap was a first class surgeon in the army, but he has gone all political."

It was only some years later that I realised who my companion had been. Alan Parks was elected to college council two years after me and, as chairman of the Joint Consultants Committee for five years, he was certainly put in a highly medicopolitical hot seat. He succeeded me as president of the college of surgeons in 1980, before his untimely death in office two years later. We had many a good chuckle over the Ogilvie incident in the knowledge that Heneage's dismissive remark in 1948 did not represent his later opinion of me. Indeed, Heneage Ogilvie was to become one of my staunchest supporters.

Having dealt with some of the background to these turbulent times, I shall now revert to the story of our return to Barts, shortly before the start of the NHS on 5 July 1948. Many of us were sad to leave the sector hospital in which so much good work had been done for nearly nine years, but the main hospital had gradually to re-establish itself and it took more than two years before all the units were back at Smithfield. Our unit moved into the wards where I had worked as a senior dresser at the beginning of 1939. Eddie Tuckwell was now our assistant surgeon; he had succeeded Alec Badenoch. We had two excellent sisters, Anne Little in Annie Zunz and Sheila Allen in Paget, and there were many mature ex-service students among our dressers.

A month or two before the appointed day, as NHS D Day was described, we were informed that Sir George Aylwen, the treasurer (or chairman), had indicated that the board of governors would be giving three dinners in the Great Hall. One of these was for members of the senior staff and medical college professors; another for chief assistants and residents; and a third for sisters and related staff. On the day of the second dinner I was telephoned by Captain Scott, the deputy clerk to the governors, and invited to speak for the chief assistants. Scott was a retired naval officer who knew a thing or two about a "happy ship" and had, therefore, adapted well to hospital administration. On a number of occasions we had discussed the impending state takeover of the hospitals and both of us were unhappy about it. I told Scott that I was not the senior chief assistant and advised him to contact Cedric Longland, first assistant to the professorial unit. A little later in the afternoon Scott called me again and said that Longland would prefer me to respond on behalf of the chief assistants. I reluctantly accepted and told him that I would feel bound to voice my anxiety about the nationalisation of our hospital. He indicated "off the record" that the administration would be glad if I did just that.

As far as I can remember we had a good dinner. Sir George Aylwen gave what I regarded as a frankly defeatist speech, stressing the "inevitability" of takeover by the state. I was especially angry because I knew he had struck a bargain with Aneurin Bevan that if the teaching hospitals were allowed to keep their "free monies" he would ensure that their association supported government takeover. There were many other voluntary hospitals with their own, often quite substantial, endowments and many of us thought it quite wrong that those funds would be transferred to the future regional hospital boards. Rightly or wrongly, I had a strong gut reaction against the whole exercise and I did not think it honourable that the undergraduate teaching hospitals should behave in this divisive way. In later years I cultivated the habit of keeping copies of my speeches – even of the notes made on the back of a menu when I was suddenly put in the hot seat – but I have no record of this occasion. That I was loudly cheered and certainly much displeased Sir George should not be taken as indicating that I talked sense, but I certainly spoke from the heart. News of the "rebel" Murley's speech spread around the hospital. While I was assisting John Hosford at his operation list on the following day Dr Langton Hewer, the then senior anaesthetist, pawkily remarked to my chief, "John, have you heard of the rousing speech made by a certain young man at George Aylwen's dinner last night?" It was clear that Hosford had not heard and there was much chuckling as Hewer gave a somewhat apocryphal second hand account of the event.

When 5 July 1948 arrived we all went on working in the same old way and it was hard to realise that we were in the midst of one of our country's greatest revolutions. In any case I had an immense amount of satisfying work to absorb my attention and I was also swotting for the London Mastership of Surgery, which was then still taken by examination. It was a good exercise for someone like myself, who had been away in the services for so long, to have to read the literature widely to surmount this particular postgraduate hurdle, which I was lucky to do at my first attempt. At that time we had a large batch of ex-service dressers, for whom I had a strong fellow feeling. It was good for us to have so many mature students and I am sure that the younger ones, coming straight from school, benefited by the mix. John Hosford was always a popular teacher, invariably wearing a bow tie for his ward rounds. In one three month period we had 10 dressers, all but one being ex-service. Towards the end of their appointment their spokesman, a former bomber pilot named Jack, inquired if it would be in order for them all to wear bow ties for their last ward round. I said, "Why do you ask me?" Jack replied, "Well, we weren't sure whether it might upset Mr Hosford." So I retorted, "You stood up to the German flak; why should you be frightened by Mr Hosford?"

A few days later the entire round assembled wearing bow ties. They were slightly dismayed when John Hosford appeared not to have noticed their sartorial elegance. With well concealed glee, however, he kept them on the wards for an unusually long round. At our Wednesday morning staff meeting he turned to Tuckwell and said, "Eddie, do you know what the dressers did last Monday?" Feigning complete ignorance Eddie replied, "Do tell us, John," which he then did. He had been much amused and so had all the patients and nurses.

When the surgical ward block at Barts was completed in 1932, with an operation theatre and some 50 beds in neatly paired wards for each firm, it was regarded as the last word in excellence. But this rather old fashioned arrangement, with a stack of five theatres, one above the other, was soon to prove outdated. Firstly, it was difficult to "double up" during an operation list – although Gillies and McIndoe had done this before the war in the largest theatre – and, secondly, it made it difficult to develop single recovery room accommodation. Many of the Barts staff seemed unaware of these deficiencies, but those of us who had worked under field conditions were more conscious of the need for change. We all appreciated the excellent theatre staffing, however, each unit theatre being in charge of a "pink" (so called because of the colour of the theatre sisters' uniform). Millicent Hosford, John's wife, had been among the first three appointed at Barts in the early 1930s; but the other two, like her, were rapidly espoused by Wilfred Shaw, the gynaecologist, and Alex Roche, a urologist.

In those days our outpatient clinic was on Monday mornings and, as was the Barts tradition, was run by the assistant surgeon and his chief assistant, together with the odd houseman and half a dozen outpatient dressers. There was also an arrangement whereby selected patients were brought into an adjacent large classroom for presentation at 1030 hours. During the next 60 or 90 minutes five or six of the more "interesting" cases would be presented by their students to the assistant surgeon, who was seated in a central position, and to the class (undergraduates on the left and often a number of postgraduates on the right). I remember that when Alec Badenoch joined our firm he found this arrangement disturbing. He had trained in Aberdeen and worked for some time in London but was unfamiliar with the system. Being the gentleman that he is, however, Alec soldiered on with the Barts pattern.

Although we did our best to secure "informed consent" from the patients selected for presentation, it would be presumptuous to assume that the more sensitive people were not put out by these public displays. At Barts we had come to accept the arrangement as an integral part of the practical teaching system. When I took these classes myself I enjoyed the teaching, but I gradually came to feel that this was neither an efficient nor, more importantly for shy patients, a humane method of teaching. A few years later I was much happier to be able to take just one or two students into my regional hospital surgical clinics for far more personal tuition.

Many patients not previously seen at clinics held by the assistant surgeon and chief assistant were directly allocated to the senior surgeon. I thought this practice unsatisfactory. John Hosford shared my view and on succeeding to the senior position he continued to run a personal clinic (known to his residents as "the black market clinic") on another day. Apart from that there were always a number of patients who had been seen in Harley Street and then, after the health service began, elected to come into a hospital bed, as was their entitlement. I was never aware of any queue jumping; but unless a strictly ordered waiting list is run this can be wide open to abuse in some hands. There were three operation lists each week, two for Hosford and one for Tuckwell, and we were on emergency duty each Monday and every fifth weekend. On our Monday duties we regularly admitted patients with hand injuries; this was possibly due to the well recognised lack of concentration that can occur at either end of the working week. I had become especially interested in hand surgery during my wartime plastic work and I much enjoyed coping with these cases at Barts – later too at the Royal Northern, until orthopaedic and plastic surgeons took over. Teaching was always rewarding, especially with so many mature ex-service students. We also ran two courses each year for the final FRCS in which I enjoyed the clinical case teaching. Here too we had a number of ex-service doctors, of whom some had been specialists for part of the war and a few had been unit medical officers with little or no wartime opportunity to further any specialty interest.

Having returned to the main hospital I was now able to improve our organisation in several ways. Firstly, I developed a code indexing system within the unit to permit better classification and retrieval of information about diseases and operations. Secondly, I persuaded my chiefs to attend a staff "hot air" round on Wednesday morning. It provided an opportunity for discussion of all inpatients and an interchange of surgical and related views, which was not feasible during the teaching rounds. Thirdly, I ran a regular pathology meeting with George Cunningham, who had so ably managed the pathology section of our postwar primary FRCS course. On these occasions, together with our students, we would present and discuss the recently removed operative specimens and the related microscope slides. This added a further important dimension to the dressers' knowledge of their patients. George and I greatly enjoyed these joint meetings and were sorry when they had to cease with the parting of our ways.

I continued to attend at St Albans, beginning with one clinic and one operation list each week (rated as "two sessions" at the start of the NHS) and then changing to four sessions a week by October 1949, when I finished my Barts appointment. Those four sessions, however, also covered my emergency work and I was on call every other week, a commitment which became ever more demanding as the popularity of St Albans City Hospital became more firmly established. Within two or three years of the start of the NHS it became apparent that the number of patients being treated in regional hospitals just outside London was increasing whereas pressure on the central London hospitals was diminishing. This was not obvious at first; but continuing to work, as I later did, both at St Albans and the Royal Northern I was soon able to share the privileges, and some of the problems, of being both a metropolitan and a provincial surgeon.

Within two years of the start of the NHS we had built up an impressive young staff at St Albans. Paul Stringer, who had been trained at Charing Cross and the Middlesex, became my opposite number and divided his time equally between St Albans and the West Herts Hospital at Hemel Hempstead. Arthur Rushforth, as already mentioned, transformed the fracture and orthopaedic work. Dr Linnell of New End Hospital in Hampstead (the site of the London County Council thyroid unit) had been a visiting consultant on much the same basis as Hosford. Then Peter Mills and E D H

("Tim") Cowen were appointed on a half time basis between St Albans and Hitchin. George Vilvandré, a senior radiologist who had also been on the staff of the London Hospital – until he resigned in a fit of Gallic furore – was joined by Geoffrey Weber from Barts. For a year or more I had transported all my operation specimens to Barts for histology reporting, but eventually new appointments were made at St Albans in histology, haematology, and biochemistry. These were supplemented by the additional appointment of young consultants in the ear, nose, and throat and anaesthetic departments to build up the service formerly provided by the occasional attendance of a few visiting consultants. Our buildings were old but our staff were young, enthusiastic, and hardworking. At that stage we had excellent support from Dr Macaulay (then known as "Uncle Mac"), the senior administrative medical officer of the regional board. The new hospital management committee was supportive because with a few exceptions its members had all served on the voluntary hospital committee. For a few years – until bureaucracy slowly overcame us – we were seemingly in clover.

There were certainly some difficulties in regard to former general practitioner members of the staff who had been displaced by newly appointed young consultants. Most of them accepted the situation with good grace; a few were unhappy and clearly resentful. Shortly after the start of the NHS I had been elected chairman of the medical committee, despite my rather tender years (I was nearly 32). I was determined to get the service better organised and had decided that we must all have unit secretaries, as had been the case at Hill End. My complaint to the administration promptly brought a committee member to my theatre. He was a local baronet, who waited until I had finished an operation and then listened politely to my request. He ensured that our needs were met. Indeed, I managed to persuade my unit secretary from Hill End to join me in the local hospital. She provided excellent service for some years before she began to find the workload too great. At my suggestion she took a private secretarial post in London with a distinguished orthopaedic surgeon. She later became his third wife. My next secretary stayed for over 10 years and was succeeded by three more, of whom the last was with me for six years before my retirement and then worked for my successor. Each of these ladies was hardworking and despite the low rate of pay carried out her duties superbly. In our primitive St Albans prefabricated outpatient department, erected in 1949, I had an office next to my consulting room. All patients for admission were seen by the secretary and given a firm date for operation: I never had a waiting list as such. Moreover, the unit secretary was always available to help a general practitioner with any patient who needed an urgent appointment. Thus our service was sensitive to the needs of the consumer; but we usually had to cope with too many patients.

Because of the pressure on the clinics I always tried to run them on an efficient "production line" system. I saw every new patient personally, but the histories of most patients were taken by my registrar and my house surgeon. In later years, when I had a senior house officer too, the history taking would be done in one of three other rooms besides my own. Our notes were as complete as possible; they included details of smoking and drinking habits, etc. By the time a patient arrived at my room I could check over the history, undertake the physical examination, explain the situation, arrange any necessary investigations, or recommend admission. If a patient was to be admitted he or she would report to the unit secretary for an admission date and other necessary details. We tried to keep return attendances to a minimum. I checked every such case note and then allocated selected patients to my assistants. But when a patient seemed to have been booked to attend again for no good reason I would write on the notes "Return to general practitioner or discuss with me." In this way I knew precisely who was attending the clinic, could control needless return visits, and have an overview of every patient. In later years I worked non-stop for four to four and a half hours with no coffee breaks.

At St Albans I soon organised a special cancer follow up clinic where I saw all the patients personally. I accept that continued hospital attendance is not a good thing for all cancer patients; but most of ours seemed to appreciate our continued interest and supervision. Moreover, on each visit a letter was sent to the family doctor with copies to any other doctor who had been responsible for past treatment – for example, a radiotherapist, former registrar, or previous general practitioner. I came to look upon this as a vital part of our continuing education, and I learnt more about cancer care and management from those patients than I ever acquired from any other source. If a patient preferred not to attend I always continued follow up by periodically writing to the family doctor. I eventually had some 600 cancer patients under regular supervision, most attending the clinic and the rest being followed up by letter.

To ensure maximum use of beds we had no fixed allocation to individual surgeons. Patients with less severe conditions were advised to telephone the ward on the day of admission to ensure that a bed was available. This was a necessary precaution lest the recent emergency load had been particularly heavy. But we always made a point of guaranteeing a bed for any major admission. The occasional patient with a less serious problem whose admission might have to be deferred on account of excessive emergency admissions was normally admitted for the next available operation day. The system worked well for many years; we ran into trouble only when industrial action and other "Spanish practices" eventually crept into the NHS. Even then, our problems were much less than those experienced in more militant areas of the United Kingdom. I am glad to say that virtually every young surgeon I have trained has continued this practice of planned admission for elective operation. It should be emphasised that even with such a well regulated system any busy general surgeon will have 50 or 60 patients awaiting admission on a firm date. If one starts to talk in terms of a "national waiting list," as has now become such misleading parlance in the NHS, then 1000 general surgeons would have 50 000 or 60 000 patients awaiting operation. If one then adds in all the specialty groups such as orthopaedics, gynaecology, plastic surgery, etc a well ordered "waiting list" of 300 000 is readily built up. To talk of a "national waiting list" for surgical operation is meaningless unless much fuller information is made available. I have for some years been of the opinion that many of these figures are phoney. Where there are long delays these are commonly due to inefficiency and other factors which should be easily remediable in any self respecting institution. The few genuine examples of real waiting list problems are often related to staff shortages, lack of operation rooms, precipitate bed closures, and bad management.

My appointment at Napsbury mental hospital provided me with much interesting work in the first few years. Since before the NHS the deputy medical superintendent there had always made careful arrangements for visits to patients referred for a surgical opinion. This was important as the hospital site was widespread and a well organised programme ensured that patients could be seen without my having to retrace my progress through the hundreds of yards of corridor. If their condition permitted I could transfer to the general hospital patients who needed major surgery, but most of the operating was done in the Napsbury theatre. On those occasions I was usually assisted by one of the younger psychiatrists. I was paid at a flat rate of £100 a year; but there were some county councils that then paid their visiting specialists on an item-of-service basis. For this absurd sum I was available at all times. After the NHS started the Napsbury pay simply became part of my overall sessional salary.

There were many entertaining moments at Napsbury. I recall one afternoon when we found a number of the patients watching an operation through the clear glass of the theatre window. In one of the male wards there was a patient who was in the habit of swallowing dessert spoons, most of which he managed to pass by the natural route. When I was asked to see him, however, an *x* ray had shown two spoons situated in his pelvis. Digital examination of the rectum revealed that they were just out of reach of the examining finger. I told the Irish sister to give him a gentle purge and, if she wished, a simple enema. I heard nothing further and inquired after him on my next visit to that ward. In her rich brogue the sister, who clearly had midwifery experience, responded, "Oh yes, Sorr, he had some strong contractions and delivered the spoons the next day."

Another time I was asked to see a very disturbed patient who was reported to have a large abscess in one buttock, believed to have arisen from intramuscular injection of sedative paraldehyde (then an old and very safe favourite in mental hospitals). When I arrived at the ward the psychiatrist in charge, a Dr Gladstone, reported that on applying his stethoscope to this "abscess" he had heard a distinct murmur. I was able to confirm this and congratulated him on his perspicacity for there is no doubt that most doctors would have missed the diagnosis. As a result of this astute observation I was able to plan the formal exposure, and excision, of an arteriovenous fistula in the buttock. This had formed between one of the gluteal arteries and its accompanying vein and was certainly related to a past intramuscular injection. Recovery was uneventful. I must here place on record my recognition of the high endeavours of the staff of Napsbury when I first consulted there. Mental hospitals worked under many difficulties and constraints but I was most impressed by the spirit of service at that time.

With these various commitments it will be appreciated that I covered a fair mileage, and this was to increase as a result of subsequent appointments. There was relatively little traffic on the roads in those days and petrol was still rationed for several years after the war. In the early years of the NHS I also used to make about 25 or 30 domiciliary visits each year with the family doctors. These visits were generally interesting and rewarding because there was the chance of seeing sick patients in their own homes and of discussing the problems personally with the family doctor and relatives. Some of the general practitioners were reluctant to use the service because the consultant could claim a domiciliary fee whereas they had to accept responsibility on the basis of their annual capitation payments. I was invariably accompanied by the family doctors in the St Albans area, and I never encountered any resentment there.

These discursive observations in what were largely the early years of my postwar surgical practice give some idea of the volume and variety of work at the time. But as I shall have occasion to return to various other aspects of my regional hospital work later I shall now come back to my Barts chief assistantship. In those days these appointments, the equivalent of the present day senior registrarship, were held for not more than three years. When I had been with John Hosford for about 18 months – I think it was early in 1948 – I was approached about taking on an entirely new appointment, that of surgical tutor. Professor Paterson Ross told me that this appointment would be made at Bethnal Green, a former London County Council hospital, where a Barts man with the colourful name of Pickup Greenwood was the surgical superintendent. On further inquiry I found that this was to be a predominantly teaching appointment with little clinical commitment, but Ross said that it would be "a natural stepping stone to the Barts staff." On this last point I was sceptical: I had known too many men to have been led up the garden path with vague promises of future advancement. Hosford was unable to help me since he knew no more of the true facts than I did. Bodley Scott told me that Greenwood was a Marxist, which exacerbated my natural, if reluctant, Tory prejudices. I was urged to visit Bethnal Green Hospital, and duly did so.

A week or two later, while we were scrubbing up to operate, Hosford asked me if I had visited Bethnal Green. I replied, "Yes, sir, I went there yesterday." "And how did you get on?" said John. "Well," said I, "it was a typical broken down old LCC dump and I was shown around by a pretty typical LCC service doctor – a third rate graduate from Cork." Nothing was heard for a few moments other than the sound of scrub water splashing in the sinks. Then John quietly rejoined, "You know, Murley, my mother's family came from Cork; my father's family came from Cork, and my father was a Cork graduate." I felt shattered; never had I dreamt that John Hosford was Irish. Just as I was wondering how best I could quietly disappear through the solid terazzo flooring, John continued, "But I do largely agree with you about Cork graduates, Murley." Great was my relief. A further aspect of this experience is what happened at lunch in the refectory. I was so full of the news that the Hosfords were Irish that I told Langton Hewer, Hosford's regular anaesthetist, and John

Beattie, his gynaecologist contemporary. They were both incredulous and said that they were sure I was wrong. When I told them my story John Beattie exclaimed, "Well, blow me down, I never knew that."

I duly reported to Paterson Ross and said that I did not feel that Bethnal Green was suitable for me. Thereupon he pressed me to turn up at the appointments committee and explain to Sir Alan Daly, the last head of the London County Council medical service, precisely why I did not like the idea of the job. I sensed that Ross might be using me to do some dirty work for him, but I rather brashly obliged. I did not apply for the job, but I duly appeared at the interview, declared that I was not interested, and told the committee why. I left the interview feeling certain that I had made the right decision but none too sure about my relationship with Ross.

Having brushed off the Bethnal Green offer I happily continued the remaining 18 months or so of the one appointment I had sought above all others. For some time after I left the army I had every intention of seeking a whole time professorial post. Hosford always assumed that I would take up a part time appointment such as he held. After the NHS had been in operation for a year or so he began to urge me to take a whole time NHS job, "like Norman Tanner and Avery Jones." I pointed out that Tanner and Avery Jones, previously whole timers, respectively in the London and Middlesex County Council services, had by then elected to enter private practice and take part time NHS contracts. This illustrates the changing point of view of many of us of different seniority in the evolving specialist scene at that time. The growing shadow of state near monopoly in medicine, rather than simple greed for greater earnings, gave added stimulus to many ambitious specialists to have some professional life independently of the NHS.

16 Research and a search for jobs

I completed my three year appointment with John Hosford and Eddie Tuckwell at the end of September 1949, but I was not unprepared for the future. Both at Hill End and Barts I had developed an interest in postoperative venous thrombosis and pulmonary embolism. Earlier in the year I had applied for the Mackenzie Mackinnon research fellowship, jointly sponsored by the Royal College of Physicians and the Royal College of Surgeons. As from 1 October this fellowship had been awarded to me and I had also been appointed to a Hunterian professorship at the college of surgeons. I was due to give my Hunterian lecture in March 1950 and I needed an opportunity to assemble the case material I had collected in the previous three years. I was also keen to undertake a study of venous flow in the legs following operation, and I had Hosford and Tuckwell's permission to do this work in their wards. This proved highly convenient since I also had the good will and support of my former ward sisters and nursing staff.

I was also keen to undertake a study of breast carcinoma and to that end had applied for the Cattlin research fellowship at Barts. It was awarded to me for two years, to run concurrently with the Mackenzie Mackinnon fellowship. Once my Hunterian lecture had been given it was my intention to develop the study on breast carcinoma. I had already given some attention to this and had done some preliminary planning with two of my colleagues at Barts. For the immediate future, therefore, I had quite enough on my plate, though there was always the further problem of what surgical appointments I might ultimately secure. My commitment at St Albans was still light and, with good organisation, there was no difficulty in combining clinical and research work. Indeed, this was commonly done on the professorial units but I, of course, did not have that particular backing for my own enterprise.

After finishing the chief assistant job I had the problem of adjusting to a different life style. Financially I was less well off, but I never felt any serious pressures as a result. It was marvellous to have time for thorough research of the medical literature and for writing. It was also good to have more time for my family; by then my wife and I had a daughter of $1\frac{1}{2}$ and a 3 month old son, in addition to Susan, my stepdaughter, who was nearly 7. With an upstairs study in Radlett I was able to do a good deal of reading and writing at home. In addition I had the pleasant diversion of a still small clinical commitment at St Albans; only later was this to grow to the dimensions indicated in the previous chapter.

Let me deal first with the work on venous thrombosis. Starting at Hill End I had begun to collect important examples from all over the hospital. The patients were seen in the general medical and surgical units, as well as some of the specialist surgical units. Apart from the orthopaedic cases, many of whom were inevitably bedbound by the nature of their disease, it was still customary for many patients to be confined to bed for far too long after an operation or through such medical conditions as a myocardial infarct. We had considerably more, and more serious, cases of thromboembolism than are seen today. But thrombosis and embolism are notoriously easy to miss, especially by the unprepared mind, so valid statistics are hard to assemble.

An important part of that work at Hill End entailed collaboration with the *x* ray department in doing venograms of the legs. At that time no radiologist put a needle into a vein: even with intravenous urograms it was still customary for a junior houseman to inject the contrast medium. This is so different from the work of many radiologists today. Moreover, in those days some of the contrast media were highly irritating if they escaped into the soft tissues. I started the venographic work with the warm support of Dr George Simon, who was on the radiology staff of Barts and Brompton hospitals. He was almost totally deaf, but he was nevertheless an outstanding doctor. To ensure the accuracy of his *x* ray diagnoses he would often appear in the operation rooms at both hospitals to study the living pathology. He was highly regarded by all his clinical colleagues.

Venographic study of the leg veins had been introduced largely by Gunnar Bauer in Sweden. Although it was still recognised that some of the larger and more dangerous pulmonary emboli could arise from the pelvic veins, there was an important educational aspect of venography. One of our greatest problems was to persuade clinicians that thromboembolism had really occurred. Venographic demonstration of changes in the legs, although in no way proving further propagation of the process, could be an important step in persuading the sceptics. And so it was with the numerous venograms I did at Hill End. Gradually staff in all departments began to appreciate the many possible variations on a basically thrombotic regime. I remember feeling especially pleased when Professor Ross told me how much better informed the students had now become. Apart from the problems of clinical diagnosis there was considerable dispute about the most appropriate methods of treatment. Heparin had only recently become available and my earliest supplies were sent to me by Professor Jorpes in Stockholm. We were just beginning to use the longer acting oral drugs of the dicoumarol family. It was an exciting time in this and virtually every other field of medicine.

By October 1949 I had a large collection of case notes and *x* rays. In regard to the latter, George Simon gave me an invaluable tip: "Murley, hang on to all those *x* rays yourself; they'll only get lost in the records department." With the collaboration of many of our keen dressers I had undertaken an interesting study of various blood coagulation tests in the postoperative period. Contrary to a number of publications at that time, I was able to show that there was no valid predictive test. But I was anxious to study the blood flow in the limb veins, and that was my immediate task. I did this postoperatively by two methods: (1) measuring the venous return from the legs with radioactive sodium, which was then virtually the only radioactive isotope available for such purpose; and (2) plethysmography. The first was simply and safely done with a short half life sodium, but the second was more difficult since it entailed putting the patient's foot and leg in a sealed container so that the volumetric changes consequent upon blood flow could be studied. For the radioactive sodium work I had the support and collaboration of a physicist, G M Owen, from the radiotherapy department. But we ran into unexpected difficulties during the terrible smog of 1949. That was in the days before the Clean Air Act. A killer fog descended on us for several weeks in the early winter. With so much town lighting and heating turned on during the smog, Owen was often able to record a profound drop in the voltage of the main electricity supply. Because of its effect on our equipment this voltage drop seriously prejudiced a lot of the recordings. I struggled on with the work, but I often felt that the terms of my research fellowship were, in Hamlet's words, "more honour'd in the breach than the observance."

Although orthodox laboratory facilities existed at Barts, there was little opportunity to apply physiological studies at the bedside. Well developed applied physiology facilities, which were commonplace in the United States, were not yet available in the United Kingdom. I was therefore working in an unfamiliar field; but I was fortunate to be able to do so in friendly wards. I was not at all proud of my achievements, but the project at least taught me that I was not the sort of person who would be likely to sustain a prolonged spell in pure research. The preparation of my Hunterian lecture progressed well in all other respects and I was able to cover the old and more recent literature quite thoroughly. When the great day came, in the still heavily bomb damaged college of surgeons, I had a packed house in the large museum hall which was then used for the lectures. The president, Sir Cecil Wakeley, was in the chair and towards the end I fancied that I distinctly heard him snoring. He was kind enough, however, to insist on publishing the lecture – all 45 pages with 140 references – in the *Annals of the Royal College of Surgeons*, with beautiful glossy reprints from The Times Publishing Company.

With that Hunterian lecture behind me I was able to start

my other research project. During my time on the Hosford firm I had, as was customary with most of the Barts surgeons, done the radical mastectomy operation for breast carcinoma. Moreover, having been an ersatz plastic surgeon in the army, I inclined towards C D Haagensen's variation of that operation in which wider skin removal with routine skin grafting was often done. In my student days I had not worked with Geoffrey Keynes, who had abandoned the radical operation in the 1920s and was generally regarded as an eccentric. Nor was it purely a question of "a prophet not being without honour, save in his own country, and in his own house." Keynes's work had been widely neglected and even unjustly vilified. That was something of which I had gradually become aware. But the real turning point for me came with a meeting I attended at the Royal Society of Medicine on 7 January 1948. With Sir Max Page in the chair, Robert McWhirter addressed the section of surgery on the treatment of breast carcinoma by simple surgery and irradiation. There was a packed house and Geoffrey Keynes later told me that he had been unable to get in. What especially struck me was (a) the uncomfortably hostile atmosphere in which Mc Whirter's paper was received; (b) the lack of any truly constructive discussion; and (c) the manifest inadequacy of the alleged statistics of Sir Stanford Cade and Sir Gordon Gordon-Taylor, who spoke for the radical school. Indeed the best punchline of the evening came when Duncan Fitzwilliams, a St Mary's surgeon, having pointed out that certain of Gordon-Taylor's figures were too good to be true, went on to say: "So the best advice we can give any woman approaching middle age is to develop a stage 1 breast carcinoma; but, above all, to go to Sir Gordon Gordon-Taylor for radical mastectomy. Thereby her prospects of survival will better those of her cohorts in the same age group who have never had cancer." It was a telling blow as our later studies were to show. Some years afterwards I heard from Maurice Ewing (formerly of Edinburgh but then at Hammersmith) that he was one of the few surgeons present who spoke to McWhirter after the meeting. I have recently heard from Robert McWhirter of someone else who spoke to him – a London surgeon, whose name he had forgotten, who expressed much interest in his paper and invited him to his nearby house so that they might have a quiet discussion. The hostile and irrational reaction of many doctors to the seemingly unconventional is a recurring feature of history.

I was then half way through my chief assistantship at Barts. Although I had not been converted by that meeting I had been given furiously to think. Pressure of work and of other events, such as the arrival of the appointed day on 5 July, did not allow much time for a second research interest, but the problem continued to bother me. I speculated that the answer might even lie in our own Barts records. I had become more and more impressed by the efficiency of our cancer follow up department, which had done some impressive tracing of patients "lost" during the war. My old friend and contemporary Richard Terry became cancer registrar after finishing his chief assistantship with Dr Geoffrey Bourne. He agreed with me that the hospital records were largely complete. The real question was: could any valid conclusions be drawn from a retrospective study of those records? None of the surgical staff seemed enthusiastic about the idea, and Walter Levitt, who had been in charge of our radiotherapy department in the past, was distinctly sceptical. After moving to St George's before the war Walter had been thwarted in his endeavours to develop a department there. Temporarily disillusioned with medicine he became a barrister-at-law, but after the war he did part time radiotherapy at Barts, and established a private practice. Meanwhile Mr I G Williams, FRCS, a Middlesex man, had been appointed radiotherapist in charge of the Barts department.

Glynn Williams, a quiet and friendly Welshman, was some nine years older than I. He was always helpful and approachable. On discussing the matter with him I discerned that he was willing to help. Moreover, we had appointed a medical statistician at Barts a few years earlier. The first incumbent had moved on to a Medical Research Council job and was replaced by Michael Curwen, a Cambridge mathematics graduate of roughly my own age who had been at Cambridge with one of my brothers-in-law. I began to call Glynn and

Michael "my two mammary collaborators." By the beginning of 1949 we had agreed on a fruitful line of inquiry which only awaited appropriate clearing of the decks of other commitments.

The planning of our project was, thanks to Michael Curwen, almost immaculate. We chose the period 1930–39 inclusive because we would be able to determine 10 year survival figures overall, and even 15 year survivals for those patients treated in the first half of that decade. There were more than 1600 case notes in the files, but many related to patients who had been referred for radiotherapy after operation at other hospitals. We therefore decided to confine our efforts to those who had been treated throughout at Barts – some 1042 in all. The indirect and ethical tracing of patients through the good offices of the then Ministry of Food had proved highly successful. The ministry refused, most properly, to give us the patients' new addresses but was prepared to forward the letters from the follow up department, thus leaving any further decision to the patient. This is the only evidence I can quote in support of the occasionally beneficent effects of bureaucracy. We were therefore reasonably confident that we might be able to fulfil the five clear objectives of the project. To satisfy ourselves about the extent of "observer variation" in collecting information from the hospital records Michael gave us a preliminary exercise. Using carefully prepared sheets we each recorded the relevant data from 100 cases. We were then tested against each other and, indeed, against our own earlier performance. Once we had passed this test Glynn and I were let loose on the 1042 case notes. It was a labour that took us many months and I am astonished that Glynn, with all his departmental responsibilities, continued so valiantly to support me. For some years he did joint consultations with me on all my St Albans radiotherapy patients. I clearly remember one day in 1952, during our research, when he asked, "Reggie, when did you last do a radical mastectomy?" After a moment's thought I replied, "I think I did one about six months ago, and that must be my last."

In those precomputer days all the information from the

sheets was transferred to punchcards in Michael's department of medical statistics. The cards then went through the Hollerith sorting machine and Michael studied every possible permutation and correlation of the data. The editor of the *BMJ* was keen to have the final paper, but before submitting it we assembled our preliminary data for a meeting of the Paget Club (a hospital rersearch club) at Barts. Glynn talked from the radiotherapy angle and I gave the comparative figures for different methods of treatment. In our audience we had Reginald Vick, who had never done anything but the radical operation, and Geoffrey Keynes, who had never done one at all in the period under review. Both were emeritus surgeons. Our conclusions were quite simple: (1) in terms of survival there was nothing to choose between different methods of treatment; (2) in terms of complications there were serious disadvantages to radical surgery; and (3) a higher local recurrence rate with certain forms of less radical treatment did not prejudice overall survival.

Glynn and I, at the invitation of Professor Frank Stammers, visited Birmingham shortly afterwards to give a repeat performance. I well remember "Pon" (Alphonsus Liguere) d'Abreu – who later succeeded Stammers in the chair of surgery – saying, "Thank heaven we can give up radical mastectomy with a clear conscience." Our definitive paper appeared in the *BMJ* in 1953 and stimulated a slowly growing interest in more conservative surgery. Whatever may have been published since in the way of prospective trials, or of allegedly randomised prospective trials – though many would question their ethical compatibility with fully informed consent – has not altered our early conclusions. It was a source of satisfaction to me that Dr George Crile Jr of Cleveland, when I met him for a second time in 1955, adopted a basically Keynesian philosophy. However much the arguments may have swayed back and forth during some of the ensuing years I have always been pleased to have played this small part in spreading the worldwide acceptance of Keynes's teaching. In this connection I often like to remind people that although the economic doctrine of "my clever brother Maynard," as Geoffrey sometimes called him, has fallen into disrepute, the wisdom and humanity of his younger brother's breast teaching are now widely accepted.

Those two early research subjects have proved of absorbing interest throughout my professional life, and I am glad that I chose to put aside some two years for this work. During those two years, from the autumn of 1949 to that of 1951, I had not been seriously concerned about the future. By the time my research grants ceased my work at St Albans was taking up rather more than half my working week, but I was paid only for four sessions a week – four elevenths of full time salary. I shared a house surgeon with Arthur Rushforth, the orthopaedic surgeon, and Stringer shared a houseman with Morgan-Jones, the general practitioner surgeon. Because Stringer had to cover Hemel Hempstead Hospital too he did one week's duty a month at each hospital; I covered alternate weeks at St Albans and Morgan-Jones covered the fourth week. We started with the services of a resident surgical officer. But Dr Macaulay was keen to have a proper "firm" set up, as in the teaching hospitals, so by 1952 we had two surgical registrars. I had expressed concern about this staff establishment since I was anxious about the problems our registrars might have in securing promotion. For this reason we began with one or two Australians and New Zealanders who would ultimately be returning home. After this tentative start I was determined only to select British candidates so long as I felt confident that they had the potential to become consultants. Happily, for 30 years we had such excellent United Kingdom applicants that each one who became my registrar moved on to senior registrar and consultant appointments.

During the second year of my research projects the assistant directorship of the surgical professorial unit at Barts became vacant and I was an applicant. Keynes and Paterson Ross had both been assistant directors, one moving into consulting practice and the other succeeding to the chair. Thereafter every later assistant director had moved on to a general surgical appointment either in London or the provinces. Clifford Naunton Morgan had held the post when I was a dresser and had then become assistant surgeon on one of the general firms. It was clear that two of the three shortlisted applicants on this occasion had similar intentions, but it was said that Paterson Ross was, perhaps understandably, seeking someone with professorial intentions. Selwyn Taylor had recently taken one or two sessions at the Belgrave Children's Hospital at Clapham and was keen to retain that connection, whereas I was more interested in a part time appointment than an academic one. John Kinmonth had recently completed a year of research with Fiorindo Simeone in professor Churchill's department at the Massachusetts General Hospital and he was firmly committed to an academic surgical future. In the circumstances it is not surprising that Kinmonth was appointed, and that he subsequently succeeded George Perkins in the chair at St Thomas's Hospital, where he had an outstanding record.

In the course of my Barts research I had also been keen to go to the United States, where my brother-in-law, Oliver Garrod, was on a Rockefeller scholarship in 1951. He had a year with professor Loeb at the Columbia Medical Center, where he did some valuable endocrine research before returning to a lecturer post at Hammersmith; he was later appointed consultant physician at Barnet. I had applied for a Rockefeller scholarship in 1950 but was unsuccessful; however, Dr Herald, one of the staff at the Medical Research Council, wrote to me: "You came very close indeed to pulling off an award." I then applied for a British Postgraduate Medical Federation fellowship. Alas, here too I was thwarted because a sharp fall of the pound against the dollar compelled the federation to suspend the funding of United States fellowships for several years.

By the time I completed my research, in the autumn of 1951, I was in need of additional hospital sessions. I did not worry much about private practice, which for most young specialists was sparse in the early years of the NHS. I had always managed to pick up some private emergency work since my chief assistant days at Barts, and I had one or two senior colleagues who allowed me the occasional use of their consulting rooms in Harley Street. But a contemporary of mine, Edward Corsi, had inherited 95 Harley Street on the death of his elder brother, Henry, who had been a dermatologist at Barts. He suggested that I should share his rooms and, from 1953, I did this for an initial rental of 160 guineas a year. This was increased to only £200 a year in 1962. We had good accommodation at the back of the house, just above the room which Reginald Payne had rented since the 1930s. I became sole occupier, paying £400 a year when Corsi retired in 1963. My annual rental was £650 in 1969; £900 in 1972; £2000 in 1979, and £4000 in 1982 – changes which show the effects of inflation. Just after I moved from Harley Street in 1983 the going rate for the same premises was £6000. Few medical fees increased at anything like the same rate in that period. Thus those in private practice were made far more clearly aware of the economic facts of life than those in the health service.

In the early years of the NHS a few of the London undergraduate teaching hospitals had built up firm links with some of the bigger regional hospitals. The link between Middlesex Hospital and the Central Middlesex (a former MCC hospital) was a notable example. Barts had been tardy in following suit; but early in 1951 Ivor Lewis, a distinguished general and thoracic surgeon at the North Middlesex Hospital, decided to move to his native Wales. His job was advertised and various members of the Barts staff made it known that the medical college was keen to forge a link with this large and busy Edmonton hospital. Although the post had been advertised as full time, the hospital administrator and staff had been told that there would be no objection to the successful candidate taking a maximum part time contract. A number of my senior colleagues, one or two on the staff of North Middlesex, pressed me to apply even though I was unhappy with the terms of the advertisement and wanted to ensure that I could remain part time with a right to some private practice. Having been reassured on this point and told that it was unnecessary to mention the matter at the interviewing committee, I applied and was appointed from half a dozen or so shortlisted candidates.

On my next visit to the North Middlesex Hospital, before starting work, the group secretary asked me if I wished to be maximum part time or whole time. I said that I had applied only on the former basis and he assured me that there would be no difficulty about this. Prudently, as it turned out, I did not immediately resign my St Albans job. Experience had taught me to be cautious amidst the growing bureaucracy and I was still uncertain regarding the final contract. Moreover, Francis Avery Jones, having successfully established himself at the Central Middlesex before and during the war, had told me that he thought I would be wiser to build on my St Albans foundations. That advice had been backed by Alan Hunt, John's younger brother, a surgeon at Barts and the Cancer Hospital. He told me how Cecil Joll had always emphasised that he had derived much better and more interesting surgical work from his provincial hospital (Aylesbury) than his London appointments. And so while waiting to have my new job confirmed on a part time basis I continued to work at St Albans too. I was able to cope comfortably with both hospitals, but I had to work very hard.

When I had been at North Middlesex for two or three months there were rumours that the North East Metropolitan Regional Hospital Board was not prepared to give me a part time contract. I was telephoned by Dr George Graham, a Barts physician member of the board. He told me that I was "very foolish" not to take a whole time contract. We agreed to differ. The senior medical officer of the board, also a Dr Graham but unrelated to George, telephoned me to say that if I would not agree to a whole time contract the post would be advertised again. Sir James Paterson Ross, in writing to me about my application for the postgraduate fellowship in the United States, hinted at my "quarrel" with the regional board; I sensed his possible displeasure. I stood my ground. The post was readvertised with a choice between maximum part time and whole time work. I duly put in again and was on an almost identical shortlist. The Australian senior registrar who had been rejected previously was then appointed. This was Keith Moore, who had been a prisoner of war in Italy and who I had known in the army at Aldershot. Although I was angry with the board, I did not begrudge Moore the job and there was no ill feeling between us. He took the appointment part time so I was at least vindicated in having persuaded the regional board to fulfil a onetime principle that candidates should be given a choice of contracts. This all happened shortly after my mother's death just before Christmas 1951. For the first time in my life I developed classical duodenal ulcer symptoms, with nocturnal and hunger pain for the next few weeks. Daphne and I took a skiing holiday at Mürren in February 1952 and the ulcer symptoms quickly abated. I had personally experienced a neat demonstration of the relationship between stress and peptic ulceration.

The promised firm association between North Middlesex and Barts never materialised. Many years later Barts and Hackney hospitals were linked together in the reorganised City and Hackney district. Perhaps, as things turned out, fate had been kind to me.

Shortly after our return from Mürren I was tempted into applying for the chair of surgery at the University of Winnipeg, which, according to the advertisement, might be filled on either a whole time basis or with some private practice. Still smouldering from my North Middlesex experience I applied for this chair on a part time basis, with Lord Horder and Sir Heneage Ogilvie as my referees. Horder had replied to my request:

> My dear Reggie,
>
> In reply to your letter, by all means make any (legitimate!) use of my name that you wish. But I am v. sorry to hear of your decision to leave us, tho' I must confess that, were I at your age and stage, I should do the same.

In the event – and perhaps luckily for me – they appointed a Canadian to the chair on a whole time basis. My father, who knew Winnipeg well, had warned me that I might be rather shocked by the climate there. A few years later, in Toronto, I chanced to meet the man who had the job, and when I mentioned that I had been an applicant he said, "I sometimes wish that you had got the job!" In view of the later Canadian problems with socialised medicine and "Medicare" I am glad that I stayed here and tried to sort out some of our own difficulties.

17 Selection committees I have known

Many young specialists of my generation had difficulty in finding consultant appointments at that time. It was those a little senior to me who had fared best, for they had qualified several years before me and taken higher qualifications before the war. When peace came a number of staff vacancies arose through the retirement of those who had delayed their departure. Moreover, at Barts those three newly appointed men took chairs of surgery elsewhere to create further unexpected vacancies. I was too young for all this, and it was fortunate that I had established the tenuous St Albans connection when I was at Hill End. While I was working on my research projects Ralph Shackman approached me on behalf of Ian Aird, the professor of surgery at the postgraduate medical school, to ask if I would be prepared to take up a whole time appointment in vascular surgery at Hammersmith. But I was as reluctant to confine myself to a single field of surgery as I was to accept a whole time appointment. So I declined that offer of an appointment without competition.

I shall now give an account of my sometimes entertaining experiences on both sides of the table at a number of selection committees.

Because I had a consultant appointment at St Albans I often represented the medical staff on the regional board appointment committees. I also acted as a medical representative for the board for staff appointments at other hospitals. Occasionally too, while seeking to secure additional sessions, I was an applicant for surgical vacancies at other hospitals. More than once I found myself on a selection committee with people who had recently been interviewing me. I had helped in the selection of two ear, nose, and throat surgeons, an anaesthetist, and an orthopaedic surgeon at St Albans. The ear, nose, and throat committees had been straightforward, but the orthopaedic one was fascinating. We had a shortlist of five or six candidates. One was a former registrar of Jackson Burrows who was acting as locum for him at St Albans and two of the others happened to be senior registrars to Reginald Watson Jones of the London and to Philip Wiles of Middlesex and the Royal National Orthopaedic Hospital. It so happened that our own staff and the regional board medical member, Plewes of Luton, favoured a Barts man who had been doing the locum work since Jackson Burrows retired to make way for a younger man. Failing that candidate, Plewes and I favoured Arthur Rushforth, the man eventually appointed, for we had to agree that Rushforth was certainly more experienced than the locum and we were prepared to support him if the others did not favour the Burrows man. In the course of the interviews Wiles, who clearly did not favour Watson Jones's man, kept on asking him why, having avoided military service and worked as a missionary in India during the war, he had decided to return to England afterwards. This clearly upset Watson Jones, so when Wiles's senior registrar (a South African Marxist) came in Watson Jones said, "Mr 'X,' there must be thousands of natives in your home country who need skilled attention; surely you should be working there?" Wiles looked quite furious about this. After interviewing all the candidates the chairman, Sir Fred Messer, a Labour MP, asked if the committee would like to narrow the field by excluding anyone. Wiles and Watson Jones agreed, one proposing and the other seconding the removal of our Barts man. Plewes then recommended exclusion of Wiles's senior registrar; this was promptly seconded by Watson Jones. I then recommended exclusion of Watson Jones's man and this was enthusiastically seconded by Wiles. And so we were left with Rushforth, a highly trained and suitable candidate with a sometimes awkward stutter; he served the hospital faithfully for 35 years. It had been a "hairy" committee, but justice was done.

In marked contrast to the behaviour of those two distinguished orthopaedic surgeons, each of whom had been so bent on excluding their rival's trainee, was that of two senior anaesthetists when we were making a joint consultant anaesthetist appointment between St Albans and Hemel Hempstead hospitals. On this occasion too we had a Barts applicant who was a superb anaesthetist but who had repeatedly failed the examination for the Diploma in Anaesthetics (this was before the FFARCS qualification). The faculty and university assessors were Marston of Guy's and Bernard Johnson of the Middlesex, each of whom had his own trainee among the applicants. Marston, perfectly correctly, said that he did not think that his faculty board would consider it proper if the Barts man was appointed without his diploma. But he was graceful enough to say, "If this man is as good as Mr Murley says, which I have no reason to doubt, then he will surely get his diploma and secure a good job." We therefore reluctantly excluded that candidate – who soon passed his diploma examination and was promptly appointed to a staff job at Barts. By then we were left with four candidates, including Marston and Johnson's own trainees. At that stage, with immaculate good manners, each of these assessors agreed that the remaining candidates were of more or less equal merit and that they thought it only appropriate that the hospital representatives should decide who should be their future colleague. The Hemel representative and I then made the final selection, which the committee confirmed. Experience of those two committees taught me a great deal about the proper and more or less disinterested responsibilities of a college or university assessor.

Between 1950 and 1957 I believe that I applied for seven other surgical appointments and was shortlisted for four of them. There was a vacancy at the Cancer Hospital (now the Royal Marsden) in 1952 for which each candidate had to offer some thirty *printed* applications, such as had generally been *de rigeur* before the NHS. There was a shortlist of five or six and the selection committee was friendly. Peter Greening (three years or more senior to me) was appointed. At about the same time there was a vacancy at St Thomas's and I was one of 36 applicants, every one of whom was interviewed before Marshall Pullen, a local candidate, was appointed.

Heneage Ogilvie (once again friendly with me) was on the committee and later told me that there were so many good candidates that he had thought it unfair to attempt to shortlist them. I had applied for vacancies at Bath (where a man four years my senior was appointed) and the Queen Elizabeth Hospital, Birmingham; but I was not shortlisted for either job. But with large numbers of applicants for both of these posts how could any of us declare that shortlisting was not fair?

But my most notable experience of sheer jiggery-pokery was when I applied for an undergraduate teaching hospital vacancy shortly after my North Middlesex Hospital debacle. The post of assistant surgeon to the Royal Free Hospital was advertised at the time of Rodney Maingot's retirement from the staff. No further details were given in the advertisement or in any other official handout. I was one of more than 30 applicants, each of whom was required to provide many copies of his application. It was made known that applicants should call on members of the medical and surgical staff, such as had been *de rigeur* with most voluntary hospital posts before the NHS. This entailed the expenditure of a certain amount of time by each staff member, and of a great deal more time by the candidates in trying to arrange convenient appointments. I remember a brief encounter with Maingot himself in the car park at the Royal Free, a visit to a paediatrician in Kensington, and various other visits up and down Harley and Wimpole streets. Sir Daniel Davies, then Royal Physician as well as a close friend of Aneurin Bevan, I knew slightly from the Hunterian Society, of which we were both members. I was impressed – as I feel sure his patients were meant to be – by a fine display of royal photographs in silver frames. I certainly cannot recall his precise questions, but I did note with passing curiosity that Maclaggan, one of the ear, nose, and throat surgeons, and the then dean, Dr Katharine Lloyd-Williams, an anaesthetist, asked me whether I had had any experience of neurosurgery. I told each of them that apart from having dealt with a number of penetrating brain wounds when working with the "unholy trinity" during the war I had no special experience. I later learnt from two of the other shortlisted candidates that they had been asked an identical question by the same two staff members.

In due course the day for the official interview arrived. The shortlist consisted of Hugh Lockhart-Mummery of Westminster, Maurice Lunn of Barts, myself, and Radley-Smith of the Royal Free. I give the names in alphabetical order because that is the sequence in which we were seen. I followed Lockhart-Mummery and Lunn and, like them, was interviewed for about 20 minutes. Miss Barry, then senior surgeon, was in the chair, and I noted that every doctor member of that committee was on the Royal Free staff, with the exception of Sir Arthur Porritt, who represented the Royal College of Surgeons. The dean was representing the North West Regional Hospital Board, of which she was a member, and it was curious to see an ear, nose, and throat surgeon (Maclaggan) there. My interview by various members of the committee had proceeded on entirely conventional lines with no odd questions; the chairman, Miss Barry, then asked me if I had any questions. I immediately perceived my chance to expose any possible jiggery-pokery to the only independent member of the committee, so I responded, "Yes, Miss Barry, I do have one question, or rather I have two questions. First, is it the intention of this committee that the individual appointed should be of a particular specialty? Failing that, is it the intention of the medical staff that the successful applicant should develop a particular specialty?" As I completed those questions I looked straight at Arthur Porritt, who was also looking straight at me. There was a perceptible pause before the answer, and I thought I saw Miss Barry give a distinct gulp: "Mr Murley, this is a general surgical vacancy, though, of course, each member of the staff has his or her own surgical hobby."

When I returned to the waiting room Radley-Smith was called in, so for the first time the outside candidates were free to talk. As Radley-Smith left the room Maurice Lunn pointed his thumb towards the door and said, "Of course, he's getting the job." Lockhart-Mummery then added, "I was at a party last night where a member of the Royal Free staff told me that Radley-Smith *had* been appointed." He continued in gently ironic style, "But I had to tell him that the interview for the vacancy was tomorrow!" It was then that they both confirmed that they too had been asked the "neurosurgical" question by Maclaggan and the dean. Maurice Lunn said that he had worked in an army neurosurgical unit in India during the war but had done no peacetime neurosurgery, and Lockhart-Mummery had told them he had no such experience. When I told them the question that I had asked Miss Barry they were much intrigued and wondered what the college assessor might say. Radley-Smith shortly returned to the room and there was a slightly awkward spell as we finished off the almost cold tea and remains of the sandwiches. The four of us then sat there for what seemed an unusually long time while the committee deliberated. Poor Radley-Smith was getting more and more fidgety and discomforted until he suddenly blurted out, "I feel I owe you chaps an explanation: I was invited to put in for this job." Thereupon we all gently reassured him and said that we had indeed already heard that. But still we waited until Miss Barry came to the door and called Radley-Smith in. We were about to go when she returned with Radley-Smith and called me in. On re-entering the room I discerned a tense atmosphere; Miss Barry drew up a chair for me and asked me to sit down. She said, "Mr Murley, I am told by the committee that I owe you an explanation. We are recommending Mr Radley-Smith to the board of governors to develop neurosurgery. But had we been appointing a general surgeon I am asked to tell you that you would certainly have been appointed." I looked hard at Arthur Porritt and could see that he was angry. Of course I should then have said, "In other words Miss Barry you told me deliberate lies in answer to my two questions"; but for once I was lost for words and simply gave her a dignified nod and wave of the head to indicate my astonishment.

"Lynn" Lockhart-Mummery and I then went into a neighbouring pub where we had a couple of pints of beer. The same evening I was telephoned by Arthur Porritt, the official representative of the Royal College of Surgeons, who said that he wanted me to know that he had totally disapproved of the committee's decision and would record his complaint with the president, Sir Cecil Wakeley. He added that he doubted whether it would do much good and he reckoned that I was lucky *not* to be appointed to the staff of a hospital which could behave like that. While we were in the pub Lockhart-Mummery and I had conceived the idea of sending a telegram to the chairman of the board of governors – in those days a convenient method of communication which I often used when sorting out inveterate problems with the Ministry of Health and other organs of bureaucracy. This telegram was duly despatched from my home the same evening:

To chairman, Board of Governors, Royal Free Hospital

Are you satisfied with the recommendations of your advisory appointments committee of today?—Murley.

About three weeks later I received a pompous note from the clerk to the governors:

Dear Mr Murley,

In reply to your telegram, my chairman has directed me to say that he is satisfied with the recommendations of the advisory appointments committee.

It was a shabby and discreditable affair of which that hospital staff should have been ashamed.

On a lighter note, at about that time I also applied for a job at Middlesex Hospital. The advertisement was for an assistant surgeon with proctological interests. I had spent two years as a clinical assistant at St Mark's Hospital – six months with Clifford Naunton Morgan and the remainder with O V ("Ossie") Lloyd-Davies, with whom I had greatly enjoyed working. I first called Clifford, who said he would be pleased to support me. I then telephoned Ossie, who, I had heard, had two or three times been rejected when applying to the Middlesex. I asked him if he would be putting in again. He said, "I have *had* the Middlesex and am certainly not applying; but don't ask me to be a referee as I have already agreed to referee three applicants." I was one of seven or eight shortlisted; two days before the appointments committee

Cliff excitedly telephoned me to say that the Middlesex staff had just invited Lloyd-Davies to put in for the job. The interviews were due to start at 5 o'clock and I had difficulty parking my car. I arrived in the waiting room before 5.30 to find that all the other candidates – who included Lloyd-Davies and at least three of his former St Mark's residents, Cedric Longland of Barts, and Emlyn Williams of Hampstead General – had already been interviewed. I was immediately ushered in to the committee and apologised for being late. I was speedily reassured that I had not kept them waiting. The chairman, Lord Astor, then asked the committee if they had any questions. Not one was asked so he himself then said, "Mr Murley, I see that you were in France during the war." Deeply mystified by this question, I replied, "Yes, sir, among many other places." I wondered whether I had somehow upset the committee but Longland reassured me that every one of them had been whisked in and out in the same way. I am sure that none of us could have disagreed with the committee's recommendation that Lloyd-Davies should get the job. Indeed I am certain that we would all have agreed that if they wanted an expert colorectal surgeon he was by far the best man.

In the late autumn of 1952 Sir Lancelot Barrington-Ward and Mr Frank Saner retired from the staff of the Royal Northern Hospital and a single post was advertised for four sessions a week, including one session at Wood Green Cottage Hospital where Sir Lancelot had also worked. I was on a shortlist of some 10 candidates, once again including Lockhart-Mummery (eventually of St Mark's and St Thomas's) and Emlyn Williams (of Hampstead General which later merged with the Royal Free). I was successful and was delighted to join the staff of this splendid hospital. Originally founded as the Great Northern Hospital in 1856, the Royal Northern had had as distinguished a surgical staff as any London hospital although, like Gordon-Taylor and Mitchiner, a number later left when appointed to posts at undergraduate teaching hospitals. Hamilton Bailey had recently retired because of mental illness, but as junior surgeon I was to share a registrar and houseman with Robert McNeill

Love and Alex Roche on a happy firm. William Gabriel, also of St Mark's, was senior surgeon and he shared a senior registrar and a second house surgeon with Alan Small, a graduate of Otago University, New Zealand. Bill Gabriel was a splendid if somewhat solemn man who wrote me a warm welcoming letter and was always a loyal and conscientious colleague. I counted myself fortunate for we had a splendid *x* ray department, then in charge of Dr L S Carstairs, and an outstanding histopathologist, Dr P M Peters. Although the hospital had not been well known in the past for its physicians we soon came to have a group of four excellent ones: W E (Bill) Clarke, a cardiologist and very much a "doctor's doctor"; Charles Foster Cooper, general physician and gastroenterologist; David Geraint (Gerry) James, outstanding dean and sarcoidosis authority; and C W H Havard, a splendid general physician and first class endocrinologist.

At the beginning of this chapter I referred to one job I was offered without advertisement and it seems appropriate to end with another. A year or two after my appointment at the Royal Northern I was visited by the vice-chancellor of the then newly founded University of Ghana at Accra. He said that they were seeking a suitable individual to become dean of the medical school and professor of surgery. I told him that I did not think it would be practicable for a single person to take on both these responsibilities in a new medical school. I was puzzled that he had come to me for advice. He surprised me by saying that he hoped I would consider the offer. I replied that had he made such an offer a few years earlier I might have been foolish enough to accept, but that, apart from the practical objections I had already raised, I now had a family of five children and, moreover, I would not trust Dr Nkruma (the then president of Ghana) further than I could throw him. The vice-chancellor seemed hurt and responded, "Dr Nkruma is a very fine man." I concluded the interview by saying, "Well, sir, you are entitled to your view and I to mine." Subsequent events in West Africa supported my own assessment of the situation; but it is a sobering thought that had this offer been made a year or two earlier I might have accepted. The Walter Mitty complex is, alas, present in all too many of us and I can think of a number of colleagues who went to similar jobs and got into all sorts of trouble. It was only several years later that I heard how a near contemporary of mine at Barts, Dr Hugh Morgan, then professor of medicine in Khartoum, had been promised the chair of medicine at Accra. After resigning his appointment in Sudan he was informed that the university of Ghana had now decided to appoint an American professor of medicine. Fortunately Hugh's vacancy in Khartoum had not yet been filled so his university reappointed him; but only in the nick of time, for a week later his original appointment would have been filled.

18 Making the health service work

When I started work at the Royal Northern Hospital in January 1953 I was 36 years old and by then I had a maximum part time contract. A year or so earlier my commitment at St Albans had been increased to six sessions, and four sessions were added in the Royal Northern group. My bailiwick included St Albans City Hospital and Napsbury in Hertfordshire, together with the Royal Northern and Wood Green Cottage Hospital in London. Before long I was, each week, seeing as many as 40 new outpatients and coping with four operation lists, including a great deal of major surgery, and it was not unusual for me to dictate and sign a hundred or more letters. I had good medical secretaries in each of my main hospitals and I introduced the same case coding system into my office at the Royal Northern that I had been using at St Albans. This greatly facilitated the retrieval of information for research and for the preparation of the papers I would publish in the ensuing years. When I look back on it all now I am astonished at the amount of work I got through and at the way I thrived on it. Indeed, I was soon to realise the truth of Reggie Payne's 1949 prediction that the "service will be carried on the broad shoulders of the professions."

All the buildings at St Albans were old, except for the prefabricated and hutted outpatient department at the Mid Herts unit, which soon proved far too small, despite the opening of additional clinics for paediatrics and gynaecology at the former county council hospital. But during the first few years of the NHS there had been a radical improvement in both senior and junior staffing of the hospital. I have always thought that this was one of the most important contributions made in the early years of the NHS. It was this improvement that received commendation from my old chief, John Hosford. I, too, having been there for more than a year before the NHS, was in a strong position to recognise the significance of these changes. Whereas Dr Macaulay, as senior administrative medical officer of the North West Metropolitan Regional Hospital Board, was instrumental in helping us in those early years, his influence, and especially that of his successor, steadily diminished. It was because we could take some of our early problems direct to him that a number of teething troubles were overcome. Later on the whole organisation became more and more bureaucratic, as is inevitable when there is only one source of central funding.

The buildings at the Royal Northern Hospital also were old and our operation theatres there were primitive. We did, however, have the St David's private wing. When it was opened, in 1929, it was the first private wing in the country. It originally had 75 private beds, but these were reduced to 50 private and 25 amenity beds shortly after the appointed day. The weekly charge for a private bed was £19.10*s* when I started; but it had risen to more than £750 by 1980, when I retired from the NHS. That wing was open for use by any established consultant in the London area and we never operated a "closed shop" for our own staff. The St David's and University College Hospital private wings were the only NHS ones in London regularly to permit this. Moreover, our own two private theatres often provided a useful overflow facility for some of our general hospital work. The amenity beds, conceived with the NHS and originally costing no more than £1 or £2 a week, were intended to provide the non-private patient with single or double room accommodation.

Both my main hospitals illustrated the supreme importance of having a good medical staff and the lesser importance of the buildings. The slow rate of improvement in both hospitals, however, later proved to be a source of disappointment and this was especially true at the Royal Northern. The political slant of the board was very much to the left, regardless of the party in power. Moreover, there was sometimes prejudice against the former voluntary hospitals, of which we were often especially conscious at the Royal

Northern. Yet had funding of the Royal Northern been related to the amount of work done – assuming an item-of-service insurance basis rather than the annual "blanket" budgeting of nationalised medicine – without doubt we would have gone from strength to strength. The number of outpatients seen, inpatients admitted, operations performed, and the general turnover greatly exceeded that of the former London County Council Archway group on nearby Highgate Hill. In contrast, I had been able to observe the frequently inefficient use of beds in larger hospitals when I worked at the North Middlesex, where some ward sisters tried to keep patients in so that the bed occupancy figures might be increased. My early discharge policy had been unpopular, particularly with my male ward sister there. I stress these points to emphasise that we had already begun to recognise the economic disparities between different parts of the health service. I was in a good position to observe these through working concurrently in several different places. I was also able to see the surprising difference in health patterns of the populations served by my provincial and metropolitan hospitals. But I shall return to this subject later.

My home in Radlett was conveniently placed between my two main hospitals, and the elective work was neatly arranged so that I could make the most expeditious use of both time and resources in each place. I was at St Albans all day on Tuesday for a clinic in the morning and operations in the afternoon; on Thursday morning for a ward round and follow up; and on Friday morning for operations. Sometimes I was there on Friday afternoon or Saturday morning too; however, I was able to switch my locus according to the workload. I did my outpatient clinic at the Royal Northern on Monday afternoon, and it was followed by an evening staff meeting. I operated there on Thursday. I saw private patients at 95 Harley Street on Wednesday morning and then consulted and operated at Wood Green in the afternoon. My private operations were usually done at the Royal Northern on Monday morning and at St Albans on Saturday. The resident staff and registrar at St Albans were free to work with the orthopaedic surgeon on the days when I was in London; likewise, my staff in London worked with McNeill Love or Alex Roche when I was out of town. Not only did all this "slot" in comfortably but our registrars and resident staff enjoyed the experience of working concurrently with different consultants. I was on emergency call on alternate weeks in St Albans and every Thursday and every fourth weekend at the Royal Northern. There was never a dull moment. When we look back on it all now – and by "we" I mean my former registrars and house staff as well as myself – we recognise these as the vintage years of the NHS. Everyone worked with enthusiasm, and pay disputes and militant unionism were unknown. One hates to misuse, or overuse, the word "dedication," but only an organisation with truly dedicated staff could have operated so well under government near monopoly and centralised bureaucracy. Even those of us who had harboured serious doubts about the nationalisation of medicine were puzzled by the seeming smoothness with which the system operated. But, as Reggie Payne had so surely predicted, this was the lull before the storm.

From the family point of view we had settled very happily in Radlett. Our house, in a quiet road, had a pleasant garden and backed on to a nine hole golf course with easy access through our own gate; but it was many years before I took up golf. I still played squash and there was a court at the end of the road. In summer I had an occasional game of tennis at the Goodisons just a few doors away. There I played with Nicholas Goodison, recently chairman of the stock exchange, and with his father and another visitor. Mr Goodison senior rarely introduced anybody, so a little research was often needed to find out who one's partner or opponent might be. By then Daphne and I had a family of four: Susan, now aged 8½, and three of our own children – a daughter and two sons – all of whom had been born at home and delivered by one or other of our two general practitioners between May 1948 and June 1951. Shortly after our arrival in Radlett a kindly neighbour had given us a beautiful labrador-cum-red-setter bitch; she had a happy six years with us before she developed a kidney carcinoma and was put down by the vet. Susan had started school nearby and was usually delivered and fetched on the back of Daphne's bicycle. There was only one problem: with five bedrooms and one used as a study, and with an au pair girl too, we were beginning to fill the house, so that Gavin (b. 21.6.51) had to sleep in the dining room. A few months after Gavin's birth my mother died in a nursing home in Bath where Dr George Kersley was treating her for rheumatoid arthritis.

Because of a lack of suitable pay beds at that time in St Albans I used to admit private patients to Stanboroughs Hydro, a Seventh Day Adventist hospital in nearby Garston. By good fortune I happened to do a prostatectomy on a Radlett man who had lived there for some years. He was a professional photographer of houses and gardens and I asked him to let me know if he should hear of any suitable larger house which we might buy. A few weeks later a large envelope arrived with a small advert pasted in the middle of a card, plus six large photographs of a lovely garden. My patient explained that he knew the house well: it had been converted from two cottages and had great possibilities for further conversion. He had photographed the garden for a gardening magazine and calendar. We inspected the house just after I was appointed at the Royal Northern: the owner, recently widowed, said that it was a family house and that she would like our family to live there. She was a member of the Plymouth Brethren and left a number of biblical texts in the house for our edification. Our first house, bought for £6000 just $5\frac{1}{2}$ years before, was sold for £6250; the new one cost £6800 and the solicitors' charges (Withers & Co) were £237. Those were the days before inflation began to take off.

A year or so after the birth of Jennifer, our first child, Daphne and I had started to take a spring holiday on our own and we continued to do so for a number of years. Each time our old Barts midwife, nurse Wooderson (half-sister of the former world champion one mile runner), would take up residence with our au pair. In April 1953, just before we changed houses, we went to stay at the Poldhu Hotel at Mullion, south Cornwall. One evening, when Daphne was sewing curtains for the new house, we were tickled to learn that the other guests had thought we were a "honeymoon couple." Had they known that Daphne was two months pregnant they might also have thought that there had been a shotgun wedding. We moved house just after our return. I am ashamed to admit that Daphne and the au pair organised the whole thing while I "relaxed at work" as the saying goes. At our new premises we had two acres of garden, plus an acre of wood and dell for which previous owners had paid a "peppercorn" rent. With playing fields behind us and the green belt stretching away to the south it was an ideal spot for both family and professional life. I remember that when I inspected the garden through the back hedge before buying the property I said to myself, "It will give me a coronary." I subsequently survived two.

I soon got to know nearly all the family doctors in St Albans, Harpenden, Radlett, and neighbouring parts; in contrast, one met very few of them in London. In an attempt to improve the situation I sent a letter to each London general practitioner before his patient was admitted for elective operation, telling him of the date of admission and operation and inviting him to visit us. After five years I had persuaded no more than a handful of doctors to call. After two or three years at the Northern, however, in addition to a staff meeting every Monday evening I had organised a regular monthly postgraduate meeting, starting in February 1956. In honour of our most famous physician, who had died in 1955, I suggested that we should call this "The Horder Club." The idea was warmly supported by my colleagues and the Horder family. Thus was instituted a regular function which was well attended by consultants, junior staff, and general practitioners. Our visiting speakers included many outstanding doctors from all over the country and also from abroad. Looking through old programmes I see listed Edward Muir, Richard Doll, Charles Fletcher, Norman Ashton, John Butterfield, John Gillingham, Sheila Sherlock, John Hunt, Donald Ross, Andrew Forrest, Philip Evans, Christopher Booth, Stanley Peart, George Crile Jr, and John Loewenthal – to name but a few.

In the St Albans area I did occasional NHS domiciliary visits with the family doctors – never more than 25 or 30 a year. These provided an opportunity for assessing the more difficult emergency and elderly patients, and for getting to know the general practitioners. Nevertheless, I often felt that it would have been better had the patient been required to make some contribution for this service as a guarantee of responsible use. It was uncommon to be asked to make domiciliary visits in London, but I recall one delightful octogenarian Ulsterman in Haringey who would often skip up and down the stairs ahead of me; he was one of the old school who always handled his generally quite humble patients with great charm. A number of our St Albans area doctors would call on their patients when they were admitted to hospital, and this too gave our resident staff and registrars a chance of getting to know them. Apart from that, it was common for meetings of the local division of the BMA to be held at the hospital, as well as periodic clinical meetings. Later we were able greatly to improve the facilities for these postgraduate meetings at both hospitals. A good feature of St Albans Hospital was that the consultants, registrars, and residents shared a dining room. A valuable exchange of ideas took place there. At the Royal Northern we had a small luncheon room for senior staff close to the residents' dining room. This was before a new communal dining room was built on the top of our remarkable circular ward block. In the 1890s the hospital governors had built a conventional rectangular block as well as this circular ward block to find out which shape would prove more suitable for nurses and patients. The dining room on the top of this circular block was built out of free monies in the 1960s – an example of the limited amount of independent building that was possible after the appointed day.

Since I am here concerned with the subject of making the health service work, it is important to consider the state of general practice in the early years of the health service. Radlett had about 8000 inhabitants when we first moved there and there were three separate practices: a single handed man, two lady doctors, and a three man group. This meant roughly 1500 patients for each doctor in a district where practice had been predominantly private before the NHS. The three man group worked extremely hard and two of the partners told me that they were determined not to let their patients feel that the service was any less good under nationalisation. But I was impressed by the steady build up of demand under the new free-at-the-time system. I recall one occasion when I was taken on a domiciliary visit. Tom Mitchell (who was our own family doctor) explained that the patient, although registered with him on his NHS list, wanted me to see her privately. He accepted that she was entitled to a private domiciliary visit, but said that the health service capitation system was hardly geared to this type of practice. Although he was a conscientious and dedicated doctor, well qualified with an Edinburgh MD and FRCP, he spoke of giving up practice and changing to a medical post with a drug company. He said, "I do not think this is fair for my wife and the children." I did not then know that he was suffering from occasional angina. I saw this same sign of severe stress in a number of other first class family doctors, and I especially remember one in Harpenden and another at Dunmow in Essex. Both the Radlett and the Dunmow general practitioners died from myocardial infarctions within the next few years, but the Harpenden doctor was lucky enough to survive an infarct. I cannot avoid the conclusion that in these highly conscientious doctors all three heart attacks were brought on by stress.

The early years of the health service generally saw more contentment among specialists than general practitioners. Moreover, many senior specialists who had previously worked for an honorarium at voluntary hospitals, or for a relatively low salary at local authority hospitals, found themselves substantially better off, despite the fact that in some instances there was less private practice after the appointed day.

It is no exaggeration that general practitioners were conscripted into the NHS by the threat of loss of compensation for the goodwill of their practices. Most of those in better class areas, some of whom lost much of their former private practice, suffered a substantial fall in income. But many general practitioners in inner urban areas with large lists, and sometimes with lock up premises, were financially better off. Indeed I can recall a number of general practitioners in districts like Dalston and Islington who lived in Hampstead or Highgate and left much of their nightwork to the casualty departments near their practices. That is a problem which will never be properly solved until the patient is in a position to exercise greater consumer choice and pressure. The lot of health service general practitioners in better class areas was to change after the Danckwerts award, the general practitioners' charter, and other later improvements which were skilfully extracted from successive governments of different persuasions by that "trade union" so much admired by Sydney and Beatrice Webb – the BMA. But this was all achieved in the days before the BMA and the Royal College of Nursing came to be classified *de jure* as trade unions. It is especially piquant that the industrial relations legislation which effected this transformation was implemented by a Tory government under the premiership of Edward Heath.

From the point of view of junior trainees, preregistration housemen, senior house officers, and registrars, the wide variety of experience available in regional hospitals gave many of them a built in advantage over the main metropolitan hospitals, where clinical teams gradually narrowed their interests. For anyone who had been working in the hospital service before the appointed day it was fascinating to see the gradual change in the balance between central and peripheral hospitals. In the early days our house staff came from many different places in response to advertisements in the medical press. At that time there was no compulsion to take a house appointment before entering general practice and it was unusual for even quite good hospitals to have more than two or three applicants. Once a full year of compulsory preregistration resident jobs became obligatory the universities were responsible for vetting the regional hospital vacancies. Despite the rich experience available in many such hospitals, and the keenness and ready availability of most consultant staff to do the teaching, some of the early university inspectors were sceptical of the training potential in the regions. Within a few years, however, as a result of the increase in the numbers graduating, it was not unusual for the universities to be pressing us to accept more resident staff than we needed. That was certainly our experience at St Albans. Well before the health service the Royal Northern Hospital, particularly on the surgical side, had always had a magnetic attraction for residents and registrars. Thirty years later more and more of the regional appointments were tied to one or two of the undergraduate teaching hospitals to try to ensure a more orderly appointments system after graduation. At both my hospitals, throughout this period, we were normally in the happy position of acquiring excellent house staff. Furthermore, as our reputation spread through the "grapevine" so the popularity of these appointments increased.

Providing my house staff were keen and hardworking I was never prejudiced about what their ultimate intentions might be. Indeed, I think I was even more interested in those who were targeted on general practice or a physicianly career since there was a greater challenge in helping them to see the relevance and potential of our surgical craft. I recall with benign amusement a number who came to me dead set on a physicianly life who later saw the virtue of being, in Moynihan's words, "a physician condemned to the lifetime practice of surgery." With much improved radiology and pathology services, more expert biochemistry, ready availability of fine needle biopsy and ultrasound techniques, surgery became more and more satisfying in both intellectual and technical content. Gone were the days when, as a surgical dresser, I might see two or three patients listed for "exploratory laparotomy" in a single operating session. Precision in preoperative diagnosis and in "making the patient safe for surgery" – another Moynihan aphorism – rightly became *de rigueur*. Moreover, contrary to the frequent contention that the span of general surgery is steadily shrinking I was able to practise a far more varied range of surgery than most of my former chiefs.

To ensure that my resident staff were quickly and fully instructed in the basic elements of our surgical service I always had each of them supplied with "Notes for guidance" at the time of their appointment. These notes emphasised the importance of keeping careful case records; giving the fullest information possible to patients and relatives; liaising closely with the staffs of the radiology and pathology departments, where possible *discussing* investigations with them – and not forgetting to insert that little word "please" on all requests for investigation; liaising closely with the anaesthetists; exercising economy in ordering special investigations and in prescribing; avoiding the "blunderbuss" use of antibiotics – which should normally only be prescribed after discussion with the registrar or me; writing *promptly* to the general practitioner – preferably before the patient was discharged; and, in the sad event of a death, arranging and attending the necropsy.

An important part of the junior doctors' training in the past had come from the experienced ward sister. Those of my generation have nostalgic memories of the many excellent women who taught us; but with the more rapid turnover of staff, and especially the progressive bureaucratisation of nursing, the experienced senior ward sister has become a rarity. This largely stems from the notorious Salmon report, which created progressive grades of "nursing officer" and gave the highest pay to those in administrative roles – who sometimes wore two piece suits and sat in offices. It is vital that nurses who carry the heaviest clinical responsibilities, whether in the wards, intensive care, recovery, special investigation, or theatre units, should be among the most highly paid. There are now, in 1990, signs of a move in this direction, welcomed by the Royal College of Nursing but bitterly opposed by the more militant trades unions to which, alas, a tiresome minority of nurses now belong.

The registrar training pattern in my two hospitals varied because of the different staffing. At the Royal Northern the appointment shared between two general surgeons and a urologist was highly popular. Alas, one of my later urological colleagues insisted on running his own service and thenceforth never had as good a registrar for urology. At St Albans the registrar was shared with my orthopaedic colleague; the appointment proved exceedingly popular because, in two years, it provided a breadth of experience in what we liked to think of as the "generality of surgery." All of those men have now been appointed to consultant posts, mainly in general surgery, but three are now plastic surgeons and one is a neurosurgeon. Through my wartime spell in plastic units I am convinced of the importance of the basic techniques of plastic surgery in the generality of surgery. Every St Albans registrar was given training in free grafting of skin, in the use of rotation and transposition flaps, and in the principles of neat repair and suturing. It was always fun to assist them with their early work in this field and to show them that 90% of plastic surgery, as indeed of most specialties, is basically simple. Dick Battle, my last distinguished plastic chief during the war, had often irreverently remarked, "Plastic surgery is a technique rather than a specialty." I would often say to my trainees, "If I was capable of doing this at the age of 27 without my final FRCS then you, at the age of 28 *with* the fellowship, can certainly do it at least as well, if not better." My orthopaedic colleague Arthur Rushforth and I always made certain that our trainees were taught how to burr a skull for the evacuation of an extradural clot since experience had shown that when this was not done patients all too often perished on their way to a neurosurgical unit. We only lost one such patient, a woman; although I was available at home on duty a fault in my telephone – which gave an unanswered ringing tone while not in fact ringing – prevented me from being reached in time, so she died on the way to a neurosurgical unit.

My first assistant at St Albans remained a registrar appointment until the day I retired. But at the Royal Northern, in the mid-1970s, I decided to use the services of the senior registrar because of my growing outside commitments at the college of surgeons and the BMA. Our registrars were always hand picked, and as we had no linked appointments for further advancement they knew that their future was in their own hands. We would appoint a British candidate only if we thought he had the ability ultimately to make the grade. In the absence of a British candidate of first rate potential we would select one from the Commonwealth. In fact, I only had three of the latter – one Australian and two New Zealanders – in 34 years. From about the late 1960s the senior registrars at the Royal Northern were joint appointments with the Royal Free Hospital. During my later years I also had senior house surgeons at each hospital; normally they had passed the primary FRCS.

For the latter half of my professional life I had a two theatre facility for operation lists at each hospital and this was an enormous help from the point of view of technical training and supervision. It had been a struggle to get those theatre suites built and, as will later emerge, we did not get all that we needed. The registrars were responsible for case note summaries and, in collaboration with the unit secretary, they maintained our code index of diagnoses and operations, which was fundamental to the easy retrieval of case records for research and other purposes. In each hospital I had been coding my notes for some years before this became part of the record service. But even then we continued our own office index: it was more readily available and often more accurate than the central index. I tried to see the histology slides of all my patients at both hospitals, and we had a regular fortnightly review of pathology specimens and histological sections at St Albans. We made a point of being present at the necropsy of any of our patients who died, and we had regular death reviews at both hospitals from the early 1950s. For our St Albans meetings we often had necropsy reports on more than 80% of those who had died, but the proportion was usually lower at the Royal Northern. I attribute this to the fact that we were generally dealing with a better informed and educated public in the St Albans area. Moreover, because there were no hostel facilities we often admitted former cancer patients for terminal care and their relatives were usually only too ready to help us by giving permission for the examination. By the time of my retirement I had on file some 30 years of these records, of which we had frequently made use in later clinical research. The registrars and house staff took part in regular clinical presentations and educational sessions at the postgraduate centres. For those few registrars at St Albans who did not have the final FRCS, and for the senior house officers, I arranged coaching sessions and set them specimen examination questions. With my unit on duty alternate weeks at St Albans, and with a one in four rota at the Royal Northern, we were always extremely busy. There was never a dull moment. Notwithstanding the inevitably growing frustrations of a nationalised service, the first quarter century of the NHS was challenging and exciting. I often told my staff, "Medicine is a demanding mistress, and few of us should want this otherwise."

19 Travel broadens the mind

Six and a half years of war largely spent in some 14 foreign lands, with friends and foes of many nations, convinced me of the truth of the maxim "Travel broadens the mind." There had been the added bonus of meeting members of my own and of allied professions who I might never have met in peacetime. And so it was to be after the war. I cannot claim, like Robert Louis Stevenson, to "travel for travel's sake." Indeed, since the war I have travelled abroad largely for professional and family reasons. But I have always been happy to return home. It was not always so, for I can remember how unsettled I felt after so long away in the services.

Through not having learnt to ski in my early years, and because I have little intrinsic skill at the sport, I never became one of those surgeon skiers who enjoy regular postgraduate courses in various delectable resorts. But Pontresina provided a fine locus for my honeymoon, and the only ulcer symptoms I ever had – which were brought on by job stress – were relieved by a skiing holiday in Mürren. In 1948 a summer holiday at Dinard with our two daughters had somehow been managed on my then meagre earnings; it had also subjected me to the embarrassing gratitude of one of my wartime amputees, Major Emile Comparot. The day before we returned home we hit a pothole and one torsion bar on our 1946 1½ litre Riley snapped through. But the mechanic at a local garage worked much of the night to fashion and replace the damaged part for no more than £20. It was my praise of this man's efforts that led our freely bilingual hotelier to say that the mechanic displayed *debrouillard* (literally, "clearing the fog"), which he chose to translate as a "capacity for improvisation." Alas, I lack that linguistic equivalent of "perfect pitch" which magically gives certain people the ability rapidly to comprehend words spoken in a foreign tongue. But, having been blessed with a good memory, I have never had much difficulty in storing a vocabulary (sometimes quite large and often quite useless) of foreign words.

During the war I had struggled to learn Palestinian Arabic; made use of what schoolboy French I could remember; gained a smattering of Polish; tried to learn Italian from one of those "made easy" books; and relied on my modern side and science remove German, with some updating. The only serious attack on an unfamiliar language I have made since 1965 was the completion of a Linguaphone course in Portuguese at the time when we began to visit Portugal twice a year. Nevertheless, I am a poor linguist and have mainly confined myself to English. So let me start with my first postwar visit to the United States, from 26 April to 19 July 1955.

I had worked hard at St Albans for eight years and at the Royal Northern for more than two. Dollar exchange problems had frustrated my earlier plans for a year's research in the United States, but I was now determined to shake myself out of the threatening NHS groove; establish North American contacts; study as much as possible of the growing edge of surgery; and, I hoped, return enriched by my travels. Sir Heneage Ogilvie – once again a firm supporter – said, "Reggie, America is too strong meat for some of the younger men. At 37, you are just old enough for it all to be a splendid tonic." Sir Arthur Porritt, strictly more practical, gave me three basic introductions which have served me wonderfully in a life of surgery: George Crile Jr of Cleveland; Howard Gray of the Mayo Clinic; and Englebert Dunphy, then of Boston. Although I had already met Crile at the Hunterian Society in London, and was later to develop a warm friendship with him, it was from these introductions of Arthur's that my strongest American surgical roots and branches developed.

No travel grants were available from the NHS in those days, so on the security of my modest investments my bank manager gave me a £600 overdraft. I booked a cheap passage on a Dutch ship to Boston but, in the event, sailed to New York on the French liner *Liberté*. It was a surprise treat when my father, living in New York, secretly switched my travel to first class both ways; I learnt of this only shortly before my departure. He told me that this might be one of the few opportunities I would ever have of savouring such means of transatlantic travel. How right he was, for I have never since done so. From 2 May I had three weeks in New York at my father and stepmother's apartment on E 74th St, Manhattan. Each morning I usually set off "at sparrowfart" (as we said in the cavalry) to visit the New York hospitals and surgeons with whom I had already made contact. The head and neck, colonic, and breast services at the Memorial Center were my first port of call; I shall not catalogue the names of the many surgeons I met. With Hayes Martin I saw a number of "commando" operations for head and neck cancer; I learnt for the first time of the combined smoking and alcohol connections of pharyngeal and related cancers. At that stage of my career it was invaluable to see a large amount of radical cancer surgery in the colorectal and breast fields, and I was forcibly reminded of the truth of that aphorism "The undergraduate questions are what? and how? but the postgraduate questions should be when? and why?" Having myself abandoned radical mastectomy I was intrigued to meet Frank Adair, who told me that at the time of my visit he had 16 private radical mastectomy patients under his care. I also met and had a spirited argument with Jerome Urban, who was then practising a supraradical breast removal. In this connection I shortly met and made firm friends with C D Haagensen of the Columbia Medical Center; he was another advocate of radical mastectomy and a good friend of my mammary collaborator, Glynn Williams. We politely "begged to differ" on this subject. I was much impressed, however, by Haagensen's utter dedication to his mission, even though I dissented from his philosophy. In striking contrast to Adair, he confessed that he had done only some 16 radical mastectomies, privately, during the past year. He said, "Many of my patients are middle class women of modest means and I tell them to come into the Dellafield [City Cancer hospital alongside Columbia university] where I help my first assistant to do the operation." I saw him do just this. The procedure took five hours and was performed with meticulous care and a routine Thiersch graft. Heneage Ogilvie, in typically irreverent style, had once said to me, "Reggie, is American blood so precious that Haagensen must do the operation so slowly, and then end up with the axilla resembling a plate of caviare with all those little black silk knots?" Heneage was often highly dismissive of American surgery, and especially of its slowness in some centres, but he did advise some of his friends to watch one New York surgeon (whom I did not see) doing an abdominoperineal excision of the rectum in 30 minutes.

Haagensen introduced me to Cecil Loeb, the splendid professor of medicine with whom my brother-in-law, Oliver Garrod, had worked. I met Cornelius Rhoads at the Sloan–Kettering Research Institute, which had been founded in the heyday of profitability of General Motors. I was much impressed by its generous funding. My records show that I attended the bone tumour clinic at the Memorial Center and the general, neurosurgical, and endocrine services at the New York Hospital. The professor of surgery at the latter, Frank Glenn, said they had so many private and semi-private patients that it was difficult to give adequate surgical training. He asked whether I had the same problem and was surprised when I told him that 95% of British patients seemed quite happy to sign a consent form which specified: "I understand that no undertaking has been given that this operation will be performed by a particular surgeon." I had not previously realised what advantages we had under the NHS from the surgical training point of view. As the late Arthur Dickson Wright was wont to say, "In days gone by people like me used to go abroad to practise on their natives, but now the foreign doctors come here to practise on ours!"

I squeezed in a lot of sightseeing in New York, especially at the weekends, and my father and stepmother entertained me at a number of fine restaurants. After a boat trip round Manhattan Island with an Irish guide who had kissed the Blarney stone, my stepmother, herself a New Yorker, said that I knew more useless things about the city than she had picked up in a lifetime. The only money I spent in those three weeks went on street cars and boat trips. Towards the end of May I moved to Boston where I had some excellent digs in Symphony Street with an elderly couple, the McAllisters, who had been highly recommended to me by Howard Eddey of Melbourne. He and his wife stayed there a few weeks after me. As an economy measure I limited myself to light breakfast in a drug store and a good evening meal. My visits were mainly to Massachusetts General, Peter Bent Brigham, and the hospitals of the Lahey Clinic, at each of which I had one or more contacts. I watched a lot of vascular, thyroid, pancreatic, and biliary surgery and, after seeing Dick Cattell do three common duct repairs in 24 hours, I felt that I had picked up many useful tips. My visit was only a year or so after Cattell had repaired Anthony Eden's common duct. Contrary to what was sometimes said in England, he told one of us that this had been a difficult repair because a considerable length of common bile duct had been removed at the first operation. I enjoyed much hospitality in and around Boston with Ed Hamlyn of the Massachusetts General Hospital; Rich Warren of Peter Bent Brigham; and Ruth Meehan, Professor Churchill's secretary, who was a good friend of John and Kathleen Kinmonth. When my old school friend John Kinmonth died in 1982 Kathleen married Rich, who had been widowed about a year before. Indeed the Warren and Kinmonth families both had cottages in County Cork for many years and shared a Block Island fibreglass yawl for ocean cruising.

I did all but one of my intercity journeys by train, mainly because I saw more of the country that way. On 5 June I took the train to Rochester, Minnesota. I arrived in the evening and was warmly greeted by Howard ("Howdie") Gray and made a welcome house guest for the next two weeks. The Grays already had Bob Horton (ex-Guy's) from Bristol with them. We were shortly joined by Ian and Eleanor Fraser of Belfast and then by Lawrence Abel's son Keith. Howdie and Wint (real name de Weenta) were charming hosts, strongly Anglophile and always befriending British visitors. We had early breakfast on the lawn each day and returned to a splendid dinner (with no alcohol) each evening. Howdie was a Baptist, and grace was always said with the company holding hands around the table. At the first meal I was caught unawares and was surprised by the hands on each side of me. After grace Howdie would tuck his table napkin around his neck and start telling one of his many amusing stories.

Bob Horton and I did a good deal of joint visiting and saw an immense range of surgery done by Howdie Gray, Jim Clagett, John Kirklin, Waltman Walters, and John Waugh. These were the very early days of open cardiac surgery and I saw Kirklin repair three atrial septal defects by the old "well" technique. By present standards the method was primitive – but it was remarkably safe in Kirklin's hands. Cardiopulmonary bypass had only just been started, but a day or two later we saw Kirklin do his sixth operation by this technique. The patient was a 15 month old baby with ventricular septal defect and weighing only 15 pounds. Although bypass work had begun elsewhere in the United States, it was a great experience to see this early use of the huge (by present day standards) Mayo–Gibbon pump. When I inspected this machine afterwards with Kirklin I remarked on how simple the design was. John was greatly pleased and said that he got tired of people who said they thought the pump was complex. Kirklin, the son of a Mayo radiologist, had been selected for cardiac training and then returned to the Mayo to start the open heart surgery there. He built a considerable reputation in this field and later moved to Birmingham, Alabama.

I was enormously impressed by the all round work at the Mayo. The technical standard of the surgery was no better than the best I had seen in Britain, but the back up for research, records, interspecialty consultation, and postgraduate education and training was superb. I recall that the surgical science building had far better animal operation rooms than we then had in most British hospitals for human surgery. Howdie introduced me to a number of the physicians, including Philip Hench, then a recent Nobel prizewinner in medicine. I had been keen to meet Berkson, their medical statistician, because I knew of him from my earlier breast research with Williams and Curwen. But I was not greatly impressed, firstly, because he dismissed the recently published work of Doll and Bradford Hill, saying that he did not accept that carcinoma of the lung was related to smoking; secondly, because he supported, and the Mayo still practised, radical mastectomy. I chaffed him about his views on both subjects and particularly chided him about lung cancer. When I jokingly suggested that he must be in the pay of the cigarette manufacturers he cheerfully responded, "Sure, you could be right. That chap leaving my office as you came in was from one of the tobacco companies." Another disappointment for me at the Mayo at that time was the thyroid surgery, mainly done by a man called Black. As the resection of each lobe was completed we were astonished to see the patient woken from light anaesthesia and made to phonate to prove that the recurrent laryngeal nerve was intact. Apart from these two points I was impressed by the high standards, as well as by the all round efficiency and humanity of the clinic.

One weekend at Rochester Howdie and Wint took the Frasers, Bob Horton, and me for a weekend trip on the Mississippi. We set out from Lake City in their large two engined cabin craft and moored in their favourite backwater for the night. Just before the evening meal we found that the dinghy had come adrift and was nestling in some rushes. I offered to dive in and collect it, but Howdie said, "Hold it, we'll just power her over to the side." He started one engine and we moved to the dinghy. I picked up the nylon painter and made her fast. Howdie said, "I hope that's a good knot, Reggie." "It's a fisherman's bend," I replied. When we retired after dinner Bob Horton and I slept on two bunks beneath the forward hatch; the two couples were in the after cabins. I quickly fell asleep but, after a rich meal, I had a vivid "falling" nightmare that I had often experienced in childhood. This time, however, I was in a dinghy which was hanging vertically from the stern of an airborne boat. I saw the painter rapidly slipping from where it was secured to the parent boat, and as the dinghy fell I kicked out sharply with both feet against the bulkhead. The loud thump woke everyone aboard. Bob, in the lower bunk, and Howdie, from the next cabin, called out, "Are you OK?" I laughed and told them of my dream. There were a few chuckles about this at breakfast but the incident was soon forgotten as we returned to Rochester the following evening. A day or two later, after a fortnight of the most wonderful hospitality and kindness I have ever experienced from two complete strangers, Wint dropped me at the station for the next stage of my trip.

I took the train from Rochester to Chicago, where I arrived at 8 in the evening to have dinner with my old friend Richard Terry and Elizabeth, his wife. He was one of those old Barts friends who had joined the Territorial Army with me before the war. He had been determined to accept only a London teaching hospital medical consultant appointment; and because he was disappointed at his lack of progress towards this goal he had moved to Chicago. Although he had already been qualified for 14 years, on arrival there he had to do one year of residencies before getting registered. He told me that he had never enjoyed anything more than going back to surgical and obstetric residencies with the advantage of his experience as a physician. He was a superb clinician and an outstanding teacher and we were all sorry when he left England. Owing to the warmth of Richard and Elizabeth's hospitality, and some delay in getting to the station, I only just caught my train to Toronto, shortly after midnight. Sadly, this was the last time I saw Richard alive. He died only a few years later after perforating a carcinoma of the stomach.

I was due to give a paper on breast carcinoma at the combined meeting of the British and Canadian medical associations in Toronto, and earn a few pounds reporting the surgical section meeting for the *BMJ*. My old friend Hal Slemon met me at the station. He had, of course, been a neurosurgeon in the RAMC with me but was now a general surgeon at Toronto Western Hospital. He had kindly agreed to accommodate my brother-in-law, Alistair Frazer, and me for the meeting, which lasted three days. I spent a further week there visiting Toronto General Hospital and the Children's Hospital; and I paid a brief call to our former neighbours in Radlett who had emigrated less than a year before. I also had the pleasure of meeting Professor McKinnon, a medical statistician, who had upset many of his North American colleagues by pointing out that the precise method of treatment for breast carcinoma did not affect survival. He was absolutely right, but his views were far from welcome at that time.

Towards the end of June, after 10 days in Toronto, I took a plane to Cleveland. It was the only internal flight I made during my three month tour. I had been booked into a cheap hotel by Fiorindo Simeone. George Crile, whom I had met before in London only briefly, called on me the next morning and said, "Reggie, this place looks like a brothel. Why don't you come and stay with Jane and me while you're in Cleveland?" Thus began a close and cordial friendship which has lasted to the present day. We had lengthy discussions on breast carcinoma and innumerable other surgical subjects. I was made welcome at the Cleveland Clinic, where the standard of work impressed me just as much as that at the Mayo. Moreover, the Cleveland Clinic had its own hospital beds in a composite set up whereas the Mayo had that ingenious competitive arrangement of beds in both St Mary's Roman Catholic and the Methodist hospitals. Apart from the wide range of general operative surgery which I watched, I was especially interested to see their arterial bank and the excellent peripheral vascular work then being done by Dr Humphries. I was also impressed to see Dr Kolf at work with his earliest artificial kidney. The clinic was giving free treatment to a poor negro who had been transferred from a downtown hospital.

There was a heatwave for much of my time in Cleveland and on 6 July I entrained for New York, spending two days at my father's apartment before visiting Charlottesville, Virginia, for three days with Douglas and Molly Nicoll. I boarded the train at Pennsylvania station for a journey through Philadelphia and Baltimore. I noticed that everyone in the carriage was black and assumed this to be common when travelling to the "deep south." Molly met me at Charlottesville and said, "Oh, I couldn't see you at first. Were you in the black section?" I had not realised that they still had racial segregation on the trains. Douglas and I, contemporaries at Barts, had been born on the same day. He had worked for a while with me at St Albans after the war. One day, during an orthopaedic meeting in London, a visiting American orthopaedic surgeon said, "Dr Nicoll, we could do with you in the States." So he emigrated and never looked back. He had a splendid department at the University of Virginia Hospital, attached to Jefferson's old university, and he lived at the charmingly named Whippoorwhill Farm, some miles outside Charlottesville. Indeed, I had noticed his postbox on a pillar some miles from his home, where it was strategically placed to ensure that his postal address was within the required 10 mile range of the hospital. This was a high pressure social and professional visit in extremely humid weather. The house was hit by lightning three times on the first evening and the lights were fused for several hours. Dougie and Molly were both mad about horses, and I found that the stable was rather larger than the house.

I spent one night with the Haagensens in their lovely house at Englewood, New Jersey, overlooking the Hudson River on the other side of the George Washington bridge. I was back in my father's New York apartment the next morning, 11 July. As generous hospitality had left me with more of my £600 than I had anticipated I went on a shopping spree. At Tiffany's I bought a brooch for Daphne and at Macy's some toys for the children (two boys and three girls by then). I gave my father a parting present of Churchill's war speeches, after a splendid dinner with him and Irene at one of their favourite restaurants. The next morning my father and Irene whisked me down to the quayside to board the *Ile de France* for a luxurious trip home, and the gain of another five pounds in weight.

At 37 I had experienced what was, perhaps, the most rewarding professional trip of my life. I had made many new friends, renewed some valuable old friendships, and acquired a vast amount of valuable knowledge. Had I spent a year doing research in the States, like Oliver Garrod during his Rockefeller scholarship, I would have had only the last month for travelling. Like him, I would probably have spent the time sightseeing and could never have learnt anything like so much as I did in my concentrated three month tour. As Heneage said, I had gone at the right time and America had not proved "too strong meat" for me. It gave me a vision of the "growing edge of surgery" which has remained with me throughout my working life. My work at the Royal Northern had been covered by a senior registrar and that at St Albans had been ably looked after by Hugh Lockhart-Mummery, who was then still awaiting his first consultant appointment. I had not worried about the loss of private practice; and although I had received no grant towards my travelling and other expenses my NHS salary had continued as paid study and ordinary leave. For that I was certainly grateful.

Only a few weeks later we were on holiday with our children at West Wittering when Arthur Porritt telephoned to say that Howard Gray had just been drowned. We later learnt that to celebrate Wint's birthday Howdie and Wint had taken a weekend boat trip on the Mississippi; they moored at the same place as they did when I was with them. As before, the dinghy came adrift. This time Howdie did not start the engine; instead he dived in. Seconds passed, and then minutes, and still he had not reappeared. Wint thought at first that he might be playing a trick on her. Then, desperate, she realised that he really had disappeared. She had never handled their large cruiser on her own before, but she took it back to Lake City. There she met a Mayo physician, Hermann Moersch, and his wife. They returned with her to the mooring place; but Howdie was not found until the next day. It was never certain whether he had drowned through being caught by some underwater vegetation or whether he had had a heart attack. His death, at the age of 54, was a great loss for the Mayo. Moreover, it was a sad loss for surgical visitors worldwide and especially those from the United Kingdom. But at the Royal College of Surgeons of England we now have a unique memorial to him. His British friends and his Mayo colleagues subscribed for the purchase of furniture and many finely bound books of reference, historical works, and encyclopaedias which now grace the Howard Gray Library in our Nuffield residential college. And on a wooden lectern there is a large "Father Brown" bible, which Wint herself donated. Some might wish to attach a supernatural quality to my Mississippi dream, but I am entirely unsuperstitious. Nylon painters have a reputation for slipping and I rather fancy that

Howdie's nautical knots may not have been as secure as his surgical ones. During the last 30 years I have spent many profitable hours reading and writing in the Howard Gray Library.

My next overseas professional visit, this time with Daphne, was to New Orleans, Houston, and Jamaica in January 1962. Although I had been invited to join one of the large surgical travelling clubs a few years earlier I had not accepted. For, with growing family and professional commitments in both the NHS and private practice, I had thought it too difficult to eke out the time and find the money for regular trips with the same group of colleagues. Perhaps too, though gregarious, I am not one of the "clubbable" types who likes to mix too often with the same people. But there was a loose knit group, going by the name of the Ambroise Paré Club, which required no regular commitment. It was organised by a surgeon, Maurice Lee, and a dental surgeon, John Bunyan (a proud and charmingly eccentric descendant of the author of *Pilgrim's Progress*). They had decided that it would be good for relationships with our West Indian colleagues if some surgeons from the home country supported a meeting of the Association of Surgeons of Jamaica. It was a good thought and proved to be a happy occasion, organised by Maurice Lee and led by Arthur Dickson Wright, who was then a vice-president of the Royal College of Surgeons. To widen the scope of our visit Maurice had arranged for us to spend a few days in the southern United States. We had two days in New Orleans. There we visited the Ochsner Clinic and Professor Oscar Creech's Tulane University unit at the Charity Hospital. The contrast between the huge municipal hospital (3500 beds), with a relatively impersonal service, and the highly personal and consumer oriented private clinic was striking. I was astonished at the amount of vascular surgery being done in the Charity Hospital, and equally astonished by the fact that when patients were undergoing surgery at the Ochsner Clinic their relatives, seated in a comfortable visitors' lounge, were kept informed every 15 minutes of the progress of the operation. When I questioned Alton Ochsner himself on whether this was desirable or necessary he promptly replied,

"Well, the relatives certainly seem to appreciate it."

On our last evening in New Orleans there was a delightful buffet supper party at Alton Ochsner's house, where we were joined by his sons and grandchildren. Dickson Wright could be a variable after dinner speaker, but on that occasion he made one of the funniest speeches I have ever heard him produce. After an opening reference to nationalised medicine, he introduced us as "eight poor civil servants with only three wives between us." He declared that our two nations might understand each other better "but for the language barrier," and then went on to give several entertaining examples of the totally different meaning of the same words on opposite sides of the Atlantic. When he was being served with cold chicken that very evening he had asked for "some leg and a bit of breast" and his hostess had said "Mr Wright, in the States we call that 'the white meat'." We were due to leave early the next day, and while settling our accounts we spotted Dickson Wright chuckling merrily to himself at a neighbouring counter. He had just bought a magnificent orchid for Mrs Ochsner and was writing a note for attachment thereto: "Pin this on your white meat – or where you like!"

We moved on for another hectically busy two days at Houston, chiefly to visit Michael de Bakey and Denton Cooley, who were then still (just!) on speaking terms, and their colleagues George Morris and Arthur Beall. There was an abundance of vascular surgery going on and a fair amount of cardiac work, but it was little compared with the immense cardiac throughput of later years. From the point of view of vascular surgical technique this visit was of great value, but I thought that the indications for some of the procedures were rather different from generally accepted British practice. There are two sides to this equation, however, and one must always allow for the fact that American patients tend to be more enthusiastic about surgery than their British counterparts. We were given a rich feast of short papers delivered by different members of the group. It mattered little whether one agreed with every detail, for the sheer variety and exciting pace of the vascular work there were immensely stimulating for those of us accustomed to the more staid and less thrusting conditions at home. It was only shortly before our visit that Cooley had undertaken what was then believed to be the first successful pulmonary embolectomy on cardiopulmonary bypass. With typical American enterprise the whole procedure had been filmed. Denton said that the most difficult part had been getting the medical photographer out of his bed in the middle of the night. From the time when I first saw the heart and lung machine used at the Mayo in 1955 I had been looking forward to the day when we might successfully salvage some of our patients with massive pulmonary embolism. So, on my return home, I reviewed all the pulmonary emboli recorded from 10 years of our "death" meetings at St Albans and then evolved an appropriate strategy. It was from this work that we were able to contribute three of the earliest successful pulmonary embolectomies on bypass in the Brompton Hospital series. Ultimately, with the introduction of the thrombolytic drugs, it became possible to salvage many of these patients by what I called "medical embolectomy." I cite this as but one example of the many ways in which a visit to the United States never failed to stimulate me or reawaken my interest in a variety of subjects.

We spent our last afternoon in Houston visiting the MD Anderson Cancer Hospital. This was well designed and, like the other hospitals on the Houston campus, a relatively small institution. It was interesting to hear that it had been decided to model the set up on our own Cancer Hospital (now the Royal Marsden) with joint surgical and radiotherapeutic clinics.

After those lively few days in New Orleans and Houston we moved on to the warm and balmy climate of Jamaica where we were made welcome by our black and white West Indian hosts. The surgical meeting was held in the sumptuous Marrakesh Hotel at Ocho Rios, where we stayed for three days. Professor Walter Mackenzie of Edmonton, Alberta, was there as Arthur Sims commonwealth travelling professor. I was one of several who contributed surgical papers, and we had an enjoyable time before moving on to the University College Hospital at Kingston. There Daphne and I stayed with Peter and Anne Weston. Peter, one of the lecturers in surgery, had been John Hosford's house surgeon at Hill End shortly after my return from the war. I was lucky enough to have two English former gastrectomy patients on the island, with whom Daphne and I enjoyed some special hospitality. I had operated on them at the Royal Northern within the previous two years and was pleased to see them both well nourished and consuming normal food. On our last day at Ocho Rios we had an early morning swim in the Caribbean. That same evening we landed in New York, with the streets deep in snow, and enjoyed the hospitality of my father and stepmother for two days.

My stepdaughter, Susan, then 19, had left for Canada shortly before our departure, but we had five other youngsters, aged between 5 and 14 years, still at home. The only way we managed to absent ourselves for such trips was usually by calling upon the services of the admirable and indefatigable Nurse Wooderson, who, together with our many au pair girls from a variety of nations, always held the fort, whether for our spring holiday or the occasional professional visit. For this particular trip Nurse Wooderson was not available and so we had another lady to stand in with the au pair. When we look back on it all now we can but marvel at our good fortune in being able to rely on such excellent support.

But I have omitted one vital part of the story of this overseas visit. On the morning we were due to depart our fifth child, Hilary, then aged 8, had her first epileptic fit. We were in two minds about what we should do: whether to go ahead with seeming insouciance or cancel everything and possibly create more tension. It was decided for us by Douglas Saunders, our splendid family doctor for many years. Having seen Hilary and administered a sedative, he firmly advised us to carry on. All was well until shortly after our return, when there was a second fit. Hilary's godfather, my contemporary John Gillingham, a distinguished neurosurgeon and professor of neurological surgery in Edinburgh, had given us valuable and optimistic advice a few years earlier when her mental handicap was first recognised. After the diagnosis of epilepsy had been confirmed, and appropriate treatment had started, John suggested that Dr Desmond Pond should see Hilary, and this he did. Desmond, a distinguished psychiatrist and later president of the Royal College of Psychiatrists, had done some early work on epilepsy and electroencephalography. Many years later, only two years before his death, and when he had recently been knighted, Desmond and Helen Pond came to lunch with us and met Hilary again. They were greatly impressed by the progress she had made despite her mental handicap. By then she was aged 30 and had been on phenobarbitone and epanutin treatment for 22 years. In the meantime she had managed to hold down a part time job and had become a moderately competent skier both on snow and water. Happily, there have been no fits for many years.

My innumerable later overseas visits to many parts of the world, whenever possible accompanied by Daphne, have brought immense pleasure and cemented many friendships. But it was those earlier trips, at a younger and more impressionable age, that helped to teach me how best to utilise my time and energy.

20 The Fellowship for Freedom in Medicine

After the meeting at the Royal College of Surgeons in April 1948 it became clear that there were to be no amendments to the 1946 Act before the appointed day. In June Lord Horder sent letters to the *Lancet* and the *BMJ* inviting the views of any who were concerned about the practice of medicine in this country following the collapse of the BMA's resistance to the unamended National Health Service Act. The response to that invitation was unexpectedly prompt and large. At first letters came from those who had not joined the service, but these were soon followed by a growing number from those who were in fact working in the NHS. Horder nominated six colleagues, three general practitioners and three specialists, to analyse the replies with the help of a small staff.

A month or so after the appointed day, in the late summer of 1948, I was invited to join a small group for dinner in an upstairs dining room at the Etoile restaurant in Charlotte Street. Apart from Lord Horder, the company included Dr Reginald Hale-White, Mr Reginald Payne, Dr George Rossdale, and Dr E C Warner, then dean of Charing Cross Hospital Medical School. I believe that one or two others were present, but I cannot now remember who they were. Our task was to devise a suitable name for our new organisation before holding an inaugural meeting. Fellowship of Freedom for Medicine? Fellowship of Freedom in Medicine? Fellowship for Freedom of Medicine? All of these and a few others were discussed, but Tommy Horder soon persuaded us that it must be the Fellowship for Freedom in Medicine. Only in this way was the message accurately conveyed that our concern was for the freedom of both doctor and patient within their very special relationship.

And so, as the letters continued to roll in, the name of the new body was decided. The response became so overwhelming that a further six doctors from specialist and general practice, including representatives from the provinces, were added to the group to deal with the replies and to ensure that they were acknowledged. An inaugural meeting was held at Caxton Hall on 13 November 1948 and I was among the 700 doctors present. They had come from all over the country and were a representative cross section of each branch of the profession. More than 1700 had by then sent letters of support.

In a sober and stirring speech Horder told the meeting of the remarkable response to his letters of invitation. Having referred to the Special Representative Meeting of the BMA, which had thrown away its last chance to resist the dragooning of the profession, he went on to say:

> It is nearly four years ago that I began to utter warnings about the inevitable consequences of a successful attempt to nationalise Medicine. This was in an address to the Cardiff Medical Society. I have been persistently and, I fear, tiresomely speaking my mind on the matter ever since. The Minister of Health – speaking to a mutual friend – called me an "incontinent romanticist." I have pleaded guilty to the adjective (speaking, of course, figuratively) but, as I prophesied, events have proved that the substantive should have been "realist."

He ended his address:

> I am still an optimist. This meeting inspires me. We who are here are the custodians of Medicine for our patients. Let us look to our charge. At this moment it needs all our vigilance and all our care.

At that inaugural meeting certain resolutions were discussed and passed:

> (i) That as this body is deeply disturbed by the way outside influences may affect the quality of Medicine in this country, it is determined to do everything in its power to render the highest standards of practice possible in the future.

That was proposed by Dr Lindsay W Batten, a distinguished

private doctor in Hampstead, and seconded by Dr A C E Breach of Orpington.

(ii) That this Fellowship is not in opposition to any other existing medical organisation, but is ready to further any efforts they may make towards the maintenance of medical freedom.

This was put from the chair by Horder and seconded by Dr A V Russell of Wolverhampton.

An executive committee was appointed with instructions to

1 Draft a constitution for the Fellowship;
2 make it known to the profession that this body now exists as an independent organisation, determined to work for a high standard of medical practice and for the freedom of the profession as being in the best interests of Medicine;
3 examine anomalies which have arisen in medical practice as a result of the National Health Service Act; and
4 analyse all constructive suggestions received from its members.

The meeting authorised an executive of 20 members as follows: Lord Horder (chairman), Dr R Hale-White (vice-chairman), Reginald Payne (treasurer), with Drs G H Rossdale and E C Warner as honorary secretaries. The initial nominations for the executive were Dr Barbara Abercrombie (Liverpool), Dr A C E Breach (Orpington), Dr S F L Dahne (Reading), Dr D R Goodfellow (Manchester), Dr G M Goodwille (Attleborough), Dr A V Russell (Wolverhampton), Mr Campbell Shaw (Bournemouth), and Professor K D Wilkinson (Birmingham). All this and much more is recorded in Bulletin no 1 of the Fellowship for Freedom in Medicine, published in November 1948.

Shortly after the meeting I was invited to join the executive together with Mr Norman Lake of Charing Cross Hospital and Etherington-Wilson of Torquay. This was recorded in Bulletin no 2 of January 1949. I was then just 32 years old and in my second year as a surgical chief assistant at Barts. Many members of the staff there, as former junior colleagues of Horder's, had joined the fellowship and I was not then aware of any antipathy to me because I had nailed my colours to the mast even before the appointed day.

Bulletin no 2 included a list of the five objectives which had been carefully thrashed out at the first meeting of the executive which I attended. These were:

1 To insist upon the preservation of the highest standards of medical practice.
2 To protect the public and the medical profession from State Monopoly in Medicine.
3 To preserve the ethical and professional freedom of the individual doctor in the service of his patients and to maintain the status of the general practitioner, including his financial security.
4 To oppose all encroachments by the State on the independence of medical educational institutions and to maintain the academic freedom of all teachers of Medicine.
5 To define the limits of State Medicine so as to protect the rights of the public and of the medical profession in relation to all types of independent practice.

To these was later added a sixth: to support and protect the character, status, and interests of the medical profession generally.

The executive met fortnightly for several months and then settled down to a monthly routine, but the formation of an amending acts committee meant much additional work for some of us.

A second general meeting was held at Caxton Hall on 19 February 1949 with about 500 present. By then the membership had risen to 2340, and from a temporary address in Westminster Palace Gardens our offices had moved to 45 Nottingham Terrace on the south side of Marylebone Road. There we had two large comfortable rooms and our office affairs were in the capable hands of Miss Cynthia Sharvelle, then working as Teddie Warner's private secretary but willingly doubling up for us. She was shortly joined by one of her friends, Miss Maccormac, and the organisation was well served by these two industrious ladies.

One vital early task was to prepare an account of the events leading up to the nationalisation of medicine while those events were still fresh in our memories. This work was suggested by Horder at one of the first executive meetings and wisely allocated to Dr A C E Breach, who did the most thorough research. The script was checked by our lawyers and the account was eventually published in August 1951. The following is a short extract from the preface to *The Medical Surrender* (July 1948).

The account which follows of the events leading up to the nationalisation of medicine in this country was prepared in the latter part of 1948 while these events were fresh in the memory of those who shared them. It was intended to compile an historical record that could be available for reference. Certain names appear more frequently than others, but the account has been written objectively and with no personal bias.

In response to many requests from our members we have now decided, with a sense of due responsibility, to make the record available, especially as it appears that the profession is likely to face a new crisis in the near future. Many of those on whom the onus of leadership rested in 1948 have left the stage; their places have been taken by others who had little share in the doings of those tragic days. It is to these new leaders in particular that we offer this record, that it may be a warning to them, and help them to avoid the pitfalls into which their predecessors stumbled.

I am often filled with nostalgia as I look back on those days. I had never worked with Lord Horder as a student because he retired from the staff when I was still in my preclinical years. But I now had an opportunity to get to know him well. He was an excellent chairman for a lively and pretty independent minded group of people. Born on 7 January 1871, Thomas Jeeves Horder was already 77 by the appointed day, but he was in full possession of all his faculties with an ever ready twinkle in his eye. A few of his detractors suggested that he had only created the fellowship because he aspired to presidency of the Royal College of Physicians. But that is nonsense. Whatever ambitions he may have harboured in that direction in prewar days he certainly had no ambition to take over from "Corkscrew Charlie," as he cheerfully labelled Lord Moran of Manton, the then incumbent. Furthermore, if any effective political action was to be taken in regard to the NHS this was clearly not a task for anyone to undertake from within the royal colleges.

Quite apart from the contact with Horder, I was fascinated

to be able to sharpen my wits on such an interesting cross section of our profession from both general practice and the specialties. Reggie Payne I had come to know well from our earlier activities at the college of surgeons, and later I was to rent a consulting room just above his at 95 Harley Street. He was a man of utter integrity and an excellent surgeon, as I have described in chapter 14. But he was such a powerful individualist, and so strongly opposed to the whole idea of nationalised medicine, that he resigned from the executive a year later though remaining a loyal member of the fellowship until his death in 1967. We fully respected Reggie's decision but deeply regretted his loss from the inner circle. Edward Warner, a physician at Charing Cross, was our overserious and incredibly conscientious honorary secretary. He had little sense of humour, but he set us all a great example by his industry and integrity, and I was to spend many hours with him drafting evidence for various investigating committees in the early years of the service. George Rossdale remained in purely private practice in Montagu Square until he died in his 90s. He had neither need nor cause to join the service since, so far as I am aware, he had never had any pre-NHS national insurance "panel" patients. I do not think that we had any other solely private general practitioners on the executive, apart from G J V Crosby (who had commanded one of our sister field ambulances at City Road barracks in 1939); Bill Russell of Northwood; George Rettie of London; and Patrick Wood of Ipswich, who joined the executive a few years later, eventually to be chairman. As for our membership, nearly all were working part time or whole time in the service. So much for those who labelled us as a group of private doctors hell bent on destroying the NHS.

Barbara Abercrombie did general practice and ear, nose, and throat work in Liverpool, as did Logan Dahne in Reading. A C E Breach was an excellent family doctor in Orpington who had previously trained as an engineer. He served the executive faithfully for several years and retired early from health service practice to return to marine engineering with his son. Indeed I was surprised to meet him demonstrating on his stand in the Boat Show at Olympia some years later. Victor

Russell was a splendid general practitioner in Wolverhampton; C E ("Teddie") Beare was a stalwart and ever youthful general practitioner surgeon in Dorking, and he survives to the present time. We were soon joined by Dr C E Courtney, a charming family doctor from Westbury-on-Trym, Bristol, who loved to exchange gardening news over dinner with Tommy Horder. Ronald Gibson of Winchester, later to be chairman of council of the BMA and a chief architect of the important general practitioners' charter, was also a relatively early member of the executive, but he became too preoccupied with BMA business. In this connection it is important to record that many fellowship members held positions of high trust and responsibility in the BMA, so much so that Derek Stevenson, one time BMA secretary, and Hugh Clegg, the *BMJ* editor, often said that if the fellowship had not existed it would have been necessary to invent it.

The surgical members of our executive, apart from Payne, Lake, Etherington-Wilson, and myself, later included Wylie McKissock (neurosurgeon) for a short time; A J Gardham of University College Hospital; Nils Eckhoff of Guy's; and my old contemporary C A Jackson, by then a thoracic surgeon at Harefield and related hospitals. Norman Lake had a fine intellect and Geoffrey Hadfield, professor of pathology at Barts, once told me that Lake should have been offered a chair of surgery. He was an excellent technician who did safe gastrectomies for peptic ulcer in the early days of that procedure, when he made much use of spinal anaesthesia. He was a capable precision engineer, and a precise exponent of the English language. He was not easy to get to know but was a man of great integrity with whom I was privileged to be associated. Etherington-Wilson, a Barts man, had been the first doctor in Torquay to confine himself to surgery. He had been a pioneer of light spinal anaesthesia and said that this had enabled him to do much improved abdominal surgery when there were few skilled anaesthetists available. He remarked to me in 1949 how absurd it was that, with his NHS salary added to private practice, he had doubled his earnings. Kenneth Owen of St Mary's, St Peter's, and the Royal Northern hospitals was a valuable surgical member of the executive for several years. Patrick Wood, the son of a fine family doctor in Hornsey who often called in at my Royal Northern clinics, had started in the NHS but then made a bold move into purely private practice in Ipswich, where he is still active. He was eventually to succeed "Bobby" Hale-White as chairman. I should mention that we always had at least one lawyer on our executive. Macrae Moir, of Withers and Co, our solicitors, was the first of these and he was followed by Henry Duckworth, Tom Denne, and Philip Durrance, every one of whom, as it so happens, has also been my family solicitor. Withers had looked after Horder's affairs and those of my father-in-law, and that is how I was fortunate enough to meet the partners and enjoy the benefit of their advice and friendship throughout my professional life. Another early legal and medical member was J A Gorsky, an astute north London coroner. Worthy of mention too is Gladys Sandes of the Royal Free Hospital, gynaecologist, specialist in venereal diseases, and notable anatomy teacher. She was a woman of brisk good humour and great spirit and her husband, Maxwell Alston, a kindly and thoughtful microbiologist, became honorary secretary in the 1960s when pressure of work forced Edward Warner to give up. One charming and slightly eccentric member was Donald McI Johnson, MP, formerly in general practice at Woodstock and Sutton before starting Christopher Johnson, the publishers. After clashing with Harold Macmillan and losing his seat at Carlisle, Donald became a member of the executive. In 1962 he published his own lively book, *The British National Health Service: Friend or Frankenstein?* A notable general practitioner member who, through pressure of work and later health problems, served on the executive for all too short a time was Bob Burns of Sheffield. He was a man of mordant wit and an excellent writer who published many highly entertaining papers, usually under the *nom de plume* Philip Auld. His book, *Honour a Physician*, was based upon 10 years' experience in NHS practice and was written during a fortnight's family holiday in Cornwall. As a result of his periodic jibe "that's one for the book," his receptionist had kept records of all the funny, exasperating, humiliating, and unbelievable things that had happened in the first decade of the health service. Our families happened to be staying at different boarding houses in Bude when we met on the beach. Bob was looking pale and tired. I discovered that his landlady was providing him with a nightly thermos flask of coffee so that he could sit up until the small hours churning out a chapter each night. His book was a masterpiece. Several of its reviewers doubted whether the author could possibly be a busy family doctor if he had found time to write it. Little did they know. His reviewer in the *BMJ*, Douglas Hubble of Birmingham, was distinctly upset and ended with the words, "We can only hope that Philip Auld feels better after this notable catharsis."

There are many others I could mention but I have said enough to show that we were members of an interesting team. There were plenty of lively arguments; sometimes even strong disagreements. I recall one occasion when my youthful brashness led me to argue violently with Horder over some difficult matter. Several of the others looked on with concern at my display of *lèse-majesté*. I felt guilty about the matter as I returned home; but I cannot now remember what the subject of our argument was. The very next day, however, I received a short note from Horder: "My dear Reggie, *mea culpa*, of course you were quite right and I was wrong. Yrs aye, Horder." We enjoyed seven years of his wisdom and humanity and I am only sorry now that there was neither the time nor the opportunity to get to know him more. But I recall one occasion in 1949 when, in regard to the NHS, I remarked, "Perhaps it will be better, sir, when the Tories get back in." Horder looked at me somewhat pityingly and said, "Reggie, when you grow a bit older you will learn that once a government takes anything over it makes little difference which party is in power." How right he was. Early in 1955 he was said to have "slipped a disc" when lifting a sack of potatoes out of the boot of his car. He was seen by Dr Campbell Cooke and by Ivor Robertson, an orthopaedic surgeon, who told him that he must stay strictly in bed. Horder later told me that his response to Ivor was, "It's dangerous to keep an old man like me in bed." But his son Mervyn records that he told Dr Cooke, "As you know, I am 84 and can no longer afford two weeks in bed." Whatever he may have said to others he told me that after a couple of days or so he turned over in bed and the pain suddenly went, so he promptly got up. On Saturday 15 August of the same year he was smitten by sudden severe pain in the chest. He diagnosed a myocardial infarct and called in his old friend Dr Lee-Lander. His son, Mervyn, in his biography, *The Little Genius*, gives an interesting account of Tommy's conversation with his family and a group of physicians whom he had invited from town for a performance by the Steep Players of *As You Like It* in his garden that very afternoon. Despite his illness, Tommy had insisted that the play should continue; he died in the early evening. The Steep Players had regularly done Shakespeare plays in the garden at Ashford Chace and we had attended the year before when on holiday at West Wittering.

Bobby Hale-White succeeded Horder. He was a charming man and a son of Sir William Hale-White, a Guy's physician. He had sustained a serious head wound in the first world war and I was always fascinated to watch the steady pulsation of his scalp at the site of a large skull defect. He was mainly involved in insurance practice in London and was an excellent chairman, remaining in office until November 1966 when he was elected as first president of the fellowship and succeeded as chairman by Patrick Wood. The following year Sir Arthur Porritt, a founder member, became a vice-president together with Edward Warner, but Warner died shortly afterwards.

During the first 10 years of our existence, the executive, together with the amending acts and private practice committees, prepared an impressive stream of evidence for various committees of inquiry: notably for Guillebaud, Hinchliffe, Cohen (Central Health Services Council Committee on General Practice), the Royal Commission on the NHS and that on medical education. This entailed an immense amount of work. A good example of our industriousness was the preparation of our evidence to the Guillebaud Committee of Inquiry into the Costs of the National Health Service. Instructions had been given to the executive at the annual general meeting on 21 November 1953. Our report of some 21 000 words, including detailed appendices and references, was prepared and faultlessly printed by The Press at Coombelands, Addlestone, Surrey, for publication three months later in February 1954. I wish that I could report that our energy had been suitably rewarded at the time. As with so many of the subjects we then addressed, however, the fruits of our labours have only become evident decades later. Many sound ideas spawned years ago in the fellowship, and generally inadmissible in those predominantly collectivist postwar years, have recently become more widely acceptable.

One of the great early achievements of the Fellowship for Freedom in Medicine was in securing a substantial improvement in general practitioners' remuneration. There was a strong feeling that government had ignored the recommendations of the Spens committee in this regard. The fellowship was firmly agreed in 1949 that the matter was one for independent arbitration but this was rejected by the BMA, whose General Medical Services Committee still favoured direct negotiation with the minister. But the vigorous efforts of a number of fellowship members who were also members of the BMA managed to get that policy changed. At the BMA Annual Representative Meeting in July 1950 Dr C P Wallace of Guildford (a fellowship member) proposed that the meeting should press for an independent court of arbitration. On the advice of the chairman, Dr Solomon Wand, the proposal was rejected by a large majority. But the seeds of a successful revolution were sewn at the very same meeting when Dr Barbara Woodhouse (a fellowship member), supported on the platform by six fellowship members in succession, persuaded the annual representatives that the Amending Acts Committee be reconstituted as a standing committee of the BMA. This Amending Acts Committee – with a fellowship representation of six out of 14 members – accepted the fellowship's view on the need for independent arbitration. By the following year, at the Annual Representative Meeting of the BMA in June 1951, Dr Wand and the General Medical Services Committee of the BMA had accepted the case for arbitration – a complete reversal of the decision the year before. But when Drs Breach, Russell, and Wallace (all fellowship members) put an amendment that the court of arbitration must (a) be independent, (b) have terms of reference based on Spens, burden of work, betterment factor, and remuneration of allied professions, (c) be binding on both parties, and (d) be retrospective to 5 July 1948 Dr Wand expressed severe disapproval of the amendment, which was then lost by a large majority. Amazingly, however, all was not lost. There were continued frustrations and a special representative meeting of the BMA in December 1951 pressed for an amending act to provide for a National Health Service court of arbitration, and then, on grounds of urgency, that the proposed arbitration should take place *before* any amending act.

By March 1952 the fellowship had achieved the breakthrough: the government accepted referral to an adjudicator (ultimately Mr Justice Danckwerts) with the following terms of reference:

> To determine the size of the Central Pool after taking account of remuneration from all sources received by general practitioners, in order to give effect to the recommendations of the Spens Committee, having regard to the change in value of money since 1939, to the increases which have taken place in incomes in other professions, and to all relevant factors.

The fund of fixed dimension from which general practitioners were then paid was known as the central pool. Following some controversy about its design a joke was then current in regard to the newly erected second world war memorial at BMA House. This solemn statuary consists of four symbolic figures mounted on the margins of a circular pond. The figures were said to epitomise "four general practitioners dejectedly regarding the central pool." But, to be serious, I and a number of consultant colleagues had pressed for a review of specialists' pay to be included with that of the general practitioners. The policy of the Central Consultants and Specialists Committee, however, was to wait for the general practitioners to go forward with their claim and, if it was successful, hope the hospital doctors would follow in their wake. Alas, as I had strongly suggested, this was a fatal mistake. The subsequent Danckwerts award virtually doubled general practitioners' remuneration overnight and was retrospective. But the government (then Labour) was astute enough not to amend the NHS Act as suggested and, following the general practitioners' award, governments of both complexions have avoided further reference of such matters for independent judicial review. The later setting up of independent review bodies for various categories, including the doctors, in no way negates what was then determined since we must all accept the maxim that *he who pays the piper calls the tune.*

The story of the Danckwerts award shows clearly how the Fellowship for Freedom in Medicine, in accordance with its third objective, was dedicated to the cause of the family doctor. It also shows how effectively our members operated through the BMA. It was another of our founder members, Ronald Gibson of Winchester, who was responsible for thinking up the celebrated general practitioners' charter of 1965, which further transformed the lot of the family doctor. Having devised this particular concept, Ronald set to work to implement it. In this he was extremely successful (more than 20 years later some might even say that from the patients' viewpoint he was too successful) in bettering the situation for general practitioners. It is interesting to recall that this was at the time of a Labour government with Kenneth Robinson as Minister of Health. I cannot resist quoting from *Hansard* of 17 February 1965 (column 1197) on the National Health Service (Manning). It is interesting to see that this starts with Mr Richard Wood (MP for Bridlington, a son of Lord Halifax and a bilateral above knee amputee whom I had known in the wartime Yorkshire Hussars). His opening words must, in 1989, still have a familiar tone:

> It is a matter of some regret to me that the first speech which I make in this House on the subject of the National Health Service should be made at a time when it is plain to everyone that a crisis faces the Service, some say the greatest crisis since 1948. The focal point of this crisis, as the House will be only too well aware, is the anxiety and dissatisfaction that exists among general practitioners.

He goes on to emphasise the growing financial strains on a service faced with unlimited demand but limited resources and ends his speech with (col 1200):

The Review Body set up in 1962 to advise the Prime Minister has now issued its fifth Report. The Government have accepted its recommendations and the general practitioners have made no secret of their dissatisfaction ....

He ended with an amusing reference to the notorious central pool:

Some time ago the Minister of Health declined in the House of Commons to give a description of the pool system, not because he lacked the ability to do so but because he feared, probably rightly, that most hon. Members – including myself – would lack the ability to comprehend it. If I were tempted to describe the pool system I would be deterred from doing so for precisely the opposite reasons.

In a speech beginning at 4.18 pm, completed at 4.59 pm (cols 1203–1218), and marked by the interruption of a number of honorable members, Mr Kenneth Robinson, Minister of Health, began by congratulating the right honourable member for Bridlington on his first speech in "shadow" capacity. Then, having ranged over a number of health service problems, he made this fascinating statement (col 1211):

There are many general practitioners – and they are, in general, those who suffer most under the present system – who are gearing themselves for this forward movement, but the profession as a whole is still a collection of individuals isolated from each other and from their negotiators. The result has been a lack of collective initative from which much of the current frustration must derive. The frustration is then projected on to the Minister and the Government as the obvious scapegoats. The waters are deeply troubled, and it is not surprising that destructive elements like the Fellowship for Freedom in Medicine and the Communist Party are fishing in them, exploiting and trying to maximise the dissatisfaction.

The "forward movement" to which Mr Robinson then referred was a proposed new general practitioners' contract which was published early in the following year and which stirred up tremendous opposition from the family doctors. I still have a copy of Denis Pereira Gray's detailed and pungent criticisms of that document, which he sent to me with a short covering letter. He concludes that letter by writing in reference to the suggested contract: "The more one looks at it the worse it gets." Denis is an excellent family doctor who is presently professor of general practice at the University of Exeter. Far from the fellowship's criticisms being in any way "destructive," as Kenneth Robinson then suggested in the House, it is clear that they represented the viewpoint of those of us who were deeply concerned with the progressive denigration of general practice.

I cannot recall when that particular section of *Hansard* was sent to me, but it certainly arrived too late for me to take the matter up, as I had done with a more personal matter regarding domiciliary visits (chapter 21). But the minister's linking of the fellowship with the Communist party can best be described as hilarious. Perhaps Kenneth Robinson had it in mind that the fellowship operated within the BMA like a communist cell. But he could hardly have meant this since our membership was well known and our policy and intentions were fully publicised in our bulletins and other papers. The "forward movement," to which he referred in his speech, had originally derived from the Danckwerts arbitration and was to further progress from the general practitioners' charter; both the Danckwerts arbitration and the charter had emanated from members of the fellowship. Indeed, as already indicated, Ronald Gibson's efforts may have been a little too successful. I am firmly of the opinion that at the present time our general practitioner and hospital services are insufficiently consumer sensitive.

In regard to being more sensitive to the needs of the consumer it is worth noting that within a few years of the foundation of the fellowship it was suggested that we might admit lay associate members. Many of us were uncertain but Horder was all in favour, and he chaired the first small committee until a lay chairman was elected. Later we had two or three lay members on the executive, and they gave us loyal support. We also attempted to enrol medical students but soon became discouraged about this. There was no real hostility or serious antipathy, simply a lack of interest in what we old men might be up to. Quite early on Dr Breach and I had visited one or two medical schools and we can at least claim that a subsequent member of the executive,

Dr J K Paterson of Huntingdon, derived from one of these visits.

With the regular issue of the fellowship's bulletin, evidence to various committees of inquiry, periodic policy statements, the publication of the reports of our amending acts and private practice committees, meetings in various parts of the country, and an annual dinner meeting in London, the fellowship exercised a lively influence during the first 20 years or so of the NHS. The membership never exceeded 5000 doctors. That it should later steadily shrink was inevitable. Far from being hell bent on destroying the service we had, by our early efforts through the BMA, that most influential of all British trade unions, made much of it more bearable for the profession. A quarter of a century after the appointed day the financial position of general practitioners had greatly improved. So much so that it took about that time for the last purely private practice in St Albans, originally of five partners, to fade away to one private practitioner. This was the outstanding Dr Ronald E Wilson, who died in March 1988 some 10 years after retirement. A succession of socialist governments since 1948 – under both Tory and Labour administrations – had determined that private general practice was only possible in exceptional places, like large cities, and with exceptional people, like Patrick Wood. Few of these doctors have been able to fund personal pensions which bear any comparison with those acquired by NHS general practitioners and they have certainly not done private practice for financial advantage.

A measure of the doctors' dissatisfaction by the second decade of the health service was the number emigrating to the United States and the Commonwealth. This had always been strongly denied by government departments and by pillars of the medical establishment, such as Lord Platt. It was another fellowship member, at that time a senior registrar and shortly to be a member of our executive, who, in 1962, produced the bombshell on medical emigration. When the Ministry of Health, the BMA, the royal colleges, and our undergraduate medical schools had little knowledge of this subject it was Dr John Seale who, by the very simple expedient of sending a letter of inquiry to the appropriate departments of state in the United States and various Commonwealth countries, managed to come up with an estimate which was close to the true figure. Seale's work was highly commended in a *BMJ* editorial on 17 March 1962. Although his figures were hotly denied by Enoch Powell who, in addressing the conference of local medical committees, chose to describe the conclusions as "a slander on your service," they were later confirmed by the study of Brian Abel-Smith and Kathleen Gales, undertaken with the encouragement of the Ministry and published in 1964. Seale had forseen that some of the émigré doctors might have registered in more than one state of a single country or, less often, in more than one country, and had made an estimated deduction to allow for this. The Ministry had then inquired of the medical schools where their former students were practising, but the schools did not have accurate information on more than a small fraction of their graduates. That misinformation led to Powell's precipitate denial. The later Abel-Smith inquiry, based upon a one in 10 study of British medical graduates, confirmed in 1964 that about 4000 doctors, born and trained in Britain, had left the British Isles in the previous 10 years and had not returned.

In the same year as John Seale's report hit the headlines there was yet another important report from a medical committee, set up in 1958 with an original membership of 37. This was chaired by a founder member of the fellowship, Sir Arthur Porritt, who had become president of the Royal College of Surgeons of England by the time that *A Review of the Medical Services in Great Britain* was published. Evidence had been given to the committee on behalf of the fellowship by Dr Hale-White, Mr A J Gardham, and Mr C A Jackson. Alas, I fear that the deliberations and ultimate recommendations of that committee were inhibited by the size and variety of its membership. It came out clearly in deploring the monopolistic tendencies of the NHS; but it was somewhat contradictory in calling for greater central coordination and unification of the health functions then subserved by other government departments. These and other points were criticised in a *BMJ* editorial of 3 November 1962. I shortly found myself chairing an ad hoc fellowship committee which was charged with commenting on the report. We had met twice by the end of the year, and on 10 January 1963 I wrote to Arthur to arrange a discussion with him. I had to point out that there was an article by Kenneth Robinson, then socialist MP for St Pancras, in the *New York Times Magazine* (dated 18 November 1962 and sent to me by my father) claiming that the Porritt criticisms were largely concerned with NHS organisation. Moreover, one or two left wingers were even claiming that the Porritt report negated the fellowship's views and aims. I met Arthur for lunch at the college of surgeons a little later and we frankly discussed the differences and sought ways of emphasising our points of agreement. He rightly stressed the problems caused by his committee's remaining "in labour" for four years, and he agreed with me that there was little point in devolving power to area health boards if the sole source of funding was from the Treasury. The overall impact of the Porritt report proved disappointing, but I fear that so large a committee tended to lead to some fudging of the issues, and that is no reflection on its wise chairman, who later became vice-president of the fellowship.

Another founder member of the fellowship, Dr John Hunt (later Lord Hunt), was largely responsible for the creation of the College of General Practitioners on 1 January 1953. The possibility had been discussed at the fellowship's annual general meeting in October 1951, and it came up again at the annual general meeting in November 1952. But we were all surprised when, only a month later, the imminent birth of the college was announced. I well remember an earlier conversation between Tommy Horder and John Hunt when the latter first mooted his idea. Tommy was all for an academy of medicine to unify the profession. He told John, "If you create a college you will simply start dishing out diplomas like all the others do." John's prompt response was, "Oh no, we shan't do that." Horder, as usual, was right. Although most people felt that the interests of the fellowship and the college were largely complementary, it is likely that the general practitioner membership of the fellowship was diluted by this development.

Since its foundation the fellowship had deplored the tendency of the NHS to deify the hospital and to denigrate the family doctor. In the first 15 years or so of the health service it is evident that we did much to ameliorate the conditions of general practice where, when all is said and done, there is by far the greatest contact between doctor and patient. Moreover, it absorbs a much smaller proportion of the total resources, so that high quality general practice must prove extremely cost effective. But we were always unhappy about the relentless and growing demands which must necessarily occur with any service provided free at the time. The rapidly increasing NHS expenditure, and the manifest deficiencies of the hospital development programme, made some of us more and more conscious of the economic facts of life.

A most important event in 1957 was the foundation of the independent Institute of Economic Affairs. Within a short time I had come to know Ralph Harris and Arthur Seldon well and this led on to my being invited in 1960 to contribute to a book which would compare and contrast the financing of health care in seven countries. The British health service was dealt with by Colm Brogan, writer and political analyst; Dennis Lees, then senior lecturer in economics at Keele; and myself. Apart from our three chapters concerning the United Kingdom, the book covered the health systems of Australia, Austria, France, Germany, Sweden, and Switzerland. The editor, Dr Helmut Schoeck, was trained in psychology and medicine before turning to sociology. Having worked at the University of Heidelberg (to which he much later returned), Schoeck was then professor of sociology and anthropology at Emory University, Atlanta, Georgia. The one clear lesson that book taught me was the number of variations on the theme of state medicine that had caused unforeseen problems in many countries. The notable exception was Switzerland, where the voluntary principle then prevailed. The preface was written by Professor F A Hayek, later a Nobel prizewinner. He stated: "There are perhaps few other fields in which so many admitted mistakes have been made since the late nineteenth century, and where it is at the same time so difficult to correct the consequences of a misguided earlier policy." *Financing*

Medical Care was published at the beginning of 1963 by Caxton Press, Caldwell, Idaho. It was widely reviewed in the United States, where President Kennedy was then revising his medicare and social security programme. My father, in New York, sent me an interesting review from the *Wall Street Journal* which concluded that the outcome of compulsory national health plans usually turns out to be quite different from what is expected.

Thus began my own absorbing interest in medical economics. In 1962 I wrote a paper entitled "Alternative and Supplementary Systems of Financing Medical Care," which was published in our fellowship Bulletin no 51, together with an interesting address by John Jewkes, then professor of economic organisation at Oxford. Dennis Lees gave the address at the succeeding annual general meeting and that was published in Bulletin no 53 in January 1963. This was shortly followed by the Institute of Economic Affairs' *Choice in Welfare 1963*, which incorporated the results of an inquiry commissioned from *Mass Observation* in which, for the first time, those polled had been offered a number of alternative and priced choices both in medicine and in education. After a second edition, *Choice in Welfare 1965*, was published it became apparent how genuinely concerned many people were about these matters. Moreover, the desire for wider choice was shown, though understandably to varying degree, by those of different social class and political persuasion, but the latter had far less influence than previously presumed.

A few years later the BMA was to follow the fellowship's lead. In the middle of the 1960s the NHS was passing through one of its recurrent crises, and early in 1967 the then chairman of the BMA council, Dr Ronald Gibson, invited Dr Ivor Jones, with the aid of an advisory panel, to "undertake research and inquiry into the National Health Service from its origins and indicate possible trends for the future." But this initial remit was much modified in July of that year when, amidst the growing frustrations of both general practitioners and hospital doctors, the representative body of the BMA adopted a resolution which called for the urgent preparation of plans for an alternative health service in which financial provision would be less dependent upon taxation.

Ivor Jones, a first class general practitioner in Sunderland, was a highly resourceful man of extraordinary energy, an outstanding medical politician described by Dr John Havard of the BMA as "one of the most brilliant negotiators I have ever known." His panel of 12 included nine other doctors and two laymen – a young barrister, R E Geoffrey (later Sir Geoffrey) Howe, and the noted economist Arthur Seldon. Working with uncanny expedition they had completed their remarkable report within two years. The first 185 pages skilfully review the history of health service financing both before and after the inception of the NHS and are followed by 418 pages of detailed appendices covering the organisation and financing of health care in 14 other capitalist countries as well as some behind the iron curtain. Early in 1970, when I was in my second year as an elected councillor, this report was presented to the council of the BMA. I then regarded it, and still do, as the finest analysis of health service organisation and financing I have ever read. In his preface the chairman of the panel wrote:

> It is our belief that reform of the administrative and financial structure should proceed together but that *if the one should to some degree precede the other, priority should be given to finance for, without additional money, little could be achieved by any change of administration.* (My emphasis.)

Far from asking the government to screw yet more funds out of the Treasury and the long suffering taxpayer, it was a clear call for those supplementary and alternative sources of funding which had been the subject of my earlier paper. The Ivor Jones report, *Health Services Financing*, was received with enthusiasm by a substantial minority of BMA council members but had a less enthusiastic reception from the general practitioner membership. Furthermore, shortly after its publication, and following two green papers under Crossman and Robinson, there was a general election with a switch from Labour to Tory administrations, succeeded by Keith Joseph's white paper which resulted in the disastrous 1974 administrative reorganisation of the NHS. The politicians had once again failed to grasp the nettle of financial reform of our health services, and the general practitioners were quietly becoming more comfortably cocooned by state welfare.

Alas, until very recently both the health service and education have remained in the bureaucratic grip with politicians of all parties showing little disposition for change. Paradoxically, it was the notorious "Barbarabarities of Castle" in 1974 that provoked the biggest ever development of private hospitals in Britain, whereas the first two spells of Thatcherism produced no more than a timid whisper of reform. Towards the end of 1986, in hopeful anticipation of a wind of change, the Institute of Economic Affairs set up a health unit under the capable direction of David Green, a former Labour town councillor from Newcastle-upon-Tyne, who, like all the best converts, had converted himself to the market economy by his own scholarship. The unit is independently funded and I am delighted to be a member of its advisory council. As with its parent body in the past, the unit is now turning out a stream of thought provoking papers which are promoting ever more lively discussion on health service reform. I wrote to Margaret Thatcher before the last election strongly suggesting that health and education were her Achilles heel. But the election manifestos confirmed that all political parties were still making obeisance to the sacred cow.

Not long after the 1987 general election, faced with a new funding crisis in the NHS, the third Margaret Thatcher administration set up an inquiry which has recently come up with a number of novel suggestions – credit transfer financing, independent hospital trusts, budgeting general practices – all of which are envisaged within the existing largely tax-financed framework. I recognise some of these suggested reforms, including tax relief on medical insurance premiums for the over 65s (where I have to declare my interest), as gentle steps in the right direction. But I cannot support the continued acceptance of almost wholly tax financed funding within a state near monopoly even though the government's proposals – whatever they may believe – are certain to lead to even greater health service expenditure. Nor can I accept the objections of much of the medical establishment to the idea of independent hospitals. I was aware of the promotion of the concept of general practitioner budget holders several years ago but must confess to considerable scepticism about this. After all, who of us would expect our purely private family doctor to take control of all our personal and insurance funds for consultant advice and hospital care? Even with competing health maintenance organisations (such as obtain in the United States), where the consumer is free to switch his or her allegiance – as opposed to being tied to a single budget holder in a state monopoly – many thorny problems have arisen. Witness the current suing of their health organisations for breach of contract by patients in six different states.

It was because of our shrinking membership and all these new developments that we finally decided to wind up the Fellowship for Freedom in Medicine in 1987. By then I had been its president for just over 15 years and, as a member of the council of The Freedom Association, I suggested that those of our members to whom the idea appealed should switch their allegiance to that organisation. Patrick Wood joined me as a member of the council of this association, and we are satisfied that freedom in medicine can now be best catered for in this broader context. Indeed, in July 1986, a year before we wound up the fellowship, The Freedom Association, the Institute of Economic Affairs, and the Institute of Directors jointly sponsored a symposium with the title "An Alternative Health Service."

I remain convinced, as did the Ivor Jones committee, that only by reform of the methods of financing health care can we achieve more efficient, cost effective, and consumer sensitive health services. It will not suffice to rely merely on the growth of the private sector to relieve the health service of its increasing burdens. There has to be fundamental reform within the service if the generality of patients is to approach the ideal of "everyone a private patient."

Lord Horder himself predicted that reform of the NHS might take 50 years. He was as good a prophet as any and we are now in the last decade of that period. The battle is not yet won but there are clear signs that the consumer is at last becoming better aware of the various options. Politicians must ultimately respond to changing consumer concepts, and when they do things may well become distinctly uncomfortable for many of the vested professional and trades union interests which have been spawned or maintained by 40 years of state near monopoly. I am well satisfied that by facing up to the economic facts of life we are at last in a position to achieve greater freedom of choice for the consumer. The Fellowship for Freedom in Medicine had a wholly honourable record in that regard.

21 Barnacles of the new bureaucracy

If State interference is pushed to the extent of placing our hospitals and nursing institutions at the mercy of the barnacles of the new bureaucracy, a bitter disappointment is in store for the advocates of State socialism; for we learn from the experience of Russia and other countries, where the bureaucratic system is highly developed, that instead of having hospitals without paying for them, we are likely to pay for hospitals without having them.*

Before the second world war it was unusual to visit any hospital, whether voluntary or municipal, in which there was not some building work and improvement going on. Yet, following the inception of the health service, 16 years were to pass before the first new hospital was completed at Welwyn Garden City. The much vaunted 10 year £1000 million plan, announced by Enoch Powell in 1962, had, after seven years, reached only £100 million a year. In the original plan the Royal Northern Hospital was scheduled for complete rebuilding; but it somehow disappeared from the plan. Twenty-eight years later that hospital remains essentially in its original state. If the nationalisation of medicine has achieved little in the way of new hospitals then many of those it has managed to complete leave much to be desired. Having totally opposed the air conditioning of operation theatres in the 1950s, the Department of Health has managed to waste vast amounts in capital, and still more in subsequent maintenance, for the air conditioning of entire hospital buildings – for example, the new St Thomas's, the Royal Free, and Charing Cross. Surely, too, there is something radically wrong with a planning system which allowed the completion of a building for nurses'

* For this quotation I am indebted to the late Henry Thompson of St Mark's Hospital, London. Surprisingly enough it is derived from *Suffering London* by A Egmont Hake, published in 1892.

accommodation, shared between Great Ormond Street Childrens' Hospital and the Hospital for Nervous Diseases, Queen Square, to be delayed for several years as a result of a union dispute. Department officials may say that union problems are not of their making. All too true, but the method of planning rarely protects the ultimate interests of the taxpayer who foots the bill. Nor can I forget my visit of inspection to Great Ormond Street Hospital in 1976. This visit was concerned with vetting the training posts for the FRCS examination regulations. It was explained that I could not be taken into the new cardiothoracic building because although it had been completed it was subject to a design "hiccup." That building was indeed suffering from a major design and construction defect which resulted in its opening being delayed until 27 April 1988. Whatever may have been the design or constructional faults, how much has this whole business cost the long suffering taxpayer? The opening ceremony was performed by the Prime Minister, Margaret Thatcher, during an intensive governmental review of National Health Service funding.

Let us now look at one or two quite simple projects of which I have close personal knowledge and experience. When walking through the outpatient department at the Mid Herts unit at St Albans one Thursday morning in June 1958 I observed on the floor a number of spots of what I assumed to be plaster of Paris. A nurse explained that the spots were barium sulphate from one of the morning's barium enema patients. I expressed my astonishment and called on the radiologist, Dr Weber, who told me that there were no lavatories in the *x* ray department, although he had requested these a year or two earlier. So when their examinations had been completed patients had to leave the *x* ray room and traverse a public corridor to the male and female lavatories (of which there was only one of each) that served the outpatient waiting room. Apart from the spillage in the corridor, which I had seen, it was not uncommon for patients to arrive at the closet and find it occupied. You could have knocked me down with a feather! I had worked for more than 10 years in that hospital without being aware of this situation. Dr Weber told me of his repeated ineffectual applications to the management committee and to the region. The *maximum* capital expenditure on a single project which a hospital management committee could authorise at that time was, believe it or not, £1000. The planned lavatories would cost more than this and therefore the project was a regional one.

On receiving this information I took up the telephone and, as was my habit in those days of an efficient telegraph service, sent a telegram to the chairman of the regional board: "I have to report spillage of faecal barium in hospital corridor at St Albans by patients leaving *x* ray department for OP lavatory and request immediate action to remedy this disgraceful state of affairs.—Murley." In reply I received the following letter, dated 10 July 1958, from A J Bennett, the secretary of the North West Metropolitan Regional Hospital Board:

Dear Mr Murley,

I am writing in reply to your letter [*sic*] of 25 June to Lord Cottesloe, the Chairman of the Board.

The upgrading of the *x* ray department at the Mid Herts Wing was one of 15 schemes selected from a very large number submitted by Hospital management committees from the region for inclusion in the Board's capital programme as and when finance permitted. Hospital management committees were asked to bring these schemes to an advanced state of readiness so that the work could begin with a minimum of delay when it seemed likely that the money was available.

The sketch scheme for this job has been agreed and the estimated cost is £3750. The Hospital Management committee have been asked that it should be further developed to tender stage by their Building Supervisor so that it will be in all respects ready to start when the money is available.

In view of the serious situation to which you refer regarding the lavatory accommodation, authority has been sought to carry out the provision of the lavatory accommodation – which is part of the scheme – at once and this is now in the hands of the Management Committee.

No apology, and no mention of the real problem until the last paragraph. Work on those lavatories started soon afterwards, and they were installed in splendid isolation at a site on the corner of the future extension but adjacent to the existing department. There was much chaffing of Dr Weber about his new "family two seater" as the building work went ahead. The cost, incidentally, seems exorbitant for those days as a year before this it had cost me no more than £850 to add a study and a playroom with a pitched roof to my own house.

I chanced to meet Lord Cottesloe at the Royal Northern Hospital a couple of months later. Again, what had been involved can only be described, without fear of the slightest exaggeration, as "a right cock up." During the autumn and winter of 1957–58 the children's ward at the Royal Northern, on the top floor of the long block, had developed extensive leaks through the roof. Cracks in the ceiling had gradually appeared and our surveyors found that the side walls at the top of this building (completed in 1888) had started to separate. The ward sister and nurses had strategically placed zinc baths and basins underneath the main points of leakage whenever it rained, and even the working class mothers of Holloway had decided to exercise a spot of "consumer choice" by removing their offspring – sometimes arranging for them to go to the children's unit at the nearby Archway hospital. Repeated letters to the regional board from our group secretary, Arthur Gray, had had no effect whatsoever. Some months before the St Albans lavatory problem I had been at the regional board offices with our hospital management committee chairman, Dr Drakeley (a mining engineer who was then principal of the North London Polytechnic), Arthur Gray, and one or two colleagues. We were there regarding the planning of a new outpatient department. At the end of the meeting Drakeley asked the chairman (Maurice Hackett, a brother-in-law of George Brown, MP – later Lord George Brown), "What is the board doing about our children's ward?" Hackett said, "What's the problem?" Drakeley replied, "It's falling down." "Falling down?" said Hackett. "That, sir, is precisely what I said and what I mean," said Drakeley. Hackett turned to Bennett, the regional board secretary, who declared that he knew nothing of the problem. Arthur Gray then stated that several letters had been sent concerning the matter. Hackett promptly promised to visit us; he did so two days later and scaffolding was put up around the block within a week.

I cannot remember the cost of the repairs, but it was many thousands of pounds even in those preinflationary days. The hospital paid a substantial part out of its free monies. Before the work was completed the regional board planned a reopening ceremony, but, in all the circumstances, it might have been better had they donned sackcloth and ashes at their offices in Portland Place. The ceremony in the board room was attended by the local MP, the mayor of Islington, regional board and hospital officials, and medical and nursing staff. After this the red ribbon draped across the entrance to the refurbished ward was duly cut, and after a tour of the ward we went down to the nurses' home for tea. I heard a voice asking, "Oh, is that Mr Murley?" and turned to see Lord Cottesloe. "How are things at St Albans?" he inquired. "Not too bad, sir," I replied, "the Cottesloe closets are up to their damp course and we are looking forward to your visit for the opening ceremony. We think it might be appropriate if, clothed in your lordly robes, you were to sit in one of them, pull the plug, and then declare the Cottesloe closets open." The chairman's face clearly showed his displeasure. Was it rude of me? In all the outrageous circumstances I hardly think so. It was because of situations like these, and our near incapacity to take any effective local action, that I became more and more enraged with the bureaucratic mess which politicians of all parties had so glibly imposed on us.

We had the same exasperation and delays over completion of the outpatient block – the one we had been to the board about when the debacle of the children's ward was brought up. The finished building, orientated almost due north, had a wall of glass on the west side where the consulting rooms faced the setting sun. Especially in the spring and autumn, when the sun was in lower orbit, the rooms on the west badly overheated – with temperatures reaching 85°F, or even 90°F on occasions – whereas those on the east side remained cooler. The ventilation plant had sensors in the central corridors and one can only hazard a guess at its conflict as it tried to decide how it might cool the west side and warm the east side.

Only a short time after these problems at the Royal Northern it was rumoured that the regional hospital board had decided to replace our excellent chairman, Dr T J C Drakeley.

We all strongly suspected that this was because he had been too outspoken about the scandalous delays in getting the leaking ward attended to. It was thought that he was to be replaced by Dame Barbara Brooke, so I arranged to get some questions asked in the House of Commons by Gerry Reynolds, the then Labour member for Islington, and by John Cronin, a former contemporary of mine at Barts, who was the Labour member for Loughborough. Cronin had at first been reluctant to get involved. But when he heard that the board chairman was Lord Cottesloe, with whom I believe he had once served on the London County Council, he joined in with enthusiasm; there were clearly some old political scores to settle. When the day for the Health Minister's question time arrived I took my surgical colleague, Desmond Farley, to the House as he had never been inside it before. I had hoped that things would be lively, and they certainly were. Derek Walker-Smith's deputy had been dealing with the previous questions and our two came, rather dramatically, just before 3.30 pm, when oral questions cease. The Speaker called for our questions just in the nick of time and Derek Walker-Smith strode to the despatch box. The first, by Reynolds, simply inquired whether Mr T J C Drakeley was being removed from chairmanship of the Royal Northern Hospital management committee. The answer was a straightforward "Yes." Cronin had insisted on the prefix "Mr" before Drakeley's name; as he succinctly put it, "Most of the buggers on our side are prejudiced against the medicos and if we say 'Dr' they will not realise that he is a doctor of science." The second question, asked by Cronin, was, "Would the Minister state who is to replace Mr Drakeley?" The answer, "Dame Barbara Brooke," produced an explosion on the Labour benches with supplementary questions going on for almost 25 minutes as members hopped up on both sides of the House. Desmond Farley said that he had no idea that the House of Commons could be so entertaining. Of course nothing was changed, but we felt that we had had our money's worth. Furthermore, it will be realised that I was capable of being even handed with each of the main political parties whenever I smelt dirty work by the bureaucrats. But, to be serious, we were all sorry to lose

Drakeley. He had been an excellent chairman and a friend to everyone from consultants to the most junior of ancillary staff. The whole affair illustrated the devastating consequences of bureaucratising the hospital service as well as the frustrations of those working in it.

Only two years earlier the new theatre suite at St Albans had at last been completed. Apart from the fact that the number of theatres was halved, a regional board "judgment of Solomon," after the plans were drawn, we then had terrible arguments about the number of autoclaves to be installed in the sterilising room. Because the board had removed two of our four theatres from the plan we had finally cajoled it into agreeing that the planned plaster room must also be used for surgery. Central theatre supply systems had not been accepted at that time and so we wanted one small instrument autoclave to service each of the three operation rooms. The board refused: we insisted. With the support of John Grimston, our St Albans MP, the matter went to the Minister (Derek Walker-Smith), but he declined to intervene. Because we were clearly getting nowhere I wrote to the managing director of A L Hawkins and Co, who were to supply the autoclaves, and asked him to have a third one ready "for my private use." He replied thanking me for my esteemed order and ending, "I quite understand." My wink had been as good as a nod and, pending the authority of the board, which we were still hoping for, we arranged for our surgeons and anaesthetists (nine in all, including the specialists) to agree to foot the bill. At this stage I informed Dr Fowler, Macaulay's successor at the board, that if they did not install the autoclave we would be presenting it to the hospital at the opening ceremony. In fact we had a splendid plan to back up a lorry outside, drop the tailboard, and display our very own toy. Well, once again we won. The board capitulated, the third autoclave was installed, and the board paid for it. We had also had to fight hard to get enough built in cupboards, on which I had been firmly insistent. At the opening ceremony a board official said, "Heaven knows what you will put in all these cupboards." Little did he know of what went on in an operation suite. Within a few weeks all those cupboards were full of equipment and some of the heavier stuff was overflowing into an extra area which we had strategically adapted.

Before the suite was put into use Dr Robert Blowers of the Hospital Infection and Microbiology Clinical Research Centre at Northallerton conducted tests to determine the adequacy of the ventilating plant in clearing bacteria. He was satisfied about this, but I was by no means happy about a plant which included no refrigeration facility. The importance of refrigeration is not only to lower the air temperature (which is clearly important in hotter weather) but also to reduce the relative humidity. We started to use the suite in November 1959, but during the next 18 months or so it became clear that the ventilating plant had insufficient capacity to ensure theatre comfort at all times. This was plainly a matter of considerable importance for many new theatre suites were then being planned. I kicked up such a fuss about this, with letters to the medical, local, and national press, that the whole thing had a wide airing. But I was convinced that we needed to instal some additional refrigeration units and, as a result of all the publicity, I was showered with offers from many air conditioning firms. Several of them came to inspect the premises. At that time I certainly knew very little about air conditioning, but I was learning fast. Indeed, fast enough to realise that some of these firms' representatives were talking nonsense. I had raised money from a number of our local firms, starting with the St Albans branch of Marconi's, some of whose staff had been patients of mine. In raising this money I had promised to return it to the various donors in the event of the board capitulating once again.

But things looked tougher this time when I received an even more pompous and imperious letter from A J Bennett, the regional board secretary. This included the sentence "I have to inform you that, in the event of your interfering with the Minister's property, an injunction will be served on you." After reading the letter I swallowed hard and counted 10 before resorting to my usual trick. Once again I called "Telegrams." The message was sent to the secretary of the board with copies to the Minister of Health, Reuter's, and Associated Press; for in those days you could get the telegraph office to send copies to several addressees. The meat of my message was:

Receipt of your letter is acknowledged. I now await injunction, copies of which will be sent to Reuter's and Associated Press—Murley.

I eagerly awaited the Big Bang. Nothing happened, although I did receive a nice friendly letter from Sir Russell Brock (this was some three years before he became president of the college of surgeons). His note read:

Dear Murley,

I have been following with much interest, in the pages of *The Times*, your battle with the forces of darkness and ignorance and I wish you well in your campaign.

Well, after that, Russell Brock was a friend for life. Since then I have tried to follow his example of sending a note of encouragement to those who are in trouble with the powers that be.

I answered Brock's note with a short letter in which I urged the Royal College of Surgeons to take firm action in the matter of operation theatre design and ventilation. He responded by saying that the idea had once passed through his mind and that, with my stimulation, he would now take it up with the president (Sir Arthur Porritt) and college council. Some weeks later he wrote that a committee on theatre design had been set up of which he was chairman and that they would be pleased to receive information and evidence.

I am happy to report that the installation of two simple recirculating refrigeration units into the top windows of each theatre – similar to those one sees on many buildings abroad – gave us an effective cooling and dehumidifying system which could be set to come into operation whenever necessary. Once again the regional board paid the bills and the money from our generous donors was, with their agreement, allocated to our medical library and postgraduate activities. It is worthy of note that on one occasion the hospital secretary sent me the bill for my telegrams. I had no compunction in signing the bill under the brief note, "Action taken in the public interest, charge to the public account." I heard no more about it. Perhaps there may be some naughty little goblin within me which goads me on in these matters. But I have achieved much success by firm action. That reminds me of a story about Lord Horder, who once met a colleague in the street who said, "Hello, Tommy, still fighting for lost causes?" "Yes," said Tommy, "I win some of them!"

It was in the course of our struggle over theatre ventilation that I thought it might be a good idea to try to publicise the seriously neglected state of our hospitals so many years after the inception of the NHS. To this end I wrote a letter to Richard Dimbleby at the BBC, to which I had a most helpful and diplomatic reply. He said he had every sympathy with my views but that he had to be careful about making suggestions regarding future productions. He had put my letter in the hands of an appropriate person, however, and thought I might be hearing something in due course.

Several months after this letter from Dimbleby, a pleasant BBC producer from the *Panorama* programme wrote to tell me that the BBC would like to make a record of the theatre problem to which I had referred. He visited me at the Royal Northern Hospital, where we had some of the oldest and most inadequate operation theatres in the country, with primitive sterilising room and related facilities. The hospital management committee gave permission for the production and in a few weeks an excellent programme had been filmed in and around my own operation theatre. The producer and his team warmly cooperated with us, and the producer was kind enough to allow me to vet the introductory words which would be spoken by Dimbleby, even accepting my several suggested alterations. In those days much of the programme was shot "live" and I had to attend the Lime Grove studios with an anaesthetist colleague.

It was while I was being "made up" in a chair next to Richard Dimbleby that he wished me the best of luck and went on to remark that as I probably knew – which I certainly did not – he was attending St Thomas's Hospital for radiotherapy; unknown to me he then had a malignant tumour. I recalled that we had first met in the last year of the war when, with Jessie Battle and her eldest boy, Nicholas, I had attended David Dimbleby's birthday party while spending a weekend with the Battles. Richard explained that our programme would be following his interview with the multimillionaire Nubar Gulbenkian, and that we would be interviewed by John Morgan after his own words of introduction and the showing of the prepared film. I vividly recall, firstly, how entertaining the Gulbenkian session was and, secondly, how nervous John Morgan was before and during the programme.

There was a socialist government at the time, with which Morgan was clearly far more in sympathy than either my anaesthetist colleague or I. When we assured him beforehand, however, that our criticisms of the neglected "slum" hospitals of Britain were entirely non-partisan he seemed much relieved, but many viewers observed that he appeared to be sweating profusely during the interview. This programme was well received by many friends and colleagues all around the country. At the time, my home did not even possess a television set. I cannot claim that we were rewarded by any noticeable speeding up of new hospital building and refurbishment, but there were some unexpected dividends.

The publicity we achieved in connection with our theatre ventilation problems led on to an important investigation on thermal comfort in a variety of operation suites. This was set up by Dr O M Lidwell of the Central Public Health Laboratory, with Professor R E O Williams of the Wright–Fleming Institute at St Mary's Hospital. The visits to 30 operating suites in 28 different hospitals were made by a physicist, Dr D P Wyon, and a nurse. Detailed data were collected on temperature, humidity, air movement, and radiant heat; to these physical measurements were added records of the subjective comfort of surgeons, assistants, anaesthetists, and nursing staff and other data. Our St Albans suite was included in the study and we were fascinated to observe the care with which physical measurements were made; there was even a gadget to measure the heat over the surgeon's head beneath the operating lamp. When this detailed research was completed in 1967 I was happy to learn that all my original contentions had been confirmed. The concluding paragraph of the discussion in the published paper (*J Hyg* 1968; **66:** 229) reads:

> This investigation largely substantiates the claim that conditions in British operating rooms often reach temperatures above those at which surgeons are comfortable. The average temperature observed in this series was over 72°F, nearly 6°F higher than the value most generally preferred by surgeons. A temperature of 64.5°F, which seems to be necessary if no more than 5% of surgeons are to be uncomfortably hot, cannot be attained without some degree of cooling over part of the year, even if extraneous heat is kept to a minimum.

Clearly we had been fighting for a good cause and we had not lost. What is more, the Department of Health was at last goaded into activity. In the following year a joint subcommittee on operating theatres was set up between the Medical Research Council, the DHSS, and the Royal College of Surgeons, and I was nominated as the college representative. It is the only Department of Health committee on which I have ever served, apart from a single attendance at the Central Health Services Council. At the first meeting I was encouraged to find that one or two of the engineers at the department were on my side: in fact they tried to elect me as chairman. But, recognising my reputation as a thorn in the flesh of successive ministers, I declined to accept the chair and so we then elected Dr O M Lidwell, who represented the Medical Research Council. Another reason for my avoiding the chair was that I wanted to retain full freedom of action to put in a minority report should this eventually prove necessary. It could be that I was wrong in that judgment, as will shortly emerge.

Our working party first met on 9 January 1970 and good progress was made with meetings in March, May, and July of that year. After that nothing happened for a year. Following a meeting in July 1971, another meeting was called for November, but it was cancelled. Even the chairman, Dr Lidwell, was mystified as to what was happening, so I wrote to Sir Keith Joseph, then Secretary of State, on 22 December 1971:

Dear Sir Keith,

In the latter part of 1969 I was appointed to a Joint Working Party on ventilation of operating theatres as Royal College of Surgeons representative. I attended the first meeting on January 9, 1970, of what appeared to be a promising working group of doctors and engineers. I take the liberty of writing to you now because I feel most strongly that the work of this group is not being undertaken with sufficient vigour. No meetings at all were held between July 1970 and July 1971. . . . I hope you will not take it amiss if I write to tell you how bitterly disappointed I am with the progress of this Working Party, and to suggest that a prod from the Secretary of State might do much to liven up the officials of your Department.

I am sending a copy of this letter to Sir Thomas Holmes Sellors, the president of the Royal College of Surgeons of England.

Sir Keith's reply was dated 17 January 1972 and I quote the relevant parts:

Dear Mr Murley,

I have been making enquiry into the lack of progress being made by the Joint Working Party . . . about which you wrote to me on 22 December.

I am sure you will appreciate the difficulties in arranging meetings to suit the convenience of a number of people such as yourself who have many other important commitments. This is the main reason for the delay in finalising the Working Party's conclusions, but the difficulties were aggravated by the prolonged illness of the officer who was chosen to act as Secretary of the Working Party. In spite of these difficulties I regard this delay as having been unduly protracted since the early meetings were held at reasonable intervals between January and July 1970.

Arrangements have now been made for a further meeting to be held on 9 February and I am assured that the work will now be pushed forward to a speedy conclusion. . . .

It was gallant of Sir Keith to try to defend his bureaucrats at the Elephant and Castle, but the comment at the end of the second paragraph hardly fits in with his remarks about "difficulties in arranging meetings." After a quarter of a century of nationalisation I had certainly learnt the truth of Horder's contention that it would make little difference which party was in power. But let me revert to two earlier variations on the bureaucratic theme. The first of these concerns domiciliary consultations.

I had been doing domiciliary consultations on the health service for some years without completing the "reason for visit" part of the claim form and without approving the final part which had to be signed by the general practitioner after the words: "I was/was not present at the consultation." As to the first of these points, I had always declined to enter a diagnosis on the form: the fact that this was alleged to be dealt with in the senior administrative medical officer's department did not convince me that it would be anything but a breach of confidence to enter the patient's name, address, and diagnosis on a form which must certainly be seen by clerical staff. When Dr Macaulay first wrote to me about this matter I gave him these reasons and he included in his reply these words: "however, I know you to be a man of honour and integrity and therefore I would not insist on your completing the diagnosis even if I *could*" (my emphasis). Because he had at first claimed that the diagnoses were needed for "statistical purposes" I had, in fact, offered to let him have an annual list of both provisional and final diagnoses unrelated to any names, but these he had declined. As for the general practitioner's part of the form, I would not have dreamt of visiting a patient without the family doctor and I therefore overprinted all my forms with "I was of course present at the consultation," which was then signed by the doctor.

Arthur Rushforth, one of my orthopaedic colleagues, dealt with his domiciliary forms in the same way and we both continued in that style for several years. It is obvious that neither of us was particularly attentive in studying our quarterly payslips from the regional board until one or other of us eventually noticed that for about a year no domiciliary payments had been made. I wrote to Dr Macaulay, who thereupon replied:

> Thank you for your letter . . . which anticipated one I was about to write you. You will recall our earlier agreement about the forms for domiciliary visits . . . however, the board is no longer prepared to make payments unless these forms are fully completed.

I referred the matter to the Medical Defence Union, who were my indemnity insurers. In due course their secretary provided me with a specimen letter informing the regional board that if no payment was made further action would be taken. The union followed this with another letter for my signature in which I noted that, having named a specific date, the letter ended: "If these outstanding payments are not made by then my solicitors will be *considering* further action" (my emphasis). This seemed to me to show a weakening of resolve by someone, and how right I was. A week or two passed and I had a further letter from the secretary of the union saying, "My council is prepared to support you up to the date of Dr Macaulay's letter, but not after that date." I called on the union secretary; he made it clear that he was personally in full sympathy but that one or two council members had encouraged a compromise. I noticed that no mention had been made of the union's lawyers' (Hempsons) views so I wrote to Mr Butcher, one of the partners whom I knew, to ask whether *in law* my position was not precisely the same both after and before Dr Macaulay's letter. I received an affirmative reply stating that the firm would be honoured to act on my behalf. I was delighted and sent Hempsons a postcard with the brief message: "Thank you for yours. Please deal death blow to NWMRHB." The fee was one and a half guineas. A little later I received a letter from the secretary to the regional board:

> Dear Mr Murley [all the previous ones had been "Dear Sir"]
>
> ... the board has now decided to pay you up to the date of Dr Macaulay's letter, but we await the authority of the Ministry of Health for the later payments.

I thought that last bit was just a convenient fudge, and it was. The board soon paid up for all the visits and continued to do so thereafter.

It is interesting to study *Hansard* on the above subject for 15 July 1959. There was then a Tory government and Derek Walker-Smith was minister. Dr Edith Summerskill opened the debate at 3.47 pm by explaining why Labour thought it necessary "to devote one of our Supply Days to debate important matters concerned with the health of the people." Mr Kenneth Robinson followed at 5.21 pm and spoke until 5.45 pm. Towards the end of his speech he said:

Then there is the question of the domiciliary consultations. The Minister will remember there was some concern expressed in the Report of the Select Committee on Estimates about abuses in the domiciliary consultant service, on which the Committee received certain evidence. It is quite impossible to find out for certain whether the abuse exists because there is so little control. In my own region, after this report came out, we wanted to be even more conscientious than in the past about certifying domiciliary visits for payment. The Minister placed an obligation on regional boards to satisfy themselves that consultations were necessary before agreeing to pay. *Two consultants in the region refused to give information which would enable the board to decide whether the visits were necessary, and the board refused to pay. The board was threatened with litigation and so appealed to the Minister, who directed it to pay.* (My emphasis.)

The above throws interesting light on the whole subject. How could any board decide whether a visit was "necessary" unless it undertook a detailed investigation of each case? The insertion of a diagnosis would give no protection against abuse. I had previously been a member of the board's own medical advisory committee when the officials had talked of "possible abuses." I had asked what evidence they had of abuses and the simple answer had been "none." One board doctor had suggested, however, that there might be one or two general practitioners who lined up a little package of visits for a particular consultant. I had pointed out that if there were suspicions about any particular general practitioner or consultant he or she should be specifically investigated. I had asked that my question and the answers should be duly minuted. It was not long after this that four of us who were appointed members of the medical committee of the regional board thought it important to ensure that our successors only got there by election. The chairman of the medical committee was Dr Horace Joules, himself a member of the board and a committed communist but a good and conscientious physician. The other three appointed members were all whole time consultants – Clive Sowry, physician at Edgware General; Arkley Steel, medical superintendent of Hillingdon; and Maxwell Alston, microbiologist at the Archway, Highgate – and the four of us managed to get our resolution passed unanimously. But we had not reckoned with Horace Joules and the board, who promptly acceded to our suggestion as a convenient way of getting rid of Murley and the other three troublemakers. A few weeks later we received letters from the board's chairman, Lord Cottesloe, explaining that the medical committee was to be "re-organised" and thanking us for our service. Thereupon we each sent an identical letter to Lord Cottesloe explaining that with our colleagues A, B, and C we had been responsible for putting this resolution forward. We expressed pleasure that our suggestion had been accepted but also our regret that we had been "reorganised" off the committee in this way. At the next committee meeting Dr Harwood Stephenson, one of our replacements, told the chairman that although Lord Cottesloe could not be accused of wanting a medical committee of "yes men" it was at least plain that he did not want a committee of "no men."

It was shortly after the debate in the House in which the domiciliary visits were mentioned that my attention was drawn to the *Hansard* report already referred to. So I wrote to Kenneth Robinson on 29 July giving my reasons for not divulging clinical information on the claim forms. I also gave the details of my correspondence with Dr Macaulay. On 1 August he sent me a printed card acknowledging my letter, "the contents of which have been noted." On return from holiday I wrote again to him:

> I shall be grateful if you would reply to my letter of July 29th in which I referred to your remarks in the House on July 15th.

On 23 August 1959 he replied in his own handwriting:

> 14 Hylda Court, NW5
>
> Dear Mr Murley,
>
> I ackowledged receipt of your letter of 29th July, but I did not consider any reply was called for.

I wrote a third letter on 18 September, drawing attention to my first, in which I had asked if he would tell me precisely what abuses he was referring to. No reply. So I tried again on 4 November:

Dear Mr Robinson,

I am still awaiting a reply to my letter of July 29th and shall be much obliged if you would now give this matter your attention. I wrote to you last on September 18th and, in view of the then impending election, I thought it only right to leave some time for your reply. Perhaps I need hardly say that I shall regard any longer delay as both frankly discourteous and a tacit admission of the weakness of your case.

Guy Fawkes Day at last produced a letter, in his own handwriting, from the House of Commons:

5th November 1959

Dear Mr Murley,

Before making charges of discourtesy you might look again at your original letter to me. But perhaps we take different views of courtesy. I am afraid that I do not feel under obligation to discuss my speeches in the House of Commons with everyone who chooses to write to me, particularly when they are not my constituents! [my mark]. Furthermore, in the light of our respective relationships to the Regional Board, I would regard argument between us of the kind you seem to desire as wholly inappropriate. You are of course entitled to draw any conclusions you like from my refusal to discuss the matter. In order to forestall any further charges of discourtesy, may I borrow the well-worn editorial formula and say that I regard this correspondence as closed.

In view of Mr Robinson's comments on "different views of courtesy" it may be best to give my first letter in full:

July 29th, 1959

Dear Mr Robinson,

I have studied your remarks in the House on July 15th, in particular your comments on payment for domiciliary visits (col 458), with much interest. The two consultants referred to are, of course, my friend Mr A F Rushforth and myself, but I fail to see how our case has any relevance to the subject of abuses which you seemed keen to publicise.

The facts are these. So far as I myself am concerned, I have always strongly objected to recording any clinical information at all on a form which goes to the Regional Hospital Board. Some six years ago the North West Board stopped paying me for visits. However, I continued to go out whenever I was called by a practitioner and I forwarded the signed form to the Board (always leaving blank the space "Reason for Visit"). After about a year Dr Macaulay wrote to say that he would not dispute the matter further and that all my outstanding claims would be met. He went on to say that he knew me to be a man of honour and integrity and that he would not withhold payment even if he could.

In July 1958 Mr Rushforth enquired whether I had received payment for any domiciliary visits. It was only then that I became aware that I had not been paid for almost one year, and so I wrote to Dr Macaulay again. Dr Macaulay had the audacity to write and say that my letter had "anticipated" one he was about to write to me. He further explained that, in view of the comments made in the Report of the Select Committee on Estimates, he no longer felt able to honour his previous undertaking that he would pass my claims for payment. As a member of the North West Board you will, no doubt, be aware of the subsequent steps I took to recover payment for past visits. I imagine that the Ministry (very sensibly when all is considered) directed your Board to pay up because your counsel, like ours, had advised that you had not a leg to stand on.

Your following paragraph in *Hansard* refers to "a minority who are prone to abuse the service for their own ends." I am not clear as to exactly what this means, but perhaps I might invite you to reveal exactly what abuses you are referring to. When I was a member of the medical committee of your Board we were twice presented with a review of the domiciliary visits done during the previous year. We diligently enquired whether there was any evidence of the abuses about which we had often heard from your side of the House. After Dr Macaulay and Dr Muir had made a few vague comments they were specifically charged with the task of bringing any examples of abuse (without necessarily mentioning names) to the attention of the medical committee. Not one case was brought to our notice.

Yet despite this I would not be so naïve as to imagine that, even in my own profession, there may not be the occasional knave who is prepared to rob the taxpayer. I feel quite certain that such occurrences must be exceedingly uncommon. Furthermore, the completion of the space on the form "reason for visit" affords the taxpayer no protection whatever against a determined rogue. The money (and time) spent at the Board on checking these forms must far exceed any possible savings.

In your remaining contribution to this debate you certainly make some very topsy-turvy comments on consultants. Like all socialists you display no love for anyone who has the temerity to earn his living outside the NHS, but surely it is most unbecoming for a member of the Regional Hospital Board to display such a partisan attitude on the subject of consultants. In any case, did not the special report of the Select Committee on Estimates refer to the increased cost of the domiciliary service since *whole time* consultants became entitled to payment for visits?

Reading this letter again, nearly 20 years later, I am surprised that Mr Robinson should have implied that I was in any way discourteous. He was wise enough, however, not to repeat any of his accusations outside the House; not that I was contemplating legal action, even though two of my medical colleagues had successfully sued two MPs (one Liberal and one Labour) for libel, and a third had secured substantial damages for libel from a member of his hospital management committee.

But I had a further clash with Kenneth Robinson in 1967 when he was Minister of Health. A young woman had been referred to my clinic at the Royal Northern Hospital with an all too brief letter from her general practitioner: "Varicose veins, please advise." This patient said that she had been getting some discomfort in the calf muscles on both sides. On examination she had no sign of varicose veins but I noticed that she was wearing excessively high stiletto heels, which were then fashionable. I advised her that the muscle discomfort in the calves could well be related to her high heels. She seemed satisfied with my advice, but then sat down and said, "I would like to have the photographs that were taken here." She made no mention of the nature of any clinical photographs which had been taken and I did not think of asking for further details. On looking through the considerable number of old notes in her folder I saw that she had attended several other clinics at the Royal Northern, including that of my colleague Dr Raymond Greene, but I could not see any pictures. I told her this and added, "Did you not sign the usual permission form for photography?" She replied in the affirmative, and I added, "Well, any pictures are now the property of the hospital." At this she got up and stamped out, saying, "Thank you for *nothing*!" I suddenly realised that, with her completely normal legs, she had probably used the appointment as an opportunity to ask for some old photographs, and I felt pretty angry. I called her back into the room and gave her a sharp reprimand for having come to my clinic and behaved in this way.

In the ensuing three months a number of letters of complaint arrived from the patient and the Patients Association, addressed to hospital secretary, group secretary, and regional board, alleging, among other things, that I had "violently manhandled" this lady. No mention was made of her request for photographs, even though the clinic nurse had independently confirmed this and the other points I had reported. Then came a letter from the regional board, requesting an answer for the minister within seven days. I felt furious, especially as it was commonplace for us to wait months for the ministry to answer the simplest requests. It was at about this time that the photographs were suddenly found in the patient's note file. They had been taken at the request of Dr Raymond Greene when the lady had attended his endocrine clinic complaining of excessive hirsutes. Now, I had noticed that she had a very full head of black hair and thick eyebrows, but I had had no reason to examine her abdomen. It transpired that it was the male distribution of her profuse pubic hair which had attracted attention at the endocrine clinic and which had been duly photographed. Thereupon I had the photographic department make copies of the prints. These, together with a copy of my letter to the general practitioner explaining the normal clinical findings in the legs, I put in a large envelope marked "Strictly private and confidential" and addressed to the Rt Hon Kenneth Robinson Esq, MP. With many a good chuckle I delivered this package personally to the porter's lodge of the Department of Health headquarters at Alexander Fleming House and I have little doubt that it reached the minister, but, sad to say, I had no acknowledgement. My accompanying letter was firm and polite. I told him that I was outraged to be asked to reply within seven days concerning such a phoney complaint when his own department was invariably incapable of attending to matters of real importance with any sense of urgency. He may have been furious, but he should have known that even a Tory minister would have had the same response from me.

It will be appreciated that I had reason to cross swords with Kenneth Robinson on a number of occasions and there was an interesting sequel to all this when, in 1975, he chanced to pay a visit to Oundle, his old public school. He was shown round by Barry Trapnell, the headmaster, to whom he mentioned that he himself had been in Grafton House. Thereupon the headmaster took his distinguished visitor to Grafton and introduced him to the housemaster. The latter, on learning that Mr Robinson had once been head boy, took the opportunity of introducing him to the then head boy who happened to be Tony Murley, the youngest of my three sons. Kenneth Robinson asked, "Is your father a doctor?" Tony replied, "Yes, sir." "Is he a surgeon?" "Yes, sir," said Tony again. Whereupon, without another word, the former minister took his departure. Until then I had not realised how deeply imprinted the name of Murley was on the memory of Kenneth Robinson. From all accounts he is a pleasant man and I am only sorry that he should apparently have been so offended.

22 Private practice

As a newly established young consultant in 1948, recently back from wartime service, I was, despite my instinctive gut reaction against nationalised medicine, relieved to have a basic salary from the health service with freedom to undertake private work. The feedback between the two types of practice was to prove instructive. In former times, whether we worked in voluntary or local authority hospitals, most of us were accustomed to certain financial constraints. In the early days of the NHS, before the great pharmaceutical revolution and all the other immense medical advances which promoted a rapid growth in expenditure, many people remained blissfully unaware of future funding problems. In private practice, however, few of our patients were then medically insured and so we were kept fully aware of the economic facts. Moreover, it was impossible not to be conscious of the need to maintain the same standards of behaviour in hospital as in private work. In the health service one soon became accustomed to working under increasing pressure and organising the work flow as efficiently as possible.

Doctors today may well have forgotten that most of the pay beds in our hospitals were initially subjected to limitation of medical fees. In the 85% of "controlled" pay beds the original maximum surgical fee was 50 guineas for a major operation, 25 for an intermediate one, and 10 for a minor one, with the anaesthetist's charges limited to 2 guineas plus 10% of the surgeon's fees. But there were some 15% of "no fee ceiling" beds. At first I was happy to limit my fees for most British private patients since I knew that through their personal taxation they were helping to pay my NHS salary and ultimately my pension. I felt no such constraints with foreign patients, however, but, in common with many of my colleagues, when I look back on my old records I am astonished at how low most of my fees were. Eventually, largely as a result of pressure from Department of Health officials – who became tired of trying to "police" a system of charges which had not been realistically updated for years – these restricted fee scales were abolished. By then there was a growing disposition for many doctors to conform to the scales agreed by the various provident organisations such as BUPA, PPP, and Western Provident.

Opportunities for private earnings were clearly much less for most physicians; however, it was not unknown for some of my medical colleagues to supplement their basic hospital salary by undertaking a full annual quota of 200 domiciliary visits on the NHS. In fact, much later on, in the case of certain geriatricians there was a suspicion that domiciliary consultations on elderly patients before hospital admission might be done rather too freely – an early example of "moral hazard" (by no means confined to geriatricians) later encountered in the private insurance sector, when neither consumer nor provider has a direct stake in the costs of the service.

Never did I see private patients in my health service hospital clinics, nor did I, except in the most exceptional circumstances, operate on a private patient during a routine NHS operation list. At an early stage, however, I had prepared myself for the odd patient – rare in my experience – who might consult me privately and then seek operation on the health service, and for the patient who, having been referred to my NHS clinic, would then ask to be treated privately. It was my consistent philosophy that I should recognise the patient's right to seek medical care in whatever manner best suited him or her. And although I would never encourage a patient to flit back and forth between NHS and private care, I felt bound to recognise that Aneurin Bevan had promised every Briton that he or she would be free to use the whole of the NHS or any part of it. Who are we as doctors to dictate to the public precisely how they should seek advice or treatment? Those of us with personal or family experience of illness know how vulnerable sick people can feel, and how confused they can be as to the most appropriate source of advice.

Throughout my 32 years in the health service I never had a waiting list as such; each patient for operation at St Albans was normally given an admission date by my secretary at, or shortly after, the outpatient consultation. The position was only slightly different at the Royal Northern. Likewise, anyone who consulted me privately and who asked if there was a waiting list for the NHS was told that I did not have such a list. Indeed it sometimes happened, especially in the early days when there were fewer pay beds, that an urgent case could be admitted more quickly to a public than to a private bed. All such patients were informed that the operation consent form for the public patient clearly indicated that "no undertaking can be given that this operation will be performed by a particular surgeon." It was plainly incumbent on us to make the position absolutely clear, but this was always done in a kindly way.

Nor was I totally unprepared when, not long after the appointed day, a lady from a good address came to see me at my NHS clinic about her varicose veins. Having been advised operation, to which she had readily agreed, she looked around the door as she left the room and said: "Of course, you'll be doing it doctor, won't you?" I invited her to sit down again and fished out an operation consent form from the rack on my desk. Having read it, her response was, "So this is what the health service has done." I explained to her that this form of consent, far from being due to the health service, had, in fact, emanated from an operation prior to the appointed day. In this case the patient alleged a breach of contract by a surgeon in his failure to perform a hernia operation personally. That patient, in a public ward of Folkestone hospital, discovered subsequently that the completely successful and satisfactory operation, with uneventful recovery and no later recurrence of the hernia, had been carried out by the house surgeon. The claim was regarded as trivial and the Medical Defence Union (the surgeon's medical indemnity insurers), on the advice of counsel, paid £5 into court in advance of the hearing. This was to protect the union's funds against having to pay the plaintiff's costs if he were technically successful, albeit with a trifling award. In due course judgment was given for the plaintiff and £1 damages awarded. But the judge criticised the plaintiff regarding the frivolous nature of the action. Moreover, because the union had paid into court more than the ultimate award it did not have to pay the plaintiff's costs even though he had won his action. It was only after this celebrated case, and prior to the inception of the NHS, that the Medical Defence Union recommended suitable modification of the operation consent form in 1950. I am indebted to Dr John Wall, secretary fo the Medical Defence Union, for confirmation of the above details.

An interesting corollary of the above is that because for many years there was no operation consent form specifically for private work it was not uncommon for intelligent and well educated patients – including even the odd lawyer – to sign standard NHS consent forms for their private operations. On many such occasions in private practice I have amended the form for my patients.

There are, and always were, some doctors who believe that health service and private work should be undertaken in entirely separate hospitals. But, although I did most of my private consulting work in my own rooms, I much preferred my surgery to be as "geographically whole time" as possible by concentrating operative work in my main hospitals. And NHS hospital food being what it usually is, I often felt constrained to tell my patients that although the diet might not match up to Ritz standards they would have the advantage of being in the care of my skilled theatre, nursing, and medical team and would generally not be in hospital for long.

Of course there were always a few junior doctors who did not approve of private practice, but I am not aware that any of my own staff publicly expressed such views. It was my regular practice to pay them 10% of the operation fee. In this connection one of the things I most liked about our onetime splendid St David's wing at the Royal Northern Hospital was that it gave us the opportunity to teach young doctors the economics of medicine. Indeed, as I entered that wing with any new house surgeon or registrar it was my custom to say,

"You are now crossing the threshold to that part of the hospital where the patient (and/or the insurer) is billed for every item of medical investigation, though the drugs are included in the overall account." I would then add that they must therefore avoid ordering needless investigations for which the patient would be charged. This economic discipline in the private wing could not fail to be applied by any sensible resident on the general side of the hospital too.

In the early days of the health service when few private patients were covered by insurance such patients generally showed a healthy concern to get out of hospital as soon as possible. But with the passage of time, and the growth of insurance through the various provident organisations, many of our private patients became far less cost conscious. And when many insurers began to encourage direct billing by the hospitals we became more and more aware of "moral hazard." It is sad to find that in recent years even intelligent people in pay beds, when thus shielded from the economic facts of life, have tended to become almost as irresponsible as those in the general service. In the later years of my practice, however, when, because of growing problems deriving from the "Barbarabarities of Castle" – which I shall shortly explain – I had to do more of my work in private hospitals I regularly had the accounts department supply me with a printout of each patient's bill. This became an essential part of my continuing education on medical costs. At the time of postoperative check up I have commonly found that, as a result of direct billing of the insurer, patients have never seen their hospital accounts. I have then given them a copy of the bill and have often been intrigued to see how surprised they are by the overall costs. This surely spells out a salutary lesson on health service expenditure, for how can we expect to see more prudent use of resources when doctors, patients, and nurses are so sheltered from the economic facts of life?

Since 1955 when I made the first of a number of visits to the United States and Canada, and with my father and step-mother living in New York City, I have been fairly well informed about the situation on the other side of the Atlantic. My friend George Crile Jr of the Cleveland Clinic, always intensely interested in all aspects of medical care and medical economics, has regularly exchanged information on our two countries' problems for more than 30 years. I well recall that by the mid 1960s Dr Crile was saying that the Americans were beginning to encounter as many problems with their private insurance system as we had with our nationalised system. Many of those problems, however, were of a different character from ours. Firstly, as mentioned to me by Frank Glenn in New York, in many places there were so many private and semi-private patients that the practical training of young surgeons was becoming difficult. On my first visit to the Mayo and Cleveland clinics it was exceptional for the trainee to undertake more than the opening up and closure of operation wounds; but on my later visits it became increasingly common to see trainees undertake the same range of surgical operations as did senior registrars and registrars in the United Kingdom on health service patients – but not on private patients. One could not help remarking that the supervision of trainees in American private clinics was often far closer and more detailed than that in some of our NHS hospitals. Doubtless the same would apply here if there were any great increase in private surgery because this would lead to a larger proportion of surgical training being done in private hospitals.

A second contrast was the much earlier development of cost consciousness and of measures for effective cost containment in the United States. It was the introduction of Medicare in 1965, and later of Medicaid, rather than the growing costs of private treatment which led to this. My father, after a small stroke and one week in hospital in New York in 1967, was asked to send all his bills to Medicare. He expressed his astonishment, and in a letter to me he wrote: "I have paid so much tax in the USA that I was pleased to send them my bills; but, as a businessman, I am compelled to ask, how long can they remain solvent?" Instead of the British system of annual budgeting, the Medicare and Medicaid systems in the United States depend on direct billing by hospitals and doctors on an item-of-service basis. Such a system, where neither consumer nor provider of the service is in a direct financial relationship, can only prove excessively expensive as experience in British

Columbia has also shown. But the lessons learnt from item-of-service governmental systems elsewhere have especial significance for item-of-service private practice in Britain where, until very recently, we have largely avoided these problems.

THE BARBARABARITIES OF CASTLE

Since I have often declared that all originality is unconscious plagiarism, excepting when it is conscious or deliberate, I must be careful about claiming originality for coining the phrase "the Barbarabarities of Castle," which I apply to the attempt of a former Secretary of State in 1976 to abolish pay beds in NHS hospitals, and to the largely unforeseen result in promoting the biggest ever development of private hospitals in this country.

Mrs Barbara Castle, bless her heart, is no more or less mixed up on the subject of private medicine than are most of her socialist colleagues, many of whom are entirely in favour of medical privacy so long as they do not have to pay the market price for it. But Mrs Castle's celebrated sinus operation in the private wing of a London hospital was well publicised in the press; indeed it was the subject of some interesting correspondence between us in the *Daily Telegraph* in 1976. And when she tried to duck the issue her surgeon felt compelled to spill the beans about her having been a bona fide paying patient. And why ever not? Who am I to argue that her ultimate intention in abolishing pay beds was not to destroy private practice but simply to ensure rapid development of strictly independent hospitals? After all, she did unsuccessfully try to introduce "In Place of Strife" and it was many years before even a Thatcher government had the courage to cut some of the trades unions down to size, before moving on to the professions.

As one of those who for many years was so strongly in favour of the move to geographical wholetimeness I could only deplore the "Barbarabarities" of 1976. I should have known better; for had not Reginald Payne warned us that the service might be carried on the broad shoulders of the professions for a full 25 years, and that then, only then, would the cracks start to appear? The year 1973 had been marked by the first outbreak of militant trades unionism in the NHS, and worse was to follow. Short of the "privatisation" of our hospitals, which is not yet on the Thatcherite agenda, there is little prospect of a return to those civilised conditions in which both public and pay beds were widely tolerated under the same roof. But even if governments did have the courage to eschew their continued obsession with centralised bargaining and pay settlements, and to set our hospitals free, it is unlikely that things could return to the *status quo ante*.

In all these circumstances it would seem more realistic to deal with the situation as we find it at present, with private practice hardly encouraged within the health service and with a growing number and variety of private insurers and independent hospitals. In 1979, during my presidency of the Royal College of Surgeons of England, the Fellowship for Freedom in Medicine did try to promote proper collaboration between the many elements of the private sector. To that end I invited representatives of BUPA, PPP, the Western Provident Association, the Independent Hospitals Group, a number of leading medical men, and some of my fellow presidents to a meeting at the college. An excellent paper prepared by Mr Will Hopper, an eminent lay member of the fellowship who later became a European MP, was put forward for discussion. Will Hopper's idea was to promote a highly ethical organisation, a foundation for private medicine with charitable status, representative of all aspects of independent medical practice, which would be able to coordinate information and advice on every feature of private medical care for the benefit of patients, doctors, and nurses, as well as all suppliers and providers of such service. To set up an ethical group of high standing would clearly be of immense value to a multitude of professional and other people who have no ready and reliable source of information or guidance. At our meeting there was considerable support for this concept from the Independent Hospitals Group and from the provident organisations, with the notable exception of BUPA – the largest such provider. I reluctantly came to the conclusion that BUPA, so long as it held a dominant position in the private insurance market, tended to regard itself as more or less the epitome of what we were seeking. But times have changed: the Barbarabarities have resulted in many new entrants to the private insurance field so that the need for that ethical organisation is greater than ever.

Turning now to what our American friends describe as the doctor's "office," I have often referred to Harley Street practice, in rows of separate houses with many rooms in part time use, as failing to fulfil the requirements of modern medicine; indeed, it is more reminiscent of a now outmoded cottage industry. In my later years I was happy to move out of my Harley Street premises and avail myself of the excellent consulting facilities at the Wellington Hospital, agreeably adjacent to Lords cricket ground. With further growth of the private sector I foresee the urgent need for the development of comprehensive clinics, comparable to the Mayo and the Cleveland, where doctors will work under excellent conditions and probably on a salaried basis. It is one thing for doctors to be salaried in a state near-monopoly service but quite another for more and more of them to work on a salaried basis in independent competing clinics and hospitals where the consumer and his insurer can exercise wider and more effective choice. To this end, a year or so ago, together with two of my colleagues, Sir Edward Tuckwell and Sir Richard Bayliss, I gave support to an abortive effort to set up a private consulting clinic in central London. I have no doubt that others will soon prove more successful.

It is evident that the whole of the above is concerned with private *specialist* practice. The strictly general practice part of the family doctor's work – apart from any insurance, industrial, or school work he may undertake – is largely as a contractor *for* service under the health service. Even in relatively affluent areas many general practitioners do little private practice. Apart from the problems of dealing with NHS and private patients in the same premises, conditions in general practice have been so changed by Danckwerts, the charter, and various supplementary payments that many general practitioners cannot be bothered with private work. In the larger cities there are, of course, still a number of purely private doctors. It is my impression, although I may be wrong, that many of them earn less than their health service colleagues and that they do not enjoy the same pension benefits. Doubtless there are exceptions, perhaps when the private practice is predominantly involved with company and insurance work as opposed to everyday personal medical service. The purely private doctor is able to refer his patients to consultants in both NHS and private practice, and he normally shows no resentment about using the services of a private specialist. Over the years, however, I have sometimes discerned an element of resentment on the part of some health service general practitioners when their patients seek, or sometimes, alas, "demand," a private consultation. Such feelings of resentment, although often understandable, are hardly excusable if we accept the general premise that meeting the patient's personal requirements must be paramount.

In conclusion, it should not be forgotten that it was Aneurin Bevan who declared, "If we were rich enough we would all be private patients." Had he possibly forgotten that in his beloved Welsh valleys in days gone by it was commonplace for the miners to appoint their own "club" doctor, and to have the power to hire and fire him? Why should Bevan and his successors so glibly have assumed that, given the right sort of help by the friendly societies and, perhaps, by the health voucher, the generality of folk could not equally well have exercised proper consumer choice?

23 The medical establishment

In the later stages of my active professional life I suppose that I became one of the so called medical establishment; however, some of my colleagues have suggested that the medical establishment really joined me. Be that as it may, I can only say that I learnt a great deal and derived considerable entertainment, not to mention some satisfaction and occasional exasperation, from this experience.

I became a member of the BMA when I first qualified in 1939, but I knew little of its functions until after the war. Although living in Radlett would normally have made me a member of the Watford division, through my first hospital location with "Barts in Herts" I became a member of the St Albans division in October 1946. In those turbulent times in the run up to the NHS there were frequent local meetings on the prospective terms and conditions of service. It says much for the naïveté of doctors, if not for their grasp of the economic facts of life, that whatever may have been the intrinsic merits or deficiencies of the proposed health service they agreed to enter a state service without having the faintest idea of what they would be paid. But I shall spare my readers any repetition of that well worn theme now.

Divisional meetings of the BMA after the inception of the NHS were, justifiably perhaps, at first heavily attended whenever the question of doctors pay was up for discussion but sparsely supported on most other occasions. It is easy to criticise any organisation confronting a bloodless revolution, as the BMA then was, and with all the subsequent "flak" therefrom. Both individually and collectively we were faced with an unprecedented situation at a time when most of the young were freshly demobilised and many of those who had remained as civilian doctors had been stretched to the uttermost. All were now faced with settling down in a rapidly changing medical environment.

Apart from the local BMA meetings, it was not long before consultant and specialist committees were formed in each of the hospital regions. But as many of the specialists felt let down by the BMA, and some of them were not even BMA members, there was no disposition for the regional specialist committees to accept the BMA umbrella. It says much for the BMA – although this may simply have been due to a desperate concern for survival – that it allowed non-BMA members to serve on, and even to take office in, both the regional committees and what was then called the Central Consultants and Specialists Committee, all of which were ultimately serviced through BMA headquarters. In addition the Joint Consultants Committee was formed as a condominium between representatives from the central body and the various royal colleges. But many specialists were disillusioned with their own colleges and so there were many potential, if not apparent, divisions in our ranks. Some would say, just what the politicians and bureaucrats ordered.

I myself served on the consultants and specialists committee of the north west metropolitan region for many years after the appointed day. I was never a member of the central committee, but I did serve on the joint committee for some five years, both before and during my presidency of the Royal College of Surgeons. It will therefore be appreciated that, together with my work at the Fellowship for Freedom in Medicine, I had substantial exposure to medical politics from just before the inception of the NHS until my retirement from it. This gave me considerable knowledge and understanding of the workings of bureaucracy and parliamentary politics. But I have never been an enthusiastic medical politician, regarding much of my own involvement as an unavoidable consequence of nationalised medicine. It has always been my considered view, however, that it is no good moping on the sidelines: if you believe that reforms are needed you have to be prepared to get in on the act and work hard. Fortunately my busy involvement in this field never detracted from my clinical work and commitment; rather did I consider that it enhanced my all round surgical performance and efficiency in and outside the health service. I could never have forgiven myself for opting out and leaving this work to other busy colleagues. Of course, it is always an appealing idea to think of working in undisturbed conditions, but I fancy that throughout this postwar period there were few other countries that did not have similar problems.

By the late 1960s I was becoming more and more disillusioned with the NHS and decided it was time to try to influence events on the council of the BMA. There was a specialist vacancy in the north west metropolitan region in 1968; I offered my candidature and was elected by a large majority. The council, representative of a broad spectrum of the profession from all over the country, was then under the chairmanship of Dr Ronald (later Sir Ronald) Gibson, a Winchester general practitioner and founder member of the Fellowship for Freedom in Medicine who had been a few years senior to me at Barts. The agenda for the monthly meetings occupied a full day and entailed a large amount of preparatory reading. I soon became aware of what I had previously suspected: that there were a good many longstanding members, some of whom had been there rather too long. Moreover, in the course of debate some of them would talk again and again; it was my own strong feeling that, once having had their say, they should hold their peace until others had spoken.

The BMA committee system required the members of each committee to be elected by the Annual Representative Meeting, the BMA parliament. Names had to be put forward before this meeting and were duly voted upon by the representatives – all very democratic, but giving little such experience to councillors unless they were also elected to the individual committees. I had no objection to the widest possible representation on the so called craft and other committees, but I thought that council members needed to get some regular experience of this work as well. Service on council also confirmed my earlier impression that the BMA was far too ready to issue statements on every aspect of medicine and the

NHS. But this may partly have been due to the fact that they had an excellent press officer, Mr Thistlethwaite, a man who was always so pleasant, helpful, and unaggressive that the media were liable to plague him too often. The press officer would ensure that statements were given by some suitable official or committee member; but I always felt – and still do – that the public gets rather irked by excessive pontification from the medical profession, especially when it comes from the doctors' own "trade union."

In 1971, during my third year on council, Ronald Gibson was succeeded as chairman by Walpole Lewin, a Cambridge neurosurgeon. He was a conscientious and highly industrious man, but I found him too tolerant of the council "gas bags" who tended to spin out our proceedings. It was James Cameron (now Sir James, and Walpole's successor in the chair) who once firmly declared, "In the BMA we are drowned in oceans of democracy."

In 1970 there were two vacancies on the council of the Royal College of Surgeons. There were 24 candidates, out of which Walpole Lewin and I were successful. We had each offered our candidature in the previous two years: on the first occasion I was second on the list of those not appointed; in the second year I had missed election by a few votes; and on the third occasion I was elected with a substantial lead over Walpole. Each of us was elected for a period of eight years. This was much more to my liking; I had been appointed by the college as one of its first surgical tutors in the 1950s and had become a regional adviser in 1965. In addition I had been appointed as an examiner in pathology for the primary FRCS examination in 1968. As a result of my election to college council I did not seek reappointment to the BMA council on the expiry of my three year period in 1971. I had enjoyed the BMA work; during it I met many old friends and made many new ones. It had been valuable experience but I had had enough.

The then president of the Royal College of Surgeons was Sir Thomas Holmes Sellors, an outstanding cardiothoracic surgeon. I had known him for many years as he had been the second chairman of the consultants and specialists committee of the north west metropolitan region, before chairing the central committee and then serving for no less than 11 years as chairman of the Joint Consultants Committee. He was a perfect gentleman, an immensely industrious and most skilful technical surgeon, and anything but the archetype medical politician, though some of his more senior colleagues had regarded him as "a BMA man" when he was first appointed to council. The truth of the matter was that far too many of our older colleagues had been passive agents in the new service, often reluctant to bend their efforts to rectifying its faults.

I felt much at home at the college of surgeons, where we were primarily concerned with preserving and enhancing the highest standards of surgery in the interests of the public. Our Royal Charter and charitable status precluded direct embroilment in the terms and conditions of specialist service in the NHS, which are determined by the Joint Consultants Committee; but, apart from that, the college has a vital responsibility for surgical teaching and examining, and for the coordination of surgical training in concert with sister colleges and the various specialist associations. For many years before the inception of the NHS the college of surgeons had inspected hospitals to assess the overall suitability of training posts. Our physician colleagues began to adopt this practice much later, but now each of the colleges has important functions in this respect. Inspections occur at intervals of not more than five years and the reports of the college inspectors are collated at the board of surgical training. The threat of the withholding or withdrawal of recognition is usually quite enough to ensure that any necessary remedial steps are taken.

At one of my earlier council meetings I was surprised to learn that the undergraduate and postgraduate teaching hospitals were not subject to regular inspection. I pointed out that this was not only illogical but also unjust, since the official labelling of a hospital carried no guarantee that its residents and registrars would receive adequate supervision and training. In this contention I was supported by the president and the decision to inspect all hospitals and their training posts was promptly implemented without dissent. In my experience this was characteristic of council's approach to problems of this kind. Whereas many people referred to "teaching" and "non-teaching" hospitals, on council these were normally referred to as teaching (or undergraduate) and regional hospitals, it being recognised that the senior staff in the regional hospitals often did just as much teaching, and sometimes much more, than those in the undergraduate hospitals. Since completing my chief assistant appointment at Barts I had worked in three busy regional hospitals where we did much teaching and training for the FRCS and did a great deal of teaching for elective students. Indeed, the vintage years of the NHS were when the range and quality of work was rapidly expanding at many of the regional hospitals.

There was a striking contrast between the way council responsibilities were arranged at the college of surgeons and the BMA. The committee work at the college was organised so that council members were progressively exposed to an increasing range and variety of experience during their period of service – eight years in the first instance and a further four years if they were re-elected. A new member would usually find himself serving on two or so of the college committees. Subsequent changes ensured that each councillor learnt more and more of the college work. Furthermore, those with greater keenness and capacity for work tended to gain greater responsibility. Such a system could only ensure that whoever council eventually elected as president would have acquired considerable knowledge and experience of all aspects of the college's work.

In my own case I served in turn on the staff and establishment committee, the board of surgical training, hospital inspection, finance and general purposes, furniture and buildings, museums, fellowship election and prize committees during my first five years, moving on to various others which need no special mention here. The president and two vice presidents served as ex officio members of all boards and committees, but it was much a matter of their availability and particular interests that determined which of those they might attend. Members of council also had a responsibility for supporting and, when appropriate, chairing the statutory lectures at the college and, starting in the period of Sir Thomas's presidency, a growing number of these Hunterian and Arris and Gale lectures were held at various provincial centres. For many of us this entailed a great deal of time and travel, with the need for careful organisation of our hospital and practice commitments.

The official hospital recognition visits were always interesting as one learnt a lot about the type and quality of work going on all over the country. The regional hospital inspections in the generality of surgery were normally carried out by a single individual – although occasionally in concert with a visitor from the anaesthetic or dental faculties. But when inspection of the undergraduate hospitals began we often appointed a pair of visitors. I can vividly remember some of the earliest of these inspections. In advance of the visits we were supplied with full details of the senior and junior staffing of all services and with a detailed analysis of the annual turnover according to a preordained schedule. A first visit would usually be intensive and detailed, whereas repeat visits might be concentrated on points of relative weakness or dubiety which had earlier come to light. Although a visitor might inspect a hospital he had visited before, he was invariably chosen from a hospital outside the region. The visits always included personal interviews with the junior staff in training, invariably in the absence of their seniors; thus junior staff were free to draw attention to matters of concern for their own wellbeing and training.

Members of council would often serve as the college representative on various advisory appointments committees for consultants and senior registrars, but most of this work was done by senior consultants in the appropriate specialties. The principles to which such a college representative adhered were to ensure that those appointed had fulfilled the basic criteria for promotion, and not to force his own personal choice on the hospital concerned. It was important for the college representative to show sturdy independence by discouraging nepotism and any possible disposition to promote the "local boy," just because he was there, when there were clearly more worthy candidates. In certain hospitals, with past evidence of inbreeding and skulduggery, it was not unknown for the president and council to ensure that a suitably tough college representative was appointed to the selection committee. Sometimes, however, there was no easy way of sorting out such problems retrospectively (see chapter 17).

One of the many pleasant aspects of council life is the dining club. The club was set up in 1869. It began with periodic dinners held at a variety of hotels – starting at the Trafalgar, Greenwich – after some of the council meetings. After earlier sporadic and rather infrequent gatherings this eventually became a regular event after each (then) quarterly council. The principal aim was to bring past and present members together under more cordial conditions following sometimes adversarial meetings. With the start of the NHS and with the college's vastly extended commitments council meetings have generally been held monthly, except in the summer vacation. Moreover, because business has greatly increased, much work is now done at a less formal morning meeting of "council in committee," held before lunch and the formal afternoon council. The club continues, however, on a quarterly basis (with minute books dating back to its foundation) and has dined for many years in the fine council room of the new building completed after the second world war. At each dinner the chair is now taken by one of the more recently elected members, who is introduced for 10 minutes by another member of his own choice, after which the chairman tells us about himself for 20 minutes. It is a splendid occasion at its best; and at its worst it is distinctly revealing of some characters.

I had started as an examiner in the primary FRCS two years before my election to council, but the last four of my six years coincided with my service on council. During the second half of those six years it was customary for the more senior examiners to take part in two or three of the overseas examinations. When examining in pathology I was chairman of the board of examiners in Cairo and Khartoum in 1971 and in Colombo and Peradinya, Ceylon, in 1972. The college had been examining for some years in these centres. I was also chairman for our first primary in Baghdad in 1974 and was lucky enough to make another trip there in 1976, when some of us were able to visit the marsh Arabs whose life style has been so beautifully described and illustrated by Wilfred Thesiger.

Our British colleges have a well deserved reputation for high standards and integrity in the conduct of their examinations. Examining overseas could be entertaining and even, occasionally, dangerous, as when a Professor Shaw (an uncle of George Bernard Shaw) was shot, but not badly damaged, by an angry Cairene some years ago. Once a failed candidate in the final had taken out a gun and potted one of the college busts. I have a vivid recollection of the occasion in Cairo when I was paired off with Professor Hill (now dead) of the Royal Free Hospital. During the oral examination we were offered bribes by two of the candidates. A young man assured us that his father was "very rich" and would make it worth our while if we put him through; and a young lady, having told us that she had "failed the examination last time," explained that her husband was an influential doctor who would, likewise, look after our interests. I gaped with astonishment, but Kenneth Hill briskly responded, "Cut out that cackle. We are here to find out what you know about pathology." Fortunately both of these candidates were so bad that they had little chance of getting through. Had they passed, I suppose that some of us might have been inadvertently "refreshed," as the lawyers say. I reminded Hill of the story about the Duke of Wellington who, when prime minister, was found fuming with rage in his office. His personal secretary said, "What is the matter, your Grace?" The Duke rasped: "You saw that scoundrel who just left my office? Well, he tried to bribe me." The secretary responded, "Oh, how utterly discreditable." "Discreditable be damned," said the Duke, "he almost reached my price!"

In 1976, when I was examining in Iraq with Professor Bill Symmers, I had another interesting experience. John Lambert, our examinations officer, reported to me as chairman that instead of the expected next pair of candidates he had found four people in the waiting room. He had discovered that the extra pair were guards accompanying two examinees from prison. The guards intended to accompany the candidates, who happened to be a Kurdish man and his wife, to their vivas. I told John that on no account would we allow the guards to come in. Lambert, with his characteristic tact and diplomacy, managed to persuade them to remain in the waiting room. To our delight, and that of the other examiners, each of these candidates performed well, and passed in the other two subjects. We were all pleased to be able to congratulate them with the other successful candidates.

Apart from that disconcerting experience with the Kurdish candidates we also became aware of other political problems when examining overseas. Deans and other officials in the medical schools and health ministries were sometimes mysteriously removed from office. On a subsequent visit one's tender inquiries about some previously respected individual would be answered by vague references to the fact that he was now "working in the country" or had "taken retirement."

One dean of the medical school in Baghdad had clearly been under considerable political pressure during our first visit. I had noticed then that he was constantly fidgeting with a string of beads which, like many Arabs, he invariably carried. He was no longer in office on the occasion of my second visit, but just before I left I was pleased to meet him again at a private luncheon party, where he seemed unusually cheerful and relaxed. This time his beads were no longer in evidence and I remarked, "Where are your 'worry' beads?" He replied, with a smile, "No worry – no 'worry' beads!"

Notwithstanding all those little local problems (as Harold Macmillan might have said), the best of the overseas candidates were generally very good, sometimes outstanding. This is impressive when one allows for the fact that they were almost invariably undergoing written and oral examination in what was their second language. In Egypt, Sudan, Sri Lanka, and Iraq it was accepted that higher medical education and examination should be conducted in English. It remains to be seen how long this will continue for changes have begun to occur in the last few years. It has always been the policy of the English college that we should encourage other countries to develop their own examination and training systems. That, after all, is how the Australasian colleges severed the umbilical cord with the "home country." Some of our sister colleges have tended to follow a rather different policy. But, ultimately, it must be right and proper for other countries to become educationally self sufficient. From the point of view of access to the medical literature and the common textbooks, however, there are enormous advantages in using what has now become the *lingua franca* of medicine. At the same time we must recognise the many cultural and other pressures which operate in these countries today. Whatever the future may hold, those of us who have had the privilege and pleasure of taking part in these overseas exercises must be ever grateful for the experience.

During the period of which I write it was often difficult for overseas graduates, having passed our primary FRCS in their own country, to secure the necessary appointments in the United Kingdom to enable them to satisfy the requirements for our final examination. It was because of this that, after examining in Iraq, I later appointed two excellent Iraquis as senior house surgeons at one of my own hospitals. In the last few years, partly to solve this problem and partly to reduce the number of our own graduates with little prospect of promotion, the college has implemented an excellent training programme for duly sponsored overseas doctors.

During my progression through various college committees and these overseas visits there had been changes in the presidency. In 1972 Tom Holmes Sellors was succeeded by Sir Edward Muir, whom I had first met in Abyssinia in 1941. He was an excellent surgeon, recently retired from King's College Hospital, but still running a large and highly successful private practice. Shortly after his re-election in July of the following year he several times told his presidential secretary that he felt unaccountably tired – often an ominous sign. On 14 October of the same year, while spending a weekend with friends, he developed severe headache, quickly became unconscious, and died a few hours later from a cerebral haemorrhage. His many friends and colleagues were deeply shattered. It was the first time in the history of the college that a president had died during his period of office.

It was not until 1953 that a maximum period of three years for the presidency was agreed. For more than a century, the office of president having succeeded that of "master" in 1822, most presidents were elected for one or two years, although Sir William Savory had four, Sir William MacCormac five, and Berkeley (the first Lord) Moynihan six years. Sir Alfred (later Lord) Webb-Johnson, often known as "affable Alfred," had been elected in 1941 in the days of the blitz and he remained in office until July 1949. He was finally displaced by Sir Cecil Wakeley who, in his turn, having anxiously awaited Alfred's departure and stayed for five years, also showed some reluctance to move on. By the time of Sir Harry Platt's election in 1953 the three year period had been agreed, subject as before to annual re-election. To guard against possible future changes in the rules, council had included a carefully framed clause in the bylaws. Any move to change this three year period must be subject to three steps: firstly, the putting forward at one council of any suggested change; secondly, its further discussion at the next council; and finally, at a third meeting, council would put any formal proposal for change to the vote. The intention was to ensure that no alteration should be suddenly sprung upon the college.

The untimely death of Sir Edward Muir on 14 October 1973, just after completing his first year of office in July of that year, resulted in Rodney Smith's election to the presidency at the November council meeting. The incoming president thus lost three months of his first year and, under the existing rules, would have been re-elected for only a total period of two years and nine months rather than a full three years. Since no previous president had died in office some members of council later felt that a special dispensation might be made but others expressed their reservations. Accordingly, the rules were amended in July 1975 and at a later council meeting on 8 April 1976 the vice-presidents (Richard Handley and Richard Franklin) put forward a resolution: "That in accordance with the powers given to council in the revised Standing Rules (Section IV, para 4) the period of office served by Sir Rodney Smith as president from 20 November 1973 to 11 July 1974 be regarded as tenable in addition to the normal period of office of three consecutive years." Thus was Sir Rodney granted three years and nine months rather than the normal three years in office.

In early 1977 a special meeting of the council under the chairmanship of the vice-presidents (Selwyn Taylor and Walpole Lewin) took place to discuss a proposal that the term of the president's office should be further extended. The proposal was firmly rejected and supported only by three members.

At the succeeding council meeting on 18 March 1977 it is recorded in standard college style that: "The Council noted the receipt of letters from Fellows regarding the term of office of the President and a summary of that correspondence by the Secretary was received." It continues:

Moved by Mr M Reilly, seconded by Mr R S Handley, but lost by 17 votes to 8, the President and Vice-Presidents abstaining, "That Council endorses the tributes paid by Fellows to Sir Rodney Smith for his conduct of the affairs of the College during his term of office as President and that in the light of these representations a Formula Committee be set up to consider a change in the Standing Rules that would make it possible for Council to re-elect the President beyond the limit now imposed by paragraph 4 of Section IV of the Standing Rules."

It being clear that there was no disposition on council's part to change the rules it was thereupon

Moved by Mr G Qvist, seconded by Professor J Goligher and resolved without dissent (the President and Vice-Presidents abstaining): "The Council endorses the tributes paid by Fellows to Sir Rodney Smith for his conduct of the affairs of the College during his term of office as President; appreciates the sentiments of Fellows who have expressed a wish that his term of office as President shall be extended; but, after due consideration of all the relevant arguments, hereby records its view that it would not be in the best interests of the College to amend or revoke the Standing Rule that governs the term of office of a President."

At the next full council we were urged to consider the subject again. There was widespread discussion. Once again the proposal was rejected.

Now, in the early months of 1977, before these meetings, I had decided that it was time for us to have a provincial president and that John Goligher would be the man. I had always described him as a "true working class surgeon"; he was immensely industrious and a fine surgical technician. He had a worldwide reputation in colorectal surgery and his book on that subject is a classic, widely regarded as the best in its class. He had at first been reluctant to agree to my suggestion, but I worked on him and more or less summarised my views in a letter to him in which I wrote: "Who better for the Hunterian 250th anniversary year (1978) than a fine Irish surgeon with a splendid Australian wife?"

At that stage John replied that "in the unlikely event of the suggestion having the support of council" he would have to accept. Apart from my efforts in rooting for Goligher I was not aware of any other plans on the part of my colleagues. One afternoon I ran into John Wakeley (Sir Cecil's eldest son), who said, "Reggie, what about you for the presidency?" I chuckled slightly and replied, "You know that I'm basically a rebel and I don't think they'll want me." Nothing further was said, but in the course of a telephone call to Alan Apley about another matter I was surprised when he said, "I think you're in the running for the succession." I had done nothing to advance my claims. Indeed, having had a large myocardial infarct in 1972, two years after joining council, I had forsaken whatever visions of the metaphorical "field marshal's baton" may flit through the mind of many a new councillor.

In June 1977 council had 24 elected surgical members and a further six members elected by the dental and anaesthetic faculty boards (three from each faculty). In the event of all 30 members being present, any candidate would require at least 16 votes to be elected.

24 Bastille Day 1977

Bastille Day, 14 July 1977, unknown to us was the birthday of Ronald Johnson-Gilbert, the college secretary. His father, a former lord provost of Edinburgh, had been a pilot in the Royal Flying Corps during the first world war, when a certain A G (Peter) Wilson was his observer. Peter, previously with the West Yorks Regiment and wounded at the battle of the Somme, had taken to the air. After the war he studied medicine at Oxford, where two of his younger contemporaries were Tom Holmes Sellors and Derek Dunlop. They became distinguished consultants and Peter went on from St Thomas's to become a family doctor in Radlett, where he later delivered our last four children. With these interesting background ramifications there was some fellow feeling between myself and Johnson-Gilbert.

At the start of the meeting I was surprised when George Qvist on my right said, "Well, the best of luck to you today Reggie." John Hadfield, on my other side, said more or less the same thing. It would be an exaggeration to suggest that I could have been knocked over with a feather, but I was quite astonished.

The routine business passed without incident and, as was the custom, the secret ballot for the election of the president, to be followed by the election of the vice-presidents, came at the end of the meeting. The secretary routinely explained the procedure and papers were circulated. At the first ballot six names came up, including Selwyn Taylor, Walpole Lewin, John Goligher, Alan Parks, and myself. Those with the least votes were excluded from the list and a further vote took place; again the one with the lowest vote was excluded. John Goligher, Alan, and I were then left and John went out that time – so much for my plans for a provincial president. I had been coming up with the most votes, but only one or two ahead of Alan each time. The first of the straight votes between us showed me with a lead of one – not enough for an absolute majority. At this stage the president suggested an adjournment for tea; this was rejected. A further ballot was taken and I was either one or two ahead but still with no clear majority. The president suggested adjournment of council for a meeting next month. Ian Todd, then a junior member, strongly objected saying many councillors would be away.

A further ballot was taken and, as the votes were being counted, John Hadfield whispered, "Sixteen, Reggie, you're home and dry." Johnson-Gilbert announced the figures. "Mr president, the ballot shows that Mr Murley has the requisite majority and is thereby elected president." Rodney and I then exchanged gowns and the presidential badge was placed around my neck. Rodney returned to my seat between Qvist and Hadfield.

Seldom have I felt more shellshocked, or more strangely elated. Now I had to say a few words: "Gentlemen, when I first joined council seven years ago little did I dream that I would ever occupy this chair. I am deeply honoured." After giving Rodney his past-presidential badge we proceeded to the vice-presidential ballots. Selwyn Taylor was re-elected for a second year; but, to the astonishment of many, Walpole Lewin – also eligible for a second year – was just beaten in the ballot, being replaced by Gordon Robson, an anaesthetist and former dean of the faculty board.

As the council meeting finished it became apparent that a number of interested people had been waiting outside to hear the result. Of these the first to greet me were Robert Cooke, who had been a recent vice-president, and Margaret Harding, my charming and efficient presidential secretary. Margaret said, "You must ring your wife to tell her the news." I replied that I was due to meet her at Barts that evening. But Margaret was insistent and promptly put me through in my office. Daphne was just about to leave home and was surprised that I should ring. I announced, "I have to inform you that you are the wife of the president." There was a brief silence and an unbelieving, "*No!*" She was delighted, although we had never even discussed the possibility.

By then seated in my office, Margaret called me on the internal line to say that Sir Henry Yellowlees, the DHSS chief medical officer, had just popped in and would like to see me. Still in a slightly shocked state, I let him wait a minute or two. When escorted in, he said, "Reggie, I just happened to be passing by and called in to hear the news. My warmest congratulations." I was delighted, for when Henry had been deputy administrative medical officer at the north west region, before moving to the ministry, we had crossed swords on more than one occasion.

This being a quarterly council occasion, the dining club was due that evening. But, months before, I had arranged to meet Daphne with Raymond and Lillian Ramsay (our best man and his wife) at the annual Fountain Club party at Barts, never dreaming that I would be president of the college of surgeons. Both commitments were fulfilled: I joined the others at Barts and then came back to the college for the port and the postprandial speeches by the chairman for the evening, Geoffrey Slaney, and his introducer, Peter Bevan. One new councillor that day was John Kinmonth, who had been at school with me and who subsequently beat me and Selwyn Taylor to the assistant directorship of the Barts professorial unit. After the dinner it was an occasion for further celebration in the president's lodge, where I was joined by Daphne and the Ramsays from Barts, and by the Kinmonths – Kathleen having nipped round in a taxi to join John.

In attempting to describe my immediate reactions and responsibilities on assuming office I cannot do better than quote from my first presidential message, which appeared at the beginning of the January 1978 issue of the *Annals of the Royal College of Surgeons of England* under the title "From the President":

> Having been elected on Bastille Day at the beginning of the summer holiday period I was astonished by the amount of paper work which daily accumulated on the President's desk. This does not include more than six hundred letters and telegrams of congratulation and good wishes which overwhelmed me but which, I hope, have all been duly acknowledged.

My surprise and pleasure on election was so profound that my sleep rhythm was much disturbed for several days. On the first night, after sleeping for two or three hours, I soothed myself by listening to recordings of Beethoven piano sonatas for the rest of the night. The following night I listened to the Brandenburg Concertos and took a long walk before sunrise. After that I had more or less recovered, helped partly by the diversion of the Court and Council cricket match against the College staff club at Downe, and also by the golf match between the Council and the Dental and Anaesthetic Faculties at Highgate Golf Course.

Election to the Presidency at the end of the last council meeting of the academic year results in instant exposure to the responsibilities of office. In addition to acknowledging the many goodwill messages I found myself signing batches of applications for animal experimental licences, a task which I nevertheless regard as a personal duty and never to be replaced by a rubber stamp. In a different category are the diploma certificates, for which a well-chosen pen and permanent black ink rather than a ball-point are essential. But the signing of licence applications and certificates is but a minor part of a busy office routine. There is also a surprising amount of important correspondence and invitations to be dealt with. There are visits from a variety of folk with problems to discuss. There is also the unending deluge of Government documents; with these I had already become familiar from my service on the Joint Consultants Committee and, at an earlier date, on the BMA Council.

All newly elected Presidents must be deeply aware of how much they owe to the foundations laid by their predecessors. With eight Past Presidents still very much alive I am in the happy position of being able to avail myself of advice based upon their experience and sagacity during the last quarter-century.

Even more does a President appreciate how much he owes to the industry and allegiance of his council members, embracing as they do such a wide and outstanding spectrum of surgical and administrative experience.

As should be well known to my colleagues, I have for many years been concerned about the grave threats to personal and professional freedom and the growing danger of State monopoly in medicine. Indeed, I was one of a number of surgeons who, at special meetings of fellows of this Royal College in 1947 and 1948, sought to warn the then President and Council of what we regarded as the serious threat of State monopoly as well as the domination of medicine by bureaucrats and the viler winds of party politics. Needless to say, it gives Cassandras no pleasure ultimately to be proved right!

It has recently become fashionable for journalists and others to talk of the imminent "collapse" of the NHS, but this is a misleading concept in a service which is still surprisingly effectively propped up by professional goodwill. Indeed, dramatic collapse such as might be promoted by wholesale resignation of doctors and dentists from the service could well result in the application of urgent and effective remedial measures. But what is happening is, in some ways, far more serious: steady deterioration of professional morale, inadequate and inappropriate investment of predominantly tax-derived funds, and excessive political preoccupation with the supposed virtues of "free-at-the time" service are causing less dramatic but far more profound damage. In these circumstances it is all too easy for hard-working and formerly highly responsible doctors and dentists gradually to lose both their capacity and their determination to remedy the defects of a manifestly substandard service. Moreover, new entrants to the profession can all too easily accept poor conditions when they have no yardstick with which to compare them. Alternatively, if and when such conditions are recognised, the only options open to young doctors may be emigration or "industrial" action. Are these the sort of conditions which should be inflicted on a long-suffering and medicopolitically innocent public?

To those who regard the provision of brand new hospital buildings as the hallmark of success in a service, one can only point to the awful lessons of Sweden, a country abundantly provided with new hospitals and well-equipped special departments. I would recommend all fellows to read a recent article by Gunnar Biorck, a distinguished professor of medicine in Stockholm and a fellow of the Royal College of Physicians of London.[1] That account of increasing bureaucratisation and politicisation of the Swedish Health service closely matches many of our recent experiences, in the NHS, though the Swedes have gone farther along the road. The serious effect on medical morale and patient care has also been described in another article by Professor Philip Sandblom, formerly of Stockholm, who is now working in Zurich.[2] Both these papers are essential reading for the British doctor who has the welfare of his own country at heart.

If I have struck a somewhat sombre note in this, my first Presidential message, it is only because I feel so strongly about the damage done by a swollen and too often incompetent bureaucracy, by needless political confrontation, and by increasing trade union militancy in many of our hospitals. Fellows may rest assured that their Council is fully apprised of all these problems and that we shall do everything in our power, subject to the limitations imposed by our Royal Charter, to help remedy this situation. Whilst many are hopeful that the Royal Commission report may in due course promote some necessary reforms, I believe that it might be foolish to place too much reliance on their efforts, however enlightened their report may prove to be.

I would conclude by emphasising that we shall need eternal vigilance within the State service to protect the public and the professions whilst doing everything possible to ensure the development of a strong independent sector. Without great determination, as well as an effective yardstick against which to measure the quality of personal medical care, it will become increasingly difficult to promote high medical standards and to preserve centres of medical excellence in Britain.

1 Biorck, G (1977) *Annals of Internal Medicine*, 86, 813.
2 Sandblom, P (1976) *American College of Surgeons Bulletin*, No. 13.

It may be seen from the above that I endeavoured, among other things, to get across four messages: firstly, that imminent "collapse" (a word still used 12 years later) of the NHS was not likely – rather there would be a process of slow attrition; secondly, with due respect to Sweden, that simply spending more *taxpayers'* money should not be regarded as a solution to our problems; thirdly, put not your faith in the possible recommendations of a royal commission; and lastly (just after the Barbarabarities of Castle) I stressed the importance of an independent sector. I received no unfavourable comments from our fellows and can only hope that there was general agreement with my philosophy. It had long been my view that so long as the colleges could be seen to act in the overall interests of the public they serve our royal charters did not in any way preclude us from entering the political field. Our own college has not deviated from this course in recent years regardless of the political party in power.

I can truthfully claim that although I was stretched to the uttermost my three years as president of the college were among the most challenging and certainly the most fulfilling of my life. Within five days of being elected president, as a regional specialist committee representative of long standing, but *not* in my newly official capacity as president, I had to attend the annual hospital specialists conference in Glasgow. In the presence of the media I had good cause to be strongly critical of the socialist government of Mr Callaghan. I was startled to hear my own recorded voice in the course of the BBC *World at One* programme that same day. But I had been careful to start my contribution with the brief explanation that I was speaking on behalf of those I represented and not as president of the Royal College of Surgeons. That was one of the few occasions during the next three years when I chose explicitly to criticise the political party in power: in all honesty I could not have done otherwise. Apart from this, I had no subsequent difficulty, as president, in giving outspoken and judicious criticism of the powers that be without prejudice to the college's charitable status.

Nearly a year before, I had arranged to attend two surgical congresses in Japan, and less than six weeks after my election my wife and I left London for two days in Hong Kong, en route to Tokyo and Kyoto for the meetings of the International Cardiovascular Society and the International Society of Surgery. Both meetings were interesting and enjoyable, and we ended the visit with two fascinating days in Hiroshima with Professor Haruo Ezaki. We were home by mid-September and I was immediately involved in many college commitments. My diary for the period shows that I hosted no less than eight fund raising luncheons in the first three months. On these occasions our guests were always conducted around one or two of the research departments of the college or the Institute of Basic Science before gathering in the president's lodge. These lunches provided an excellent opportunity for both potential and existing donors to see the fine work of these departments, which have produced one Nobel prizewinner and three fellows of the Royal Society in the last 25 years.

After my election had been announced in the national press on 18 July I was surprised to find how interested the media were. Three days later Peterborough's column in the *Daily Telegraph* referred to me under the headline "Surgical leap-frog," describing me as a "redoubtable standard bearer" and also as "one of a dwindling number of old style surgical 'characters'." A few days later, on 30 July, in *Pulse International* under the headline "Surgeons adopt firebrand," the anonymous writer described me as "an intensely political animal, with an enormous knowledge of the facts at his finger tips, and an unusually competent capacity for debate. He has . . . political muscle." Penultimately it was remarked, "If Murley is not a firebrand, then he gives a remarkable impression of the part." I must confess that I had not realised that I had earned such a reputation. It was at about the same time that one of my brothers-in-law, George Paine, the then Registrar General, was reported by Peterborough to have given evidence to the Select Committee on Race Relations and Immigration. George, when remarking on the difficulties of carrying out a national census, had said, "The painter J M W Turner always hired a boat on the Thames for the two nights of the Census to avoid being counted."

It was after these reports appeared that I was approached by

World Medicine for an interview by Dr Barbara Evans, with whom I established a close rapport. I had never met her before, even though she was the wife of Philip Evans, the distinguished royal paediatrician, with whom I had written my second wartime medical paper. Her report appeared in volume 12 of that magazine on 7 September under the title "From the Sticks to the Tops." Barbara's visit was shortly followed by an invitation from Jack de Manio for a radio interview. Unfortunately he fell ill two days before this was due and then took early retirement. Some time later I had an invitation for an interview by Jean Rook of the *Daily Express*, about whom I had heard a great deal without ever reading her articles. A mutual friend promised me, however, that I could safely submit to a "no holds barred" session. She brought her photographer with her and I must confess that the succeeding two page article, although somewhat racy and, in places, slightly bawdy, was highly entertaining and certainly did no harm. I was subsequently pressed to invite her to speak at one of the college monthly dinners, where her keenest fans certainly enjoyed hearing her.

I count myself fortunate that Sir Douglas Black had been elected president of the Royal College of Physicians shortly before my own election at the college of surgeons. Although I did not know him at that time, his wife, Molly, had been at school with Daphne and this contributed to a cordial relationship with him and our senior sister college. Two weeks after my election we were both invited to lunch with Douglas and Molly at the college of physicians to meet the Sir Arthur Sims travelling professor, together with Arthur Sims's daughter Margaret and her husband, Lewis Black (not related to Douglas Black). The visitor was professor Alleyne from the West Indies, a black doctor with a Chinese wife. I recall with some amusement the moment when Douglas introduced himself to Lewis and then introduced Lewis to the West Indian professor. Lewis, an Australian, chuckled and said, "I guess that we're the All Blacks here!"

Another happy event, a few months after my own election, was when my student and wartime contemporary, John Gillingham, became president of the Royal College of Surgeons of Edinburgh. Anthony Alment, yet another Barts graduate, was at that time president of the Royal College of Obstetricians and Gynaecologists. In 1980 the three of us were invited to a celebratory dinner in the Great Hall at Barts when each was appointed to the honorary consultant staff.

After my return from Japan I continued to fit in as much of my hospital and private work as possible, but my college programme had to take priority. Private work could be adjusted to that programme; but hospital pressures were far heavier. My colleagues at the Royal Northern Hospital, where I also had the support of a senior registrar and a senior house officer, obligingly took over much of my work there, but I continued to cope with as much as possible at St Albans where I had a registrar and senior house officer. In "quiet" college weeks I sometimes still managed three weekly NHS operation lists; but I soon realised that I would have to pass on much of my St Albans work too. My colleagues there were loyal and helpful in every way and I was much indebted to them.

On 28 December, just as I was in close reach of home after taking my labrador on a stiff country walk in bitterly cold weather, I suddenly developed pain over the left breast. After my infarct of 1972 I had no doubt that this was angina. I made it to the house. A young physician friend – who himself had had an infarct when he was only 36 – was shooting pigeons in our wood and dell. He fetched his electrocardiograph from his car and put the leads on me to confirm the diagnosis of a right posterior lesion. I spent only two days in hospital and convalesced at home. With Edward Muir's having died suddenly four years earlier, the alarms rang out loudly at the college. I managed to confound everyone, however, by attending the biannual diploma ceremony 14 days later, when I shook hands with 220 diplomates from the FRCS, faculty, and MRCS examinations. Sir Tom Holmes Sellors, from his front row seat, kept an eagle eye on me; he had promised to apply prompt resuscitation should it be necessary to do so. But all went well, and after a night in the lodge I took council next day, having left Selwyn Taylor to supervise the morning meeting.

An imminent major event in the college calendar was the celebration, in the week of 13 February, of the 250th anniversary of John Hunter's birth. Before my illness Tony Van den Bergh, a writer, approached me on behalf of the BBC. He had previously made a good programme for St Thomas's Hospital, and the BBC was keen to mount a short radio play about Hunter. I was enthusiastic, as was Jessie Dobson, the past curator of the Hunterian museum. We both met Tony and were impressed by his knowledge and enthusiasm. After detailed discussion he composed an excellent script to which we made only minor changes. The producer was Greek, and we were delighted when he brought his full cast to the Hunterian Museum before the recording so that they might acquire a sense of the history. I spoke the introductory words when the play was broadcast on the morning of Monday 13 February 1978. It was a splendid start to a notable week. The same evening I gave the Hunterian Society's annual Hunterian oration at the Mansion House, taking as my subject "Some contemporaries of John Hunter." The Lord Mayor and Sherriffs attended, and a fine reception followed.

I had been lucky to be invited, nearly a year before, to give this oration and then to have the good fortune to become president of the college of surgeons. On the following day the Queen and the Duke of Edinburgh were due to attend an evening reception at the college; but when we returned to our lodge from the Mansion House Sir Philip Moore, Her Majesty's private secretary, telephoned to warn us that the Queen had a cold and might be unable to come. Early the next morning he called again with the bad news that both the Queen and Prince Philip were incapacitated. The good news, however, was that the Prince of Wales would be coming instead, accompanied by Sir Philip and his own equerry, Captain Timothy Ward. We had arranged that there would be an informal walkabout around the great hall after the presentation of our past presidents and a large group of foreign honorary fellows in the council room. This arrangement had been welcomed by Sir Philip on behalf of the Queen. The occasion proved a happy and successful one. I had made it clear that I would leave it to the royal visitors to select with whom they might wish to speak, so that I could not be accused of dispensing special favours.

The Prince of Wales much enjoyed the occasion; and the system of serendipitous selection worked well. One of the Prince's earliest encounters was with Sir Henry Osmond Clarke, KCVO, of whom the Prince asked, "And what do you do, sir?" Nobby Clarke, the royal orthopaedic surgeon, who the Prince had apparently not met, responded in his charming Dublin accent, "Well, Sorr, I spend some of my time operating on a few of your relatives." A little later my youngest son, wearing a Hawks Club tie, was also spotted and asked what he did. Anthony replied, "I am still at Cambridge, Sir, and I'm the boss's youngest son." A few paces on the Prince spotted two familiar faces from the United States, George Crile Jr, one of our honorary fellows, and Helga, his wife. They were delighted to be greeted and reminded Prince Charles that he had visited the Cleveland Clinic (where Crile worked) just a few years before. After many more encounters our visitor moved on to the splendid museum, where he met some of the Hunterian trustees and patrons as well as the conservators and the curator. It was then that I presented him with the memento for the Queen – an attractive paperweight, fashioned in heavy plastic and bearing a fine copy of the bas relief head of John Hunter from the original Tassie medallion. This had been made by one of our museum technicians and was mounted in a transparent velvet lined case. It is customary for such mementos not to be expensive or extravagant, and this particular item had been the happy suggestion of Elizabeth Allen, the Hunterian Museum curator. We finally sent the Prince of Wales on his way with a beautiful bouquet for the Queen. Some months later, at one of the college diploma ceremonies, I had the pleasure of admitting him to the honorary fellowship.

In that week there were several scientific meetings in the college; and there was a special Hunterian oration by Lord Wolfenden – the first by a layman – in the Hall of Lincoln's Inn on 16 February, followed by the Hunterian dinner at the royal college. The week ended with the Hunterian Society's annual dinner (like the college's always held as near to

Hunter's birthday as possible) at the Savoy Hotel on 17 February. Throughout the week we had on display the plaster model of a bust of John Hunter by Nigel Boonham. I later presented a bronze cast of the bust to Camden Council, in Lincoln's Inn Fields, on behalf of the college. As an enthusiastic Hunterian for the previous 30 years I could not have had a more moving and enjoyable week.

During the festival week I was still convalescing from my cardiac infarct. On the advice of Dr Walter Somerville I gave up all professional work – both hospital and private – for a full three months. Thereafter, on the recommendation of my distingushed cardiologist, I had substantial relief from my surgical commitments. My good friends and senior colleagues George Qvist and Harold Rodgers took over most of my work. George had recently retired from the Royal Free Hospital and thoroughly enjoyed acting as my locum; and Harold, recently retired from the chair of surgery in Belfast and formerly a colleague of mine at St Albans, also gave me devoted support. My trainees, and my patients, were very fortunate, and I was indebted to my hospital authorities and regional boards for making this possible.

Leaving aside the matter of my illness, the presidential workload steadily increased. Detailed statistics would be tedious; suffice it to say that my college diary shows that, apart from the routine office work, during my three years I had no less than 477 specific engagements in the college itself, including council and faculty board meetings; a further 140 working engagements at outside venues; 190 official dinners – 87 in the college and 103 elsewhere – and 173 official lunches of which 146 were at the college. Besides regular visits to the other royal colleges in London, Edinburgh, Glasgow, and Ireland, my air travel overseas was well over 100 000 miles, with Daphne accompanying me on 85 000 miles of those journeys. I also signed more than 2000 diploma certificates for the FRCS, the faculties, and the Conjoint Board, and wrote some 3000 college letters. There was inevitable and unavoidable fluctuation in the weekly workload; occasionally there were three important dinners and two or three luncheons in the same week, but there were quieter weeks when I had more time for the study of important reports and papers.

A joint meeting in London with the American College of Surgeons had been suggested in the year of the Hunterian celebrations. This took place at the Queen Elizabeth Hall, South Bank Arts Centre, in March 1979. There was a large attendance at this enjoyable three day meeting. The theme was "the generality of surgery." I attended overseas meetings with the royal Australasian and the South African surgical colleges as well as the College of Physicians and Surgeons of Canada. Our monthly dinners for fellows and members and their guests at Lincoln's Inn Fields were important events. We invited interesting speakers such as Ralf Dahrendorf, General Sir John Hackett, Archishop Coggan, Sir David Napley, Patrick Hutber, Ralph (Lord) Harris, and Cardinal Basil Hume, to name but a few.

As president I had a close association with the faculty boards of dental surgery and anaesthesia, attending all their board meetings and social events, and much enjoying their comradeship. I helped both deans with the design of their new robes. Once I suggested that the dentists and anaesthetists might prefer to hold their own independent diploma ceremonies. Both faculties declined at the time, although I knew that there were strong rumblings of separatism among the anaesthetists. Only recently has a College of Anaesthetists been created within the Royal College of Surgeons; they are still with us but no longer strictly of us. The dental faculty, founded one year before that for anaesthetics, retains its original relationship with us, but it now has its own diploma ceremony.

It was a source of pleasure and education to visit the headquarters of sister professions: the Law Society, the Inns of Court, the engineers, chemists, and accountants, as well as the Royal Society, Royal Institution, Royal College of Veterinary Surgeons, various City companies, and the medical branches of the three armed services, to highlight just a few. It would be hard to imagine any better way of learning about the relationships and interdependence of the host of organisations that form that complex jigsaw which, together with our political institutions, makes up the so called establishment.

The president and dean (later master) of the Institute of Basic Medical Sciences also represent the college on the Parliamentary Scientific Committee, some of whose meetings are of great interest. I was able to see the work of the Air Traffic Control Centre at West Drayton, of the Thames Barrage, and of part of the British Standards Institution. I had great fun attending one meeting in a committee room at the House of Commons when air conditioning was the subject for discussion. After the opening papers I stood up and said to the Tory chairman, "I must declare my interest: I am a taxpayer and, as a taxpayer, I must protest about the needless waste of public money on the full air conditioning of hospital buildings." Not many years before the DHSS had refused to provide this very necessary facility for operation theatres, yet there was profligate wastage on the air conditioning of entire buildings. As luck would have it our room overlooked the Thames, and so I said to the committee: "Cast your eyes across the river to yonder St Thomas's where two new buildings [for hospital and medical school] are now fully air conditioned from a single plant. The bill for the first year was £1.25 million and, as a taxpayer, I protest, as did the medical school when it was notified of its share of the bill." I raised a laugh. Legionnaire's disease from this source had not then been recognised.

Other specially enjoyable occasions were a splendid banquet at the Guildhall in honour of the Portuguese president, a small private luncheon with the Lord Mayor, garden parties at Buckingham Palace, and a rather amusing investiture. And at a dinner in the RAMC mess I found myself sitting opposite the Sandhurst Military Academy commandant (the father of Prince Charles's equerry, whom I had met at the college). He promptly invited Daphne and me to the next Sovereign's parade at Sandhurst. That was a stunning occasion at which we learnt that a horse really *is* ridden up the steps of the main building at the end of the ceremony.

In December 1977 I had been invited to speak at the annual luncheon of the Saints and Sinners, with the instruction to entertain them for 10 minutes. I put much hard work into the preparation of that speech and collected a large cheque for my named charity – research at the College of Surgeons. I was invited again in the following year, when I had to follow Lord Harris of Greenwich (not to be confused with Harris of High Cross) and Lord Goodman. Lord Harris ran considerably overtime which exasperated Lord Goodman, who had to cut his contribution down to six minutes; mine was slightly less. I assured Lord Goodman, however, that our charity cheques would be no smaller. Indeed on returning to the college I remarked that I had never before been able to earn at a rate of £30 000 an hour. These and all my other speeches I invariably prepared with great care, sticking strictly to a time limit – usually no more than 10 minutes – and, as had been my practice for years, I always kept copies to avoid the chance of needless repetition. Even when compelled to make an impromptu speech I usually preserved the notes I wrote on the back of the menu or other papers. That happened in Cairo in 1972 when, as examiners, we were taken to a Rotary lunch at which, during the first course, the chairman asked me what my subject was; I replied "general surgery" and he said, "No, I mean your subject for today." Horrors! I said, "Give me five minutes." After jotting headings on the back of the menu, my subject, "Understanding," gave me 10 minutes on language and international relationships (especially between Egypt and Israel), among other things.

The college work was strenuous, but I paced myself carefully and greatly enjoyed every minute of it. Nearly a year after my appointment I lost the services of the splendid Margaret Harding. Having been married for several years without achieving motherhood, she had decided to adopt a baby. Before she left I warned her that she would probably soon become pregnant; most happily, she managed this a year or so later. But again I was fortunate because just before Margaret's departure a splendid New Zealander, Kathy O'-Neill, had called on a friend at the college and heard that we needed a locum secretary. Kathy was small, good humoured and highly industrious, and had been secretary to a judge "down under" who had given her a sabbatical year between his own appointments. Kathy took to my job like the proverbial duck to water and made many good friends at the college, among whom Daphne and I are happy to be included. She later moved to Sydney with a stockbroking firm and then took a law degree before becoming personal assistant to a judge in the Court of Appeal there.

On completion of my presidency in July 1980 I was two weeks from my 64th birthday and took early retirement from the NHS. Having been elected after seven years on council, however, the rules decreed that I still had two more years to serve. That I did not gain weight during my three years as president I largely attribute to an important tip which I had learnt from Lord Home at a luncheon some years before: he claimed that one of the things that helped to keep him fit when he was Foreign Secretary was remembering to drink a glass of water with every glass of wine. Little tips like that, as well as the shrewd guidance of my physician and cardiologist, kept me active and fit then and during the next decade. I was succeeded in the presidency by Sir Alan Parks,* who, as a young man, had once shared Sir Heneage Ogilvie's sofa with me in 1948. Little did we then guess what we were in for!

* In October 1982 Sir Alan had a massive myocardial infarct while attending a meeting of the Italian Surgical Society with us in Rome. Very sadly, he died in London two weeks later.

25 Time for everything?

When the time came to retire from my NHS hospitals I felt no pangs. I had seen the vintage years and worked with many good colleagues. At St Albans they gave me a splendid farewell dinner and a present; but I managed to avoid a similar farewell at the Royal Northern because when I was elected as president of the college of surgeons they had given me a beautiful illuminated address and entertained Daphne and me to a celebration dinner. I thought they should be spared the responsibility of a further presentation to one who had been largely an absentee surgeon for three years, so I slipped quietly away.

I had decided to continue private practice as I did not want to sever all contact with patients. But I firmly resolved that, come what may, I would stop operating at 70. Geoffrey Keynes had once told me, "I did not give up surgery, it gave me up." He explained that with being away at the war until almost his 60th birthday, and with the gradual death and retirement of his referring doctors, his practice rapidly diminished. I had a similar experience: although I still felt extremely fit, I did not think it fair, without the support of a younger surgical team, to continue operative work. My last three operations were a resection of colon cancer, a thyroidectomy, and a conservative (bilateral) mastectomy for breast cancer. I went on seeing a number of my old private cancer patients, however, a few of whom still come to see me. I also continued to give second opinions where these might be helpful. Another interesting activity, for which I now had more time, was to advise on a number of medicolegal problems, where long experience can often prove especially helpful.

This limited and safe connection with clinical practice has enabled me to diminish my strictly surgical life quite painlessly. I still have useful and satisfying connections with the college of surgeons through its fundraising committee, court of patrons, Hunterian trustees, and the *Lives of the Fellows* committee, of which I now chair the last two. The Hunterian collection, entrusted to us by parliament during the Napoleonic wars, has 15 trustees by office (including the Lord Chancellor, the Prime Minister, the Chancellor of the Exchequer, and the Speaker of the House of Commons, who, unsurprisingly, have not been seen at trustee meetings for many years) and 14 by election – essentially the working members. Conditions have so changed since the trustees were set up that it would be ludicrous to expect these senior and immensely busy politicians to attend. Nevertheless, the present and the previous two Lord Chancellors have visited the museum and, like many others, have been fascinated by the unique collection it contains.

Throughout my active professional life I had supported a number of societies both in London and elsewhere, attending each of them more intensively during spells of service on their councils. I had been most active in the Hunterian Society, where I was honorary secretary for four years and then president in 1970. Far from having been released from responsibility for some of the others, as I had anticipated, I became president of the Medical Society of London in 1982 and of the Harveian Society in 1984; each required a presidential address. For these, as for the Mitchiner lecture at the Royal Army Medical College in 1980 and other occasions here and abroad, I was lucky enough to have a variety of medical subjects of lifelong interest so I did not run out of suitable material. I also spent six years on the executive of the International Society of Surgery. In addition to the biennial surgical gatherings, this required twice yearly attendance at committees in Basle with a number of interesting surgical colleagues from different countries.

Another medical occupation I had in semi-retirement was service on appeal tribunals. For a few weeks I did some medical appeal tribunals for the Department of Health; but I found these singularly unsatisfactory. For every individual who might have suffered injustice at some earlier medical assessment it became clear to me that there were a very large number of "welfare Willies" keen to extract the maximum benefit from the public purse. Many of these were rank scrimshankers. I took the opportunity of quietly withdrawing from these tribunals. On the other hand, I derived much pleasure from undertaking pension appeal tribunals, which are administered by the Lord Chancellor's department and which deal with pensioners from the armed services. After my own wartime experience I felt that this was a job to which I could apply myself with satisfaction, and so it proved, but it occupied far more time and attracted only the same daily payment as the medical appeal tribunals. The pension entitlement tribunals are made up of a lawyer chairman, with a doctor and an ex-service layman or woman, depending on the sex of the appellant. The so called assessment tribunals, however, consist of two doctors and a layman. There is a considerable volume of paperwork to study in advance of the hearings, particularly for the entitlement courts. It was interesting and especially good to find that in most cases there was little difficulty in coming to an agreed decision. Some lively and vigorous discussion and disputation could often occur in the more difficult cases. In the event of a tribunal being unable to give an agreed judgment it is obligatory to have a fresh hearing with a different tribunal, but this did not happen with any on which I served.

A sad feature of our service pension system is that the widows are not treated as generously as are those in Australia, Canada, and the United States. If one half of a married couple's disability pension were allocated to the widow when a service pensioner dies many cases of hardship might be avoided: after all, the pension (untaxed) is often an important element in the total income of the married couple and the loss of it can be sorely felt by the survivor. With the law as it stands there is no legal way of getting round the problem. But there were a few times when the medical member of an entitlement tribunal could justifiably manipulate the medical "facts" in favour of the widowed appellant with the full approval of the lay member and legal chairman. Such occasions gave me profound satisfaction, especially since Daphne – twice widowed herself – has been active in Cruse, the widows' organisation, for nearly 25 years.

Perhaps appropriately, for an aging surgeon, I find myself more and more concerned with death. The college *Lives of the Fellows* committee has responsibility for publishing, at roughly 10 year intervals, each new volume in this rolling record of our fellows' lives. For some years a strenuous effort has been made to collect curricula vitae from the fellows themselves. The information is then carefully preserved in the college library; but we are also heavily dependent upon obituaries in the medical, daily, and local press. This labour of love is undertaken by the library staff and a number of past members of council. At their best the resultant records are of immense value, but, like the compilers of all such information, we have to contend with a number of fellows and families who are slothful or reluctant to provide information. As I grow older my responsibility for writing obituaries of colleagues increases; it is sometimes a difficult task. Moreover, when an obituary is to be published in one of the more prestigious newspapers even a carefully prepared and accurate record can be subedited and then, perhaps, further cut at the last minute to make it fit in with other material on the page. That being so, it is only right that, in the national press, the author's anonymity should be preserved. I do know that it is not uncommon for obituary editors in the upmarket daily papers to receive a fair amount of "flak" from friends and relations of the dear departed.

Following the death of Sir James Paterson Ross, the late Sir Geoffrey Keynes wrote to me: "Did you approve of Jim's *Times* obituary which I wrote? . . . I told him [Paterson Ross] what I was doing, so *he* should have approved!" In another of Geoffrey's letters after Ross's death, dated 6 July 1980, not in his fine sepia ink holograph but personally typed with many corrections, he wrote, "It seems indecent the way I go on living relentlessly, while my younger friends drop off before their time." Paterson Ross, one of his "younger friends," had died aged 86, and Geoffrey was then 93.

Even more difficult, and requiring considerable research, is the giving of official addresses at thanksgiving and memorial services. I have had responsibility for a fair number of these, both for distinguished colleagues and relatives. Among the many that have given me great satisfaction I would include those I gave for John Kinmonth, Sir Thomas Holmes Sellors, and Sir Geoffrey Keynes. The detailed study of the life and work of an old friend and colleague, and the collection of anecdotes and reminiscences from family and friends, can prove rewarding in highlighting one's own inadequacies and failings. As a reverent agnostic I have derived not a little entertainment and education from several of these services. On one occasion a medical widow of strong character and good humour, who was in the process of planning her late husband's service, remarked to me with a good natured chuckle that she had been "severely catechised by the vicar" concerning the religiosity of the deceased. From her account there can be little doubt that she contributed to that clergyman's further education. The preliminary arrangements for another service underwent a slight hiccup when the priest in charge was reluctant to accept the service for one who, so he thought, had been related to atheists. But a little tactful pressure from the highest prelate in the land persuaded this priest that the religious views of the relatives, or even those of the dear departed himself, were not admissible in precluding the appropriate service desired by his family. In passing, I feel bound to remark on the curious fact that so few services of thanksgiving are held for the life and work of the many outstanding women on whose devoted service many men are so dependent. The women's lobby has been strangely silent about this.

Less serious, but often requiring much hard work, is the preparation of after dinner and other speeches, which I have usually much enjoyed. The research for many of these has taught me a great deal that I did not know, or at least helped me to sort out some of my misunderstanding of less familiar subjects. This all began with my involvement with that college meeting in 1948, which led on to further invitations. Early on, these were often concerned with medicopolitical issues; however, the range of subjects greatly widened in later years. But after listening to Arthur Dickson Wright at his very best, and then hearing him repeat so much on many later occasions, I became careful to avoid overexposure. The discipline of careful preparation, crisp editing, and keeping within a time limit is essential to continued success. For this reason certain invitations are best declined, however tempting they may at first seem. On the whole I have much preferred giving a carefully researched speech in an unfamiliar ambience – as in Dublin to the Royal College of Surgeons in Ireland, or at an unaccustomed City company – to the provision of the more lighthearted postprandial entertainment at, say, a cricket club. This is largely because my records of the former include more historical and related data of interest than do the latter. But, during the year long printers' strike at *The Times*, as guest speaker at the annual dinner of a printers' charity I did greatly savour the opportunity of firmly and politely taking the pants off SOGAT in the presence of Prince and Princess Michael of Kent. The discreet – and sometimes less discreet – trailing of coat tails can be an interesting exercise.

One of the joys of what I describe as "semi-retirement" is having more time for reading and writing. The execrable standard of my handwriting and a tendency to writer's cramp long ago led me to use a typewriter – and later to possess two electric machines. I have typed innumerable personal letters, medical papers, and formal lectures, only making use of a trained secretary occasionally for some special piece. In my NHS years I had many letters published in the *BMJ* and the *Lancet* and in the lay press – the *Guardian*, the *Telegraph*, *The Times*, even in the *Daily Mail* and the local papers; but there have been rather fewer since my retirement. I worked all these letters over carefully five or six times, searching for the right word or phrase and, with growing experience, making them as concise as possible. To me the preparation of such letters was an important exercise in clarifying my thoughts. Keeping copies of most of them in my files serves to reassure me that, at least most of the time, I was writing sense. At any rate there are none of which I now feel ashamed – even if I should be – but I can smile at some of my earlier enthusiasms and indiscretions. Three years ago, with some cursing and swearing, I mastered the use of an Amstrad word processor – sheer magic for editing and revising articles and papers, and an enormous help when there are no longer hospital and private secretaries to deal with all the personal correspondence.

It is good to have time to read the newspapers and journals, and I am now able to indulge my main reading interests in history, biography, and economics – activities which were once predominantly vacation ones. To repair all one's early ignorance in later life is not easy, but I have collected the many excellent volumes of the *Oxford History of England* and have read D M Low's abridged version of Gibbon's *Decline and Fall of the Roman Empire*. Detective stories seldom interest me, and novel reading I confine mainly to vacations and air travel. My knowledge of music is slight; but since my marriage to a spouse who, although not playing any instrument herself, had a lively interest implanted by a highly musical elder brother I have gradually come to appreciate more and more classical music, especially Mozart, Beethoven, Bach, Brahms, Vivaldi, Haydn, Elgar, and Mahler. Although I read music well enough to play the piano badly, I am incapable of humming a tune from the score; this deficiency is matched with my incapacity to tune my ear to a foreign tongue.

I have no special aesthetic appreciation of painting or sculpture; nor have I any true talent with pencil or paint brush, apart from a fair standard of draughtsmanship. For short periods, usually when on holiday, I often enjoy painting in oils, but I get paint on my hands and clothes and lack skill in mixing colours. When my college presidential portrait was painted by John Walton I was amazed at the ease with which he handled colours, all the while indulging in animated conversation. And he never got a spot of paint on himself. Others are often astonished when they see surgeons carrying out an operation while chatting away in the operation theatre. It was Daphne who suggested that John should paint my portrait, and he took infinite care with every detail. Only when it was completed did I realise how badly many other artists portray the hands; but, as John said during one of the sittings, "Reggie, there will only be three bits of you in this portrait – your head and your two hands." Everyone was delighted with the finished picture, especially the subject himself. Although the portrait was painted in the rare book room above the college library, we had chosen for the background the Hunterian ambience of the entrance hall with Weekes's fine statue of John Hunter and the busts of George III and Joseph Banks. I was wearing the tie of the Royal Australasian College of Surgeons for three reasons: firstly, my busiest spell of wartime surgical training was with two Australian surgeons; secondly, many of our casualties at that time were from the Australian forces; and thirdly, to my great pleasure and delight, that college had been the first to award me an honorary fellowship. "Every picture tells a story," as the saying goes.

Whatever may have motivated me in my youth, I think that I have rarely been inspired by altruism alone, even though I have frequently become associated with movements of benevolent or charitable purpose. I have a high regard for personal freedom and have always found it hard to accept inefficiency and bureaucracy. I recall that when I applied for an early postwar appointment one of my referees described me as having "a singular intolerance of the second rate." I took it then as a slightly barbed compliment, but he may have identified one of my main motivating forces. Having lived through the postwar period of paternalistic collectivism under both Labour and Tory administrations, I have become concerned about the growing influence of the state and the erosion of personal responsibility. Without ever having been starry eyed about the virtues of the family, I have come to have a strong and growing belief in the importance to society of family life. For this reason I was delighted a few years ago to be invited to become a sponsor of Family and Youth Concern and a trustee of its associated Responsible Society Research and Education Trust. Originally set up at the suggestion of Dr Stanley Ellison, this organisation has done splendid work in promoting the moral message in relation to family and social life. Among many of its hardworking supporters it would not be invidious to highlight the magnificent work, in both national and international fields, of its honorary secretary, Mrs Valerie Riches, ably backed by her husband, Denis. A number of excellent educational videos have been produced by Robert Whelan on behalf of the Responsible Society Research and Education Trust, the most recent being a 15 minute video, "The Truth About Aids," which is much in demand from schoolteachers who have found it far more suitable for their pupils than the longer and vulgarly explicit "government" video on the same subject. This organisation also has the firm and long standing support of a number of my old friends and respected colleagues such as Lord Shawcross, Sir Brian Windeyer, Sir John Peel, and Sir John Ellis. I am proud to be associated with them.

I was privileged, too, to become a patron of The Jagiellonian Trust, an independent charity supporting education, scholarship, and culture in Poland. Caroline (Baroness) Cox, the daughter of my former surgical colleague Robert McNeill Love, was responsible for involving me with this trust. I also support Medical Aid to Poland. Through my concern with these organisations I am able to pay respect to former Polish wartime colleagues and to my old friend Professor Witold Rudowski of Warsaw. One can but hope that a touch of glasnost and perestroika will eventually seep through to the gallant nation for which Britain went to war, but which was badly let down by us and our allies. It was Caroline also who persuaded me to serve on the health committee of the National Council for Academic Awards, a body which is predominantly concerned with the assessment and validation of degree courses where none previously existed.

Caroline Cox originally trained as a nurse and was later head of the sociology department at the Polytechnic of North London (formed in February 1971 by merging the Northern and North Western Polytechnics). Within a month of its formation the Polytechnic was plagued by student occupations and disruption of the court of governors and academic board meetings; and the trouble continued off and on until November 1974. It so happened that I had to give an address at the thanksgiving service for Caroline's father at St Martin's-in-the-Fields when she, an old fashioned Liberal turned Tory, gave me the typescript of a book she had written with two of her colleagues (one a former communist, the other a Labour party member) about the troubles at the Polytechnic. She had been unable to find a publisher. After reading the manuscript I was convinced that this ugly history must be published, so I referred her to Ralph Harris (of the Institute of Economic Affairs). Ralph not only had the book published by the Churchill Press in 1975 but also suggested the highly appropriate title *Rape of Reason*. Those of us who had known the splendid Northern Polytechnic in the days when its principal was Dr T J C Drakeley (also chairman of the Royal Northern Hospital management committee) were especially appalled by this sad saga. Caroline has since told me that she thinks that my intervention was indirectly responsible for her peerage.

Having joined the somewhat incongruously named Society of Individualists during the war and then become a founder member of the Fellowship for Freedom in Medicine, it is not surprising that I also joined Viscount De L'isle's Freedom Association, which is now so ably chaired by Norris McWhirter. Widely regarded as "right wing," as is somewhat inevitable with all such bodies, I would say that the association's charter of rights and liberties includes principles which should be widely embraced by anyone who is not besotted by notions of the implicit virtues of collectivism. Indeed, whatever may be the undoubted worthiness of Thatcherism in giving free reign to market forces there is still a significant residual element of paternalism in parts of the Tory philosophy: witness their reluctance to relax central government control over education and health care, in both of which fields governments of all complexions have been largely responsible for the growth of militant trade unionism and professional vested interests. I am conscious that some of the reforms I seek would not leave me so cosily protected from the economic facts of life as I have been during the last 40 or so years.

Concern for economic facts made me an early supporter of the Institute of Economic Affairs. I have known that marvellous body since it first began in simple and relatively primitive circumstances at Hobart Place. My friends Ralph Harris and

Arthur Seldon, working in an independently funded institute, have lived and thrived in conditions starkly contrasting with people like me who have, largely through circumstances beyond our control, lived under a government umbrella – government employees and then government pensioners. In my own small way I have been privileged to participate in some of the institute's work and to enjoy a little of its reflected glory. I was a guest at its memorable 30th anniversary dinner in 1987, and in the last few years I have served on the advisory councils of both its social affairs and health and welfare units, which have set out to promote the same questioning philosophy and scholarly approach that the parent institute has applied to so many aspects of governmental and private monopolies.

An entirely different ball game, with which I only became involved after finishing the college presidency, was to succeed Sir Tom Holmes Sellors as chairman of the Medical Council on Alcoholism. The council publishes an important international journal, *Alcohol & Alcoholism*, and a quarterly newsletter for general practitioners, which is distributed free of charge. Three excellent booklets for general practitioners, nurses, and medical students have been published; and these also are issued free of charge. The council, too, arranges regular meetings and symposia for students and professionals. Every one of these activities is now generously financed by the distillers and brewers at no expense to the taxpayer. Indeed, in 1983 I derived much satisfaction from thwarting Kenneth Clarke (the then Minister for Health) in his ill advised endeavour to "disorganise" the council into a new quango. We have Lords Porritt and Hill and Professor Harold Stewart as our patrons and Sir Douglas Black as president. One of my anaesthetists, in introducing me at a meeting, said, "What a laugh! Reggie is now chairman of the alcoholic doctors group." But, quite simply, the purpose of the council is educational: it is to promote better recognition by doctors of those patients with alcohol problems. Medical people with drink problems are guided into the skilled hands of a different organisation, the Doctors and Dentists Group.

My old friend Sir John Charnley, who had exasperated me

with his brilliance and bounce when I first met him in Cairo in 1943 – sheer jealousy on my part – died in August 1982, nearly a year before I had my left hip joint expertly replaced by Rodney Sweetnam. At about that time Jill, Lady Charnley, invited me to be president of the John Charnley Trust, an office which I was privileged to take on. My student interests and early war experience had made me something of an orthopaedic surgeon *manqué*, so I was happy to have the opportunity to do honour to a great surgeon and to his specialty, which has made such remarkable advances in the last two decades. In the five years since its foundation the trust has been able to give generous financial support to young orthopaedic surgeons seeking further experience, as well as to selected research projects. It also sponsors an annual John Charnley memorial lecture, held alternately in Manchester and Liverpool.

One interesting organisation with which I have a continuing association as representative of the Royal College of Surgeons, and in whose origin I played some part, is the United Kingdom Inter-Professional Group. In 1976, during the time of the Barbarabarities of Castle, I was telephoned by Independent Television News and invited to be interviewed during the lunchtime news. I inquired if this was intended to be a confrontation with representatives of the hospital unions and was assured that it would be a "straight interview," and "live." I asked who would be my interviewer and the reply was "Robert Kee." I further inquired, "Is that by any chance the author of *The Green Flag*, that splendid book about Ireland?" The answer was "Yes." I readily agreed. When I arrived at the ITV studios shortly before the news programme Robert Kee asked if I would object to any hostile questions about the hospital dispute which was then going on. I said that I had no possible objections and, moreover, if I could not defend my thesis it was clearly not worth airing.

I much enjoyed my few minutes' sharp sparring with Kee, and later that day my Harley Street receptionist, Mrs Jones, told me that she had received several encouraging telephone calls about the interview. Also, a number of letters and other messages of approval arrived at my home; among them was a message on behalf of the Law Society which came through a Mr Tunnicliffe, a Cambridge solicitor. He expressed some keenness to establish an interprofessional group. I had had similar ideas in mind for some time, and I readily agreed that there was a need for exchange of information between many of those professions which were faced with problems in regard to self regulation, indemnity insurance, advertising, and other important matters. I made it plain, however, that I was emphatically *not* in favour of a cosy defensive professional group, comparable to the Trades Union Congress: our primary objective must be our duty to the public we served; and if they could not be convinced of the importance of the professional ethic it was doubtful whether we would make much progress against attack from either of the main political parties.

Before I became president of the college of surgeons further discussions had been going on and the United Kingdom Inter-Professional Group came into being just before my election. Sir David Napley, a former president of the Law Society, was its excellent first chairman and the initial membership included, among others, the Law Society, Bar Council, Royal College of Surgeons, Royal College of Veterinary Surgeons, Institute of Chartered Accountants, Royal Institute of British Architects, Society of Actuaries, Society of Patent Agents, Institute of Chartered Surveyors, and the Pharmaceutical Society. The chairmanship and the secretariat has been held in turn by different professions, each for a period of three years. There have been inevitable differences between those who preferred a low profile and others who sought a more aggressive stance, and a subgroup was formed to represent some of the professions in discussions on the European Common Market. As one of those who has always favoured the low profile approach, I have never been interested in seeking office, and I remain convinced that our most useful function has been in the bringing together of professional people, often of widely differing background and practice, for the exchange of information. Valuable work has been done by several working parties on such subjects as continuing professional education, professional liability, and self regulation. Although I have seen nothing of Mr Tunnicliffe since our first meeting in 1976, I am happy to recall that each of us had a son who played in the Cambridge golf team a year or two later.

These are just a few of the many activities which have kept me busy in the last few years. But when winter is past and spring is in the air this old man's fancy still, perforce, turns to two acres of garden and a small wood. News of this evokes much sympathy from colleagues, especially when I tell them that we are lucky enough to have two gardeners, an elderly man and a younger woman – of whom I am the deputy to my much more knowledgeable spouse.

26 Faith, family, and friends

Our beloved Wint Gray, widow of Howard Gray of the Mayo Clinic, used to say, "Faith, family, and friends; on these do our lives depend." Both Howard and Wint had been stalwart friends of visitors from many nations; they were a charmingly devout couple who fully lived up to Wint's triplex aim. I have no orthodox religious faith, but I have an implicit belief in the ultimate ability of man, despite his frequent foolishness and transgressions, to achieve a state of grace. Norman Birkett, in one of those celebrated John Freeman interviews, referred to his early upbringing in a devout family, and went on to say that he would describe himself as "an agnostic Christian." For many years past, and after considerable reflection, I have classed myself as a "reverent agnostic." This has proved an acceptable religious category when entering hospital as a patient, although one staff nurse at the King Edward VII Hospital was keen to hear my further explanation. At a college dinner that great Christian soldier, Sir John Hackett, said, "My dear Reggie, an element of agnosticism is essential to any sort of belief." The whole of creation, in the distinctively evolutionary sense of that word, is so remarkable that I do not consider it irreverent to state that in regard to the concept of God I simply do not know. The longer I live the more comfortable do I feel as a "reverent agnostic."

As to my family life, however truthfully a man may describe the undoubted excellence of his wife there is always the risk that others may deem any account of her virtues as mere hyperbole. To avoid exposing myself to that risk, I shall merely state that I could not have been more fortunate in my marriage. Medicine has been my only mistress and neither Daphne nor I have taken another lover in 43 years. But, as that turbulent priest Donald Soper once said to me, "It is probably lack of opportunity which keeps most of us faithful." A busy and fascinating job therefore has its advantages. I do not, and shall not, pretend that a busy surgical life ever permitted me to spend as much time with my children as some of those who work regular office hours. I did, however, play some part in the nappy changing and bathing; but because, unlike Daphne, I had never had bedtime stories read to me regularly as a child, I was not as good as she was at reading to the children. Daphne always made sure that a child went happily to bed, whatever trauma might have occurred during the day. I remember once when Susan was at school and Jennifer and David, our own first two, were behaving impossibly after measles (a slight touch of measles encephalitis perhaps?) Daphne confessed to riding off on her bicycle and deserting them for a whole hour. She had stayed out just long enough for the youngsters to think that she might really have left them, so on her return they behaved like little angels.

I suppose that in the course of bringing up six children we had our ups and downs; but nothing so awful that could not be discussed with close friends. The paying of school fees stretched us considerably. Susan and Jennifer went to separate coeducational boarding schools. David and Gavin preferred to be day boys and went to nearby Aldenham, cycling there each day and staying to do their evening prep in the boarding house to which they belonged. The financial saving was marginal, but they were more closely involved with the school than were our day boys at Dulwich. Tony, our number six, was due to go to Aldenham, but he had elected to board at Edge Grove, the splendid preparatory school which all three boys attended. A row with the then Aldenham headmaster when the older two had already left the school and only a year before Tony was booked for entry convinced me that I should make other arrangements. Out of three other schools which accepted him, Oundle was Tony's and our own choice. Ultimately, a history exhibition to St Catharine's College, with a later switch to what I described as "the sportsman's easy option, land economy" (half the university rugby and cricket teams seemed then to be in that faculty), gave him four years at Cambridge.

And so, around the time of my own retirement from the health service, I was sometimes able to watch him play at Fenner's, or with the university golf and rugby fives teams.

Hilary, our fifth child, was very special. Her handicap, which is not capable of specific classification, was presaged by a slow start, feeding problems, and somewhat crowing respiration. When 4 years old she was knocked over by a stolen car while walking with our au pair girl. She was trapped beneath a fence on which the car came to rest in a neighbour's front garden, and magically saved by an AA motorcycle patrolman who was providentially passing by. Hilary was concealed beneath the fence, partly squashed by the weight of the car but with a post on each side of her taking some of the load. The gears were engaged and the wheels still turning as the thieves (two ex-Borstal boys) slipped away through fields at the back. The patrolman, a powerful Canadian, disengaged the gears, stopped the engine, and righted the car. Hilary, with many Tardieu's spots around her mouth (evidence of asphyxia), was admitted to St Albans under the care of my orthopaedic colleague, Arthur Rushforth. She had a number of fractured ribs but was out of hospital in 10 days. But after getting her into an ambulance the AA man had set off again and intercepted the breathless thieves as they crawled through a hedge on to another road. He brought them back into Radlett, where they were arrested. At the first hearing by the magistrate the case was referred to Hertford Crown Court, where each received a stiff prison sentence. I duly rewarded the AA patrolman and highly commended him to his headquarters.

We sent Hilary to a nearby school for the handicapped. When the other children had chicken pox she too had a fever but no spots, although she was a little breathless. Alfred Franklin, who had been responsible for her infant care at Barts, had early queried a possible "congenital heart," so we took her to Graham Hayward (Barts and National Heart Hospital) in whom I had great confidence. He said, "The heart's OK but screening shows a little shadow in one lung. Get Watkin Edwards to see her." Besides having been at school with me, "Wattie" was a superb chest physician. He confirmed the diagnosis of a primary tuberculous focus, traced one other infected child at the school, and also the source – a nice old gardener there with chronic cough and bilateral lung cavitation. All three patients were cured and Wattie described this as the most satisfactory enterprise in which he was ever involved. While still on her anti-tuberculous drugs, however, Hilary had her first epileptic fit. That also was controlled and before long, with her youngest brother away at school, she too said she would like to board. It was then that Gabbitas Thring found us a marvellous school for handicapped girls near Stroud, run by Anglican nuns. Hilary spent some six years there and was given excellent simple basic and cultural education, with visits to choir and music festivals and fine old houses. By sheer determination she learnt to water ski in Algarve and then to snow ski with the handicapped ski club.

In parenthesis it is worthy of record that some five years after Hilary's accident my then St Albans house surgeon, Robert Kennedy, telephoned to say that he had admitted a young man with severe acute ulcerative colitis. He had been the driver of the stolen car and was terrified when he found himself in one of my beds. I asked Robert to tell the patient that he would not be safe in my hands, and we arranged transfer to a colleague in another hospital.

The upbringing of a handicapped child is a challenge for all concerned, especially for the mother. No words could adequately convey how much I owe to Daphne, who has always shown unerring skill and intuition, and boundless love, in handling this problem. Our other children have played their part by showing great patience. We are, of course, much luckier than the many families with far more seriously handicapped children. But there is a sense of immense satisfaction, not to say triumph, in progressively meeting, and where possible overcoming, the successive problems and difficulties. In this long drawn out process that we have all learnt valuable lessons and our lives have certainly been enriched.

Throughout most of our married life we have had labrador bitches – a succession of four. A dog is the best possible burglar alarm, as our local PC has often remarked. But it was only in my retirement that I got to know the present bitch really well, because I had the pleasure of taking her to evening training classes. I have come to the conclusion that a better understanding of a dog's mind can be of great help in comprehending the behaviour of human beings. As for understanding the minds of human beings, I fancy that we all might benefit from exposure to the London taxi drivers' examination, as depicted in that very entertaining film "The Knowledge." Some years ago one of my St Albans house surgeons, a University College Hospital graduate, told me how he had supported his wife and two children during his student days by working as a part time taxi driver. I had found it hard to believe his colourful description of the taxi drivers' training and examination, but all was confirmed in the subsequent film. In addition to acquiring an enviable knowledge of the roads and places in central London, taxi drivers are trained to face up to the foibles of human behaviour. Many a professional man could benefit from some appropriate training on these lines. Such skill as we may have in handling difficult interpersonal relationships has largely been acquired in the hard school of experience.

That brings me to the last of Wint Gray's three principles for the good life: friends. Alexander Pope said, "How often are we to die before we go quite off the stage? In every friend we lose a part of ourselves and the best part." But Harold Balfour puts it rather more hopefully, as the guest list at Edwin McAlpine's (Lord McAlpine of Moffat) annual party now regularly reminds us:

> Though years roll on,
> If friends remain
> No year is lost,
> But each a gain.

Both these quotations lie on a spectrum of truth, but any one person's subjective position on that spectrum must vary with personal circumstances. The late Lord Horder, when in his 80s, once told me that he deeply missed the loss of his old friends. When I responded, "But what of us young ones?" he said with sadness, "Well, you are not the same as the old ones," and that must surely be true. Geoffrey Keynes, of course, cultivated many young friends and may have had the aptitude to avoid the greater sadness experienced by Tommy Horder, who had once been his more senior physician colleague at Barts.

Anyone who has been through university and medical school, and then worked in hospital medicine, has abundant opportunity to meet many people and to make a wide variety of friends. Those of us who spent several years in the armed services had further opportunities to meet many whose paths we would not otherwise have crossed. When I look back on my own life I find that I have no fewer than five friends from my school days with whom I am still in touch. The Dulwich College war record names some 120 boys known to me who perished during the second world war, of whom half a dozen or so were quite close friends. But things were far worse after the first world war. I, of course, missed the possible friendships of Oxbridge. Many of my Barts contemporaries are still around, however, and there is that added bonus of wartime contacts. As to my hospital colleagues, even though I had no serious or lasting rows with any of them they mostly remain just "good colleagues"; nevertheless, one or two unexpectedly solid friendships developed – a physician here, an anaesthetist there. There are, too, a number of general practitioners and specialists living nearby, and proximity has facilitated the chance to get to know one another better. Some of my colleagues have a special facility for cultivating friendship with their former patients, but I think that most of us would prefer not to be responsible for the continuing medical care of those we know really well; better perhaps for them to be in the hands of a highly respected colleague.

Among his special professional friends a surgeon is sure to place high on the list those younger surgeons he has helped to train. The first of mine, Norman Rothnie, senior surgeon at Reading, and John Currie, neurosurgeon at Barts, have now retired, but they and their families have remained firm friends with me and my family. There followed many conscientious, industrious, and highly competent doctors who are now scattered around the United Kingdom in Aberdeen, Ashford,

Bedford, Bristol, Cambridge, Ipswich, London, Manchester, Oxford, Winchester, and other parts, working in teaching and regional hospitals. There are others overseas in Adelaide, Auckland, Ontario, Rotorua, and South Africa. I remember them all with affection and try to keep in touch with every one of them.

We regularly see, and enjoy close friendship with, my first postwar surgical chief, John Hosford, who will be a sprightly 90 in July 1990. He and Millicent, after 25 years' retirement to Portugal, are now back in Britain. Also born in the year of the century, and only two weeks John's junior, is the equally lively Arthur (Lord) Porritt, a source of my most valued postwar American introductions and a tower of strength, wisdom, and commonsense during my years at the Royal College of Surgeons. After a goodly spell as sergeant surgeon and five years as Her Majesty's Governor General in New Zealand neither he nor Kay has ever lost the common touch. Two of my former postwar "junior" surgeons on the Hosford firm, Alec Badenoch and Harold Rodgers, also survive in their 80s. Regrettably infrequent though personal contact with some of these splendid people must be, we relish their friendship – "no year is lost, but each a gain."

A new development, and generally a happy one, is that more and more of our friends and relatives are joining the medical survivors' club. Of those with cancer it is the children that derive the greatest benefit: when a two year old great-niece of ours was found to have leukaemia 12 years ago I was able to give her grandparents and parents a message of hope. She survives to this day. The adult survivors of malignant disease are still mainly those who have been fortunate in their type of tumour and their own inherent immunity.

But it is in the cardiovascular and orthopaedic fields that so many of us have reaped the greatest benefits. Within the last few months two mature old friends of mine have joyfully survived coronary bypass operations. I say "mature" because one of them, Sir Ian Fraser of Belfast, a distinguished surgeon, is 87 years old and the other, Dr Kenneth Hutchin, is just 80. Ian Fraser (a contributor to this Memoir Club series) I first met during the war and – now I must choose my words very carefully indeed – he is probably one of the more sprightly of no fewer than three of my surviving surgical colleagues who have advanced well into their ninth decade. He, like me at a much earlier age, developed angina while walking his dog. But it must surely be a bold Irish surgeon who, like his patient, so blithely ignores the mere counting of the years. As for Kenneth Hutchin, formerly a highly respected general practitioner in Hatfield, he is still performing as medical correspondent for the *Daily Telegraph*. In celebrating his 80th birthday a couple of months after his operation Kenneth is doubly a survivor, having been a prisoner of war in the notorious Changi camp. It is incongruous to think that Kenneth's few years in Changi on a starvation diet may have mitigated the earlier stages of atheroma.

The quality of life for many of us has been immeasurably improved by advances in the orthopaedic field, but it is salutary to realise how easily we can fail to count our blessings. I remember John Charnley remarking that when there was no effective surgical treatment for hip disease, apart from joint fixation or osteotomy, many elderly and not so elderly people bore their pain and disability with admirable stoicism. Once hip replacement became possible, however, that which had been stoically borne in the past was far less readily tolerated. What John said about the hip now applies to the knees and will steadily apply to our expectations in many other conditions as orthopaedists reach those parts that former orthopods could not reach.

My own membership of the survivors' club dates from the war. How fortunate I was in wartime to survive shot and shell, and malignant tertian and cerebral malaria. How fortunate I have been since to survive two myocardial infarcts: the first in 1972, after angina on the previous morning, provoked by an early morning swim in cold water; the second, smaller, one in 1978, after walking the dog in bitterly cold weather.

I tend to forget the searing nocturnal pain in the middle of my back in late 1974, when I suspected that I had a leaking abdominal aneurysm and was whisked into hospital only to find that it was my old problem of renal stone, painlessly pissed out a month later before the start of an operation list.

More recently, while in Portugal, I had a painful recurrence of gout. I am now ready to classify my pains: ureteric colic from stone was *intermittently* the worst, cardiac pain from infarction was severe and promoted the most anxiety, whereas the pain of the last attack of gout was *persistently* the worst. It is plain that in the later stages of our lives most of us consume more medical resources than at any other period. So none should forget the little notice, seen in an infant intensive care unit, "Remember that the first few minutes of life are the most dangerous," to which some joker had added, "Not to mention the last!"

The above were the final words in the proofs that arrived on 21 March 1990. Just 12 days earlier I had had unusual angina while walking to my car after a Barts Fountain Club dinner. But a happy and expert cardiac catheterisation by Roworth Spurrell on 20 March and skilful left internal mammary artery and double vein graft surgery by Gareth Rees in the Wellington Hospital two days later gave me three or four days' leisure in which to correct the proofs. On my second night in intensive care I received a visit, and a smacking kiss, from the dean of Bart's – Lesley Rees, my surgeon's spouse. Now, safely home again on 30 March, I hope to have deferred those last few dangerous minutes of life for a few more years. I remain, as ever, deeply grateful to my colleagues and happy that we all chose medicine – that satisfying and demanding mistress.

Index